Disability Studies and the
Environmental Humanities

Disability Studies and the Environmental Humanities
Toward an Eco-Crip Theory

Edited and with an introduction by
Sarah Jaquette Ray and Jay Sibara

Foreword by Stacy Alaimo

University of Nebraska Press | Lincoln & London

Acknowledgments for the use of copyrighted
material appear on pages 623–24, which
constitute an extension of the copyright page.

Publication of this volume was assisted by
a Humanities Division Grant from Colby
College, Maine.

Library of Congress Control Number: 2017936592

Designed and set in FS Me by L. Auten.
FS Me is an accessible typeface designed to aid
legibility for people with a learning disability.

Contents

Foreword

Stacy Alaimo

While we might wish that all our ethical and political commitments would align and become so beautifully articulated as to be inseparable and synergistic, it is nonetheless often the case that historically rooted discursive and ideological formations mean that ethics, politics, and scholarship take place within more messy, vexed, and contradictory terrains.[1] Eli Clare, in his potent essay in this volume, navigates through volatile conceptual landscapes, writing that four concepts in particular, "natural, normal, unnatural, and abnormal," "form a matrix of intense contradictions, wielding immense power in spite of, or perhaps because of, the illogic." Political movements for environmentalism and disability rights have rarely converged, so it is not surprising that disability studies and the environmental humanities would have developed as separate fields. But this separation, however predictable, is hardly a neutral oversight. Mainstream U.S. environmentalism, saturated by wilderness ideals, as Sarah Jaquette Ray argues in this collection, has a "hidden attachment" to the abled, hyperfit body, which has resulted not only in scholarly and political exclusions of disability from environmentalism but also in the physical exclusion of disabled people from the secluded landscapes of national parks, as Alison Kafer argues in the chapter from Feminist, Queer, Crip that is reprinted here. Shifting from the environmental humanities to the allied field of critical animal studies reveals clashes that are even more glaring. David Mitchell and Sharon Snyder write in these pages, "It's safe to say that the relationship between disability and animality is a strained one."

Elizabeth A. Wheeler, in her essay in this collection, notes the "devastating, even genocidal history of comparing people with disabilities to animals," which makes alliances between disability rights and animal rights as well as disability studies and animal studies terribly overburdened. And yet the work of Sunaura Taylor, Temple Grandin, Dawn Prince-Hughes, and others intrepidly fosters multispecies relations. In the pages that follow, Anthony J. Nocella II advocates for a philosophy of "eco-ability," which brings together "disability theory, animal advocacy, and ecology." The account of his own protests against dolphin captivity provides a striking example.

Projects that seek to connect disability studies with animal studies and environmentalism are often fraught, as such alignments are hardly "natural" but must instead be constructed and reconstructed through multiple positions, critiques, and rearticulations. It could even be the case that the conflicts arise not just from a lack of attention or a lack of dialogue but from more obdurate differences based in constitutive exclusions and overdetermined histories. Critiquing the values of "stability" and "integrity" in Aldo Leopold's Sand Country Almanac, a classic in environmental studies, with its influential concept of the "land ethic," Kim Q. Hall writes that the "devaluation of impurity and changing bodies and places . . . has informed heteronormativity, classism, racism, ableism, and sexism." Even if we shift our attention from canonical texts of environmental ethics to more contemporary environmental justice paradigms, we find that they are propelled by the ideal of "natural," "healthy" bodies. Valerie Ann Johnson notes in her reprinted essay, "Those of us in the environmental justice community are not immune to our society's standards of health, beauty, and normality." Indeed illness and disability may be evidence that environmental injustice has occurred. Jina Kim, in "Cripping East Los Angeles," writes, "While studies of environmental racism invariably reference disability to denote environmental harm, few if any address the phenomenon from a critical disability perspective."

Examining the physical and the conceptual in/accessibility of environments, environmentalism, and environmental studies is one starting point for cripping environmental studies and forging alliances between the fields. Starting from the other direction, disability studies could be enriched by attending to multispecies perspectives and ecological systems. Sarah Gibbons, for example, suggests an alliance between the environmental value of biodiversity and the concept of neurodiversity in her essay discussing the "disconnect . . . between the concern that environmentalists express for rising diagnoses of autism" and the struggle for "equal rights" for those with autism. Biodiversity, which remains rather problematic as a scientific category, is nonetheless invaluable during this era of the Sixth Great Extinction. Biodiversity stresses the value of each species but also insists that diversity is crucial for the workings of broader ecological systems. Siobhan Senier argues in her essay on "blind Indians" that "for the most thoughtful scholars in environmental humanities, disability studies, and indigenous studies, systems are critically important." Senier explains that sustainability science and indigenous ecological knowledge enable us to understand these systems, insisting, however, that indigenous knowledge is "utterly intertwined with indigenous sovereignty" and not a "free-floating commodity, ready to be lifted by settler colonials when they feel in crisis." Indigenous thought, environmental studies, and disability studies converge within epistemologies that are immersed, entangled, embodied, and political. Similarly posthumanisms, new materialisms, and ecomaterialisms may help crip the environmental humanities and extend disability studies beyond the anthropocentric as they traverse human/

nonhuman divides, emphasize interactive material agencies, and encourage us to consider the human as part of assemblages with nonhuman species, as well as with technologies, substances, and prosthetics. Wheeler's beautiful essay, "Moving Together Side by Side: Human-Animal Comparisons in Picture Books," which concludes this collection, calls for "a 'prosthetic community,' a cluster of living beings, ideas, resources, and objects that enable disabled children's full inclusion."

Disability Studies and the Environmental Humanities takes on the difficult challenge of working within both of these fields, putting forth multiple ways of critiquing, accessing, and recasting natural and cultural worlds. Many of the essays within this wide-ranging volume grapple with volatile conflicts and contradictions that are not readily resolved. Indeed, the epistemologies, ontologies, politics, and trajectories of disability studies and the environmental humanities often diverge. But it is precisely these bold attempts—that refuse ready answers—that make this volume so significant, positioning it as an invaluable point of departure for further scholarship. Referencing Jack Halberstam's model of unlearning, or "negative forms of knowing," Jasbir Puar states that "disability studies is already successful in this vein, undoing conventional ways of knowing and knowledge of the body, of capacities, of human and species variation." But she proposes something "wilder": "an overwhelming of modes of knowing such that what constitutes knowing itself becomes confused, disoriented, dissembled."[2] Many of the essays that follow promise such productive confusion and disorientation. Kelly Fritsch, after noting the "troubling consequences for how ableism and environmental activism come together against disability, particularly when disability is framed as an individual health problem resulting from a toxic environment," asserts that "the problem is not toxicity or disability but rather our continued emphasis on disability as an individually economically quantifiable toxic condition." While I disagree that toxicity itself is not a problem, the way toxicity leaks and disperses in metaphorical and discursive directions remains an issue for many intersectional political struggles. Natasha Simpson analyzes the intersectional quandaries in the food justice movement. The food justice movement is rightfully meant to center the experiences of poor communities of color; however, it also often centers specific notions of health, which can limit its relevance and impact for people with disabilities—particularly those with multiple oppressed identities. These essays challenge us to unlearn fundamental conceptions of toxicity and health, calling us to imagine how other key terms could be recast as part of new political movements attuned, simultaneously, to disability, environmentalism, and environmental justice.

Puar's invocation of the disorienting, dissembling "wild," like Ladelle McWhorter's recasting of the term <u>deviance</u>, suggests that human and nonhuman lives be thought within paradigms that stress dynamic transformation and nonhuman agencies. Such a framework would be a far cry from predominant, managerial notions of sustainability that seek to stockpile inert "resources" to ensure the continued prosperity of the few.[3] But in the pages ahead Hall revitalizes the cold, wooden discourse of sustainability by proposing that we "crip sustainability": "To crip sustainability means valuing disability as a source of insight about how the border between the natural and the unnatural is maintained and for whose benefit. It means understanding a sustainable world as a world that has disability in it, a perspective that recognizes the instabilities, vulnerabilities, and dynamism that are part of naturecultures."

Kafer's essay explores "new understandings of environmentalism that take disability experiences seriously, as sites of knowledge production about nature." My conception of "trans-corporeality" in <u>Bodily Natures: Science, Environment, and the</u> <u>Material Self</u> emerged from fluctuating disability experiences, involving multiple chemical sensitivity (MCS) or environmental illness (EI), as it is also interconnected with something that could be diagnosed as rheumatoid arthritis (RA).[4] In Joseph Dumit's terms, MCS, EI, and even RA are illnesses or syndromes you have to "fight to get,"[5] meaning that the path to diagnosis is rocky and often inaccessible. Years ago I woke up on New Year's Day feeling severe joint pain and immobility. I managed to get to the hospital to be told by one physician that I had Guillain-Barré syndrome, while another rolled his eyes and uttered a different diagnosis: "That disease that starts with an 'M,' you know,"—as the first physician rolled her eyes in turn. "Do you mean MS?" I ventured. This incident and the years that followed intensified my interest in disability studies as well as in science studies' theories of material captures and the relations between embodied experience, diagnostic categories, and the alternative epistemologies of social movements and communities. People with MCS or EI, for example, move through the world as something akin to a scientific instrument that registers as harmful the very substances that others do not even notice or, if they do, consider to be harmless, normal, or even commendably sanitary and fresh. Epistemological quandaries are inherent in this condition, as questions of proof and dismissals of paranoia rarely recede. Kim's concept of the "epistemology of somatic witness" suggests the politics of knowledge involved in this and in many other situations of embodied knowledge production.

When both impending storms and public air fresheners cause pain, diminish mobility, and create mental fog, the "environment" cannot be readily divided into "nature" and "culture," nor are human bodies and minds separate from wider material interchanges and interactions. The nineteenth-century notion of "rheumatics" as "environmental invalids" that Traci Brynne Voyles discusses is, I would argue, part of a trans-corporeal paradigm that interconnects disability and environment. Thinking through the epistemological and political problematics of, say, diagnostics or accessibility, with the sense that one is always immersed within that which must be reckoned with, may be productively scaled up to grapple with immense problems of climate change, global environmental injustices, and extinction. The concept of the anthropocene, for example, in which the human is often imagined as a disembodied, abstract force, requires an exhaustive cripping, which could begin—"cripistemologically" in the words of Robert McRuer and Merri Lisa Johnson—by attending to "rejected and extraordinary bodies" and to the "places where bodily edges and categorical distinctions blur or dissolve."[6] This may seem a stretch, and yet thinking of humans and all other species as they exist at the permeable, enmeshed crossroads of body and place, within wider networks and interchanges, may be much more revealing and generative than imagining environments as external resources and humans as discrete agents. There are many sites, concepts, and theories that would benefit from thinking environmentalism and disability studies together. This capacious and thought-provoking collection analyzes an abundance of such sites, challenging scholars, activists, and everyone else who inhabits a bodymind within this multispecies world—wrought by neoliberalism, ableism, racism, homophobia, and other modes of exclusion and domination—to live and think in ways that are more inclusive, more fierce, and more just.

NOTES

1. I use the term articulate in the sense of connecting ideological or discursive elements, as described by the cultural studies and post-Marxist theories of Stuart Hall and Ernesto Laclau and Chantal Mouffe.

2. Jasbir Puar, in McRuer and Johnson, "Proliferating Cripistemologies," 164.
3. See Alaimo, "Sustainable This, Sustainable That."
4. See Alaimo, Bodily Natures.
5. Dumit, "Illnesses You Have to Fight to Get."
6. Johnson and McRuer, "Cripistemologies: Introduction," 134.

BIBLIOGRAPHY

Alaimo, Stacy. Bodily Natures: Science, Environment, and the Material Self. Bloomington: Indiana University Press, 2010.

———. "Sustainable This, Sustainable That: New Materialisms, Posthumanism, and Unknown Futures." PMLA 127, no. 3 (2012): 558–64.

Dumit, Joseph. "Illnesses You Have to Fight to Get: Facts as Forces in Uncertain, Emergent Illnesses." Social Science and Medicine 62, no. 3 (2006): 577–90.

Johnson, Merri, and Robert McRuer. "Cripistemologies: Introduction." Journal of Literary and Cultural Disability Studies 8, no. 2 (2014): 127–47.

McRuer, Robert, and Merri Johnson. "Proliferating Cripistemologies: A Virtual Roundtable." Journal of Literary and Cultural Disability Studies 8, no. 2 (2014): 149–69.

Introduction

Sarah Jaquette Ray and Jay Sibara

Our goal in this project is to bring into dialogue the interdisciplinary fields of disability studies and the environmental humanities. While scholars in the environmental humanities have been troubling the dichotomy between "wild" and "built" environments and writing about the "material turn," trans-corporealities, and "slow violence" for several years now, few focus on the robust and related work being done in the field of disability studies, which takes as a starting point the contingency between environments and bodies. Like environmental justice and the new materialist scholar Stacy Alaimo's (2010) theory of trans-corporeality, which insists that the body is constituted by its material, historical, and discursive contexts, disability studies challenges dominant perceptions of the body as separate from the contexts in which bodies live, work, and play.

Similarly the environmental humanities focus on issues, from food justice and migrant farmworkers to climate debt, military legacies, and green imperialism, that also concern disability studies scholars, such as the validity of a mind/body dualism, corporeal and mental health as a new form of privilege in what Ulrich Beck (1992) has deemed a "risk society" in Western culture, the impact of nation-building on marginalized populations and places, the myth of American rugged individualism, and parallels between the exploitation of land and abuses of labor. Putting these fields in dialogue means identifying what we learn by recasting these concerns of the environmental humanities in terms that disability studies scholars enlist, such as ableism, access, and the medical model.

For example, when we recognize that bodies are "becoming" or "temporarily abled," we begin to see how the prevailing use of pesticides disables farmworkers in order to provide fruit and vegetables to (make healthy) those who have access to them. Likewise the slow violence of military legacies, to use the postcolonial eco-critic Rob Nixon's term, manifest most often as physical and mental disabilities, both domestically and abroad. The myth of the rugged individual contributes to the social construction of "disability" and simultaneously, as many environmental thinkers argue, fosters the exploitation of natural resources. Work in environmental justice, in both the humanities and social sciences, has made some motion in the direction of disability studies by emphasizing toxicity and "body burdens," but it rarely draws on the insights of disability studies scholars, who assert that disability not be understood as a "burden" and who increasingly acknowledge that the ablement of the privileged often relies on the disablement of others (see, e.g., Meekosha 2011). And when environmental scholars critique the implicit white, male body of the outdoor enthusiast, naturalist, or adventurer, they fail to acknowledge the ableism these categories ultimately serve to reify (see, e.g., Braun 2003). In other words, it's not just any white male that heads "into the wild" in the pastoral fantasy; it's what Rosemarie Garland-Thomson (2013) calls the "normate" body, or more specifically what Ray calls in her essay in this volume a "wilderness body ideal."

The lack of exchange between these fields goes both ways and has at times reflected missed opportunities and also opposing frameworks that lead to tensions, as Alaimo outlines in her foreword to this collection. Though disability studies scholars show that built environments privilege some bodies and minds over others, few have focused on the specific ways toxic environments engender chronic illness and disability, especially for marginalized populations, or the ways environmental illnesses, often chronic and invisible, disrupt dominant paradigms for recognizing and representing "disability." Indeed the focus on built environments dominates in disability studies without recognizing wilderness as a constructed environment (Kafer 2013), and connections between the environment and disability, when addressed, are done so in the natural and social sciences, often without the critical lenses of humanistic fields, with the exception of Eli Clare's (1999) groundbreaking work. The humanities fosters a clearer understanding of how texts do the cultural work of ableism or resist such ableism, as well as attunement to the ways nature and space are similarly asked to do the work of social control. If, as geographers and anthropologists focusing on disability recognize, environments can be disabling, and if, as new materialist environmental justice scholars argue, our bodies are our first environments—the "geography closest in," as Adrienne Rich (1976, 212) puts it—it seems that environmental humanities and disability studies indeed have much to offer each other.

In recent years a handful of scholars have acknowledged and begun to articulate the tensions that have prevented more collaboration between these fields and to provide models for cooperation and convergence. For example, in 2013 the flagship journal for ecocriticism, ISLE: Interdisciplinary Studies in Literature and Environment, included a special essay cluster on disability and ecocriticism; an essay from that issue by Matthew J. C. Cella is reprinted in this collection. The 2014 sustainability-themed Society for Disability Studies (SDS) conference generated even more discussion, reflected here in works by Siobhan Senier and Jina B. Kim. The editors of this volume also convened panels to foster these conversations at the 2013 American Studies Association (ASA) conference on climate debt as disability; the 2015

SDS conference, which brought some authors of the essays herein together; and the 2016 ASA conference's Environment and Culture Caucus, which presented another opportunity to continue the conversation among contributors and other audiences. Moreover in 2016 George Washington University hosted its biennial Composing Disability conference with the theme of "crip ecologies."

Inspired by these early conversations and seeking to foster more, we solicited papers by graduate students and independent scholars working in the humanities or closely related fields. We welcomed broad understandings of disability and strongly encouraged submissions that take into consideration intersections not only among disability and environment but also among other categories of difference that are co-implicated in those first two terms, including race, gender, class, sexuality, and immigration or nation. We also welcomed pieces covering historical and contemporary periods as well as proposals addressing non-U.S. regions and transnational relationships. The contributors we selected from this search demonstrate in varied and sometimes unpredictable ways just how much these two fields have to offer each other.

As we looked for thematic and theoretical connections among the submissions alongside the foundational pieces, we narrowed down to a collection with a primary geopolitical focus on North America; essays that expand beyond that focus, including works by Cathy Schlund-Vials, Julie Sadler, and Anita Mannur, share a concern with tracing the disabling legacies of U.S. military, national security, and industrial impact. Thus the collection ultimately reflects our shared scholarly background, expertise, and networks in transnational American studies and will likely be especially useful to scholars and students of disability and environment working in and around this expansive field, but we expect it will prove productive for those working beyond the boundaries of American studies as well because of its interdisciplinary strengths.

Temporally the project spans the seventeenth century to the present, beginning with Senier's essay engaging the legacy of American colonization and continuing with Ray's essay tracing the history of ableism in early environmentalist thought and the wilderness movement of the Progressive Era, as well as work by Traci Brynn Voyles on the history of the Salton Sea (1920s–present), Víctor M. Torres-Vélez on the U.S. Navy's occupation of Vieques Island, Puerto Rico (1941–2004), Mary E. Mendoza on the U.S.-Mexican Bracero Program (1942–64), Schlund-Vials on the U.S. Central Intelligence Agency's "Secret War" in Lao People's Democratic Republic (1964–73), Natasha Simpson on the Black Panther Party's food justice organizing (beginning in 1969), Mannur on Union Carbide's disaster in Bhopal (1984), and Sadler on the U.S. Iraq War (2003–11), all of which provide historical context for the pieces with a more contemporary focus. The historical breadth of the collection offers multiple temporal points of entry to students and scholars and allows for analysis across historical eras, countering what some have criticized as a "presentist" focus in disability studies (Wheaton 2010, 4). Further, if we take seriously Nixon's arguments about slow violence, limiting the eras around which these essays are organized misses the point: many of the injustices these essays describe have burdened and will continue to burden bodies and minds well beyond the scope of their declared time frame.

In addition to representing several historically oriented essays, the collection deliberately contains a broad mix of disciplinary and interdisciplinary approaches in the humanities and closely related fields, ranging from literary studies to community development and medical anthropology. The selection also reflects our commitment to intersectional analysis and to including the work of emerging and independent as well as established and senior scholars.

Organization of the Book

In constructing this anthology for use by scholars and students we have created a "Foundations" section highlighting the few but pivotal contributions scholars have already made to this emerging field of fields. We separate these foundational texts from the new essays in order to recognize the early and influential work of scholars who undertook the challenge of bringing together two (and sometimes more) fields that rarely have been in dialogue. Bridging these fields entailed intellectual, political, and professional risks, without which the current collection would neither be possible nor legible. Thus we distinguish these texts not to create a "canon" or "best of" list but rather to construct the anthology as a genealogical project, an approach we hope will allow readers to analyze the development of conversations about disability and environment from the early 2000s to the contemporary moment.

Certainly other equally appropriate foundational texts exist, as do many works that focus on health, bodies, and landscape or environment, some preceding the 2000s, some contemporaneous with those included here. By reprinting these particular texts we offer variations of how these fields might speak to each other, but we do not mean to suggest that there are no other possible fruitful synergies. Because so many of the authors of the new essays draw on and extend the works in the foundational section, we believe it will benefit readers to see a lineage of thought collected in one volume. To that end we organized the foundational pieces chronologically, which reflects the emergence of these works over the past decade leading up to the present moment, a snapshot of which is found in the new works section.

Opening the "Foundations" section, Ray's 2009 essay "Risking Bodies in the Wild: The 'Corporeal Unconscious' of American Adventure Culture" builds on the work of scholars who have "challenged the race, class, and gender exclusions of early and contemporary environmentalism" but moves beyond those critiques to demonstrate the ways environmentalism and its legacies, the wilderness movement and contemporary risk culture, possess a "corporeal unconscious" that idealizes the physically fit, masculine, and white body. Environmentalism has thus defined the disabled body as contradictory to its vision of a harmonious relationship between humans and nature, further reflected in the use of ableist metaphors and analogies to describe environmental crisis. Yet, Ray contends, "despite a troubled historical relationship, environmentalists and disability studies theorists share important values" in their mutual promotion of "an increased awareness of place and of various versions of bodies in place," pointing toward the possibility of a shared understanding of "an ethical way of being in the world," a theme taken up by other writers in this section, including Anthony J. Nocella II and Cella.

Moving from a focus on mainstream environmentalist movements to environmental justice organizing, Valerie Ann Johnson in "Bringing Together Feminist Disability Studies and Environmental Justice" (2011) calls for the "merging" of these two fields in order to "confront the power dynamics" that marginalize people with disabilities from environmental justice activism and scholarship. Pointing to the implicit ableism often underlying environmental justice rhetoric, which tends to "conflate disability, disease, and environmental injustice," Johnson argues, "We need to disaggregate the possible results of environmental injustice (e.g., exposure to toxic substances emanating from landfills or hog operations that injure the body) from the person, however they are embodied." Johnson contends that people with disabilities need to be at the center of organizing to ensure that environmental justice's aims and language reflect and prioritize the issues affecting those whose well-being environmental justice claims to represent.

Mel Y. Chen's essay "Lead's Racial Matters" (2012) draws attention to a substance that has been the focus of much environmental justice activism in the United States, as well as the focus of a U.S. "panic" in 2007 regarding the threat of lead poisoning from Chinese products. Chen traces how media discourses mobilized protectionist and "contagion" discourses from earlier anti-Chinese, anti-immigrant campaigns in the United States, leading to the racialization of lead as a "foreign" and specifically Chinese threat to the health of white American children. This media narrative regarding a hypothetical threat never actually documented or proven diverted attention from the continued impact of lead on the health of low-income children of color in the United States as well as the health of Chinese workers and their communities. Chen observes that U.S. media discourses have taken up environmental justice rhetoric about lead poisoning in ways that contribute to the racialization of low-income black communities as prone to criminality because of cognitive impairments, a reminder to environmental and disability justice advocates about the risks of mainstream media coverage and co-optation of movement goals.

In "Defining Eco-ability: Social Justice and the Intersectionality of Disability, Nonhuman Animals, and Ecology" (2012), Nocella develops a philosophy of eco-ability that incorporates concerns about social justice for people with disabilities as well as nonhuman animals to "demonstrate how disability studies can take a position on the current ecological crisis." Nocella provides a useful introduction to central concepts and critiques in disability studies for readers coming in without that background, and then shows how ableism and speciesism are interrelated systems of discrimination and oppression. Interrogating the ableism in some animal liberation rhetoric, he offers a different model of engagement between animal studies and disability studies, identifying the synchrony between disability studies' critiques of normalcy and its valuations of interdependence with theorizations of ecology that similarly emphasize interdependence and diversity.

Similar to Nocella but using the tools of literary studies and phenomenology, Cella in "The Ecosomatic Paradigm in Literature: Merging Disability Studies and Ecocriticism" (2013) contends that it is possible to "deconstruct norms of embodiment while simultaneously promoting ethical treatment of the natural world." Cella introduces the ecosomatic paradigm to literary studies; this method of analysis, which synthesizes ecocriticism with the sociocultural model of disability studies, reflects what Cella describes as the "contiguity between the mind-body and its social and natural environments." He notably expands the archive of literature often studied within disability studies and ecocriticism, demonstrating the resonance of the ecosomatic paradigm across a range of works, including Nancy Mairs's Waist-High in the World, Cormac McCarthy's The Road, and Linda Hogan's Solar Storms.

Further developing connections between the social model of disability and environmental studies, Alison Kafer in "Bodies of Nature: The Environmental Politics of Disability" (2013) points to the ways disability studies' focus on built environments has "prevented [the field] from engaging with the wider environment of wilderness, parks, and nonhuman nature because the social model seems to falter in such settings." Drawing on insights from environmental studies, Kafer argues that the natural environment needs to be recognized among disability studies scholars as another built environment designed to exclude people with disabilities and people of color, along with "queer acts and practices," in order to make nature accessible and comfortable for white, middle-class, heteronormative, and able-bodied travelers. Sharing common concerns with Ray, Kafer analyzes how popular discourses of nature and environment as well as writings about nature employ ableist rhetoric and reflect ableist assumptions. She concludes with a reading of Clare's Exile and Pride that inspires her call for a "cripped environmentalism" in recognition that "the experience of illness and disability presents alternative ways of understanding ourselves in relation to the environment."

We are delighted to reprint Clare's "Notes on Natural Worlds, Disabled Bodies, and a Politics of Cure" from Serenella Iovino and Serpil Oppermann's collection, Material Ecocriticism (2014). Carrying forward his work in Exile and Pride, a book that arguably put the intersection of these fields on the radar of many environmental justice scholars, this more recent essay critiques the impulses toward health that underwrite both ecological restoration efforts and the "politics of cure" surrounding disability. Clare asks, "Are disabled bodies akin to cornfields," monoculture landscapes stripped of biodiversity and history? In this framework "disabled bodies are as damaging to culture as cornfields are to nature," a troubling analogy for both a "healthy" nature and a "diverse" culture. In the end Clare's contribution is so important because it exemplifies the messiness of putting these fields in dialogue with one another; he presses, "How do we witness, name, and resist the injustices that reshape and damage all kinds of bodies—plant and animal, organic and inorganic, nonhuman and human? And alongside our resistance how do we make peace with the reshaped and damaged bodies themselves, cultivate love and respect for them?" A politics of cure, like the ecology of restoration, is a double-edged sword. Further, as the inclusion of Clare's essay in Material Ecocriticism reflects, this relationship is not mere analogy; the material connections between our bodies and our environments cast in sharp relief the myriad ways damaged environments damage bodies, and bodies are contingent upon their environments.

These foundational works collectively identify tensions that have kept these fields of inquiry apart and point toward exciting possibilities for coming together. Importantly they model intersectional approaches to exploring disability and environment, incorporating race, class, gender, and nation into their investigations, a precedent taken up by many of the contributors in the "New Essays" section as well. Through these investigations, many of which share a common methodology of media and discourse analysis, these foundational pieces collectively demonstrate the value of humanities-based inquiries in identifying how mainstream discourses about disability and the environment have supported the interests of white supremacy and ableism, while also showing how resistant and activist discourses including environmental justice and animal liberation have still excluded or marginalized people with disabilities. Several of these works incorporate personal testimony as well as personal communications with other activists and scholars, reflecting a common methodology in environmental and disability writings that here is reworked in ways that crip the nature writing genre and ecologize the disability memoir.

We organized the new pieces in sections that foreground key theoretical and thematic points of convergence between the two fields, based on the essays that resulted from our call. Those themes allow us to make arguments within the broader argument of the volume. We chose not to organize these pieces according to discipline or chronology because doing so would overemphasize those shared dimensions of each category over the much more productive contributions that each section—organized thematically instead—makes. Since the fields of environmental humanities and disability studies both seek to be interdisciplinary, showcasing how thinkers from different fields address similar themes reveals the new insights that such cross-disciplinary dialogue can generate.

This organization is intended to facilitate intellectual engagement among the more known, foundational works and the other thematic clusters in the volume. It prompts readers to discover and explore the ways in which the earlier work has influenced new scholarship in many and multiple directions; for example, Kafer's work is referenced in new essays by Mannur, Kim Q. Hall, and Elizabeth Wheeler; each scholar takes up Kafer's work in different ways, which illustrates precisely the kind of diffusion of these groundbreaking ideas across disciplines and approaches that we want this volume to showcase. By demonstrating how these fields are converging, we aim to inspire further synergy between them. Recognizing that it is not possible to create a definitive collection covering all angles on this particular topic, we hope readers will agree this volume demonstrates the fruitfulness and urgency of ongoing dialogue between these fields and will be inspired to fill in any gaps they perceive.

The essays in "Corporeal Legacies of U.S. Nation-Building" insist that one of the most productive points of contact between the fields of disability studies and environmental justice is U.S. imperialism. The pieces in this section thus address a topic of central importance to environmental justice scholarship: the environmental legacy of U.S. military occupation. They demonstrate that this environmental legacy is a disability legacy, something few scholars in either the environmental humanities or disability studies have theorized. And they employ intersectional analyses of disability, race, gender, and nation—again a rarity in the environmental humanities and disability studies.

The essay by Senier, "Blind Indians: Káteri Tekakwí:tha and Joseph Amos's Visions of Indigenous Resurgence," is a case study foregrounding blindness in disability studies and indigeneity as key to understanding the ways in which imperialism has been and continues to be disabling. "Prosthetic Ecologies: (Re)Membering Disability and and Rehabilitating Laos's 'Secret War'" by Schlund-Vials explores the urgent current issue of injury caused by unexploded ordnance in Laos. A close reading of the visitor center, this essay proposes the concept of "prosthetic ecologies" to help us understand the twin corporeal and ecological slow violences resulting from the CIA's nine-year covert bombing campaign against Lao PDR during the longer U.S. military intervention in Vietnam and the broader region of Southeast Asia. Much disability studies scholarship on prosthesis and war injury has focused on canonical narratives from white Western literature (e.g., Mitchell and Snyder's [2001] theory of narrative prosthesis) or white U.S. veterans (e.g., Serlin 2004; Gerber 1994); like Torres-Vélez, Schlund-Vials expands this scholarship by analyzing the experiences of nonwhite, non-Western people disabled by U.S. bombings (and testings, as Torres-Vélez describes). Schlund-Vials is engaged in work that pushes disability studies in these new critical, more global directions, which Michael Davidson (2006), Helen Meekosha (2011), and others have called for. Similarly Torres-Vélez's "Reification, Biomedicine, and Bombs: Women's Politicization in Vieques's Social Movement" takes us to another site of U.S. expansion and draws on fifty interviews to analyze biomedicine's foundations in militarization and forward a gendered analysis of disproportionate harm to women, whose critiques of expert knowledge and revision of understandings of disease causality help Torres-Vélez articulate a vivid example of what he calls a "conspiracy of invisibilities." We are excited to include this piece as disability studies are often underengaged within fields like medical anthropology, Torres-Vélez's disciplinary orientation. Its inclusion reflects our sense that this lack of engagement does not result only or entirely from ableism by scholars in fields other than disability studies but also perhaps from an implicit racism underlying disability studies, which has discouraged ethnic studies scholars and scholars of color from engaging with the field (e.g., Bell 2006). Torres-Vélez suggests that disability studies might benefit from a challenge to some of the long-held tenets of the field, which may prove inadequate or even alienating to those attempting to theorize the experiences of people who have become disabled as a result of racist inequalities and imperialist violence and military occupation. Sadler's "War Contaminants and Environmental Justice: The Case of Congenital Heart Defects in Iraq" exposes precisely the kind of NIMBYism that characterizes modern "precision" warfare in the current U.S. military entanglement. Scrutinizing the "affective symbolism of the heart," Sadler rejects the depersonalization the language of modern warfare invites and shows that there is nothing surgical, precise, or clean about the U.S. assaults in Iraq. Bringing to the fore the uneven impacts of expansion and national security on bodies deemed disposable, this section shows that empire disables some people in order to enable other forms of privilege.

The next section, "(Re)Producing Toxicity," attends to the accumulations accrued by externalizing environmental costs to the highly interior intimacies of the body. Kelly Fritsch's "Toxic Pregnancies: Speculative Futures, Disabling Environments, and Neoliberal Biocapital" takes on the deployment of disability as an apocalyptic speculative future and refocuses attention on the imbrication of disability with neoliberal (bio)capitalism. The Union Carbide disaster at Bhopal calls for serious attention from a critical disability perspective, and Mannur provides it in "'That Night': Seeing Bhopal through the Lens of Disability and Environmental Justice Studies." Invoking Nixon's notion of "slow dyings," Mannur demonstrates in close readings of two non-Anglophone texts that the lethal effects of the Bhopal disaster are ongoing.

The third section, "Food Justice," brings together essays that emphasize the relationship between disablement and systems of food production and cultures of food consumption. Simpson's "Disabling Justice? The Exclusion of People with Disabilities from the Food Justice Movement" critiques the food justice movement for implicit ableism on the grounds that invisible disabilities such as food allergies make the modern food revolution inaccessible to some people. Hall's "Cripping Sustainability, Realizing Food Justice" dovetails with Simpson's essay, directing readers' attention to the mainstream food movement. Critiquing popular food writings on sustainability for excluding disability from all that is to be sustained and for promoting a heteronormative vision of sustainability, Hall's piece makes the case for an alternative understanding of sustainable foodscapes that places accessibility front and center.

The fourth section, "Curing Crips? Narratives of Health and Space," evokes the tradition of using certain kinds of palliative environments to heal or, worse, cure invalidism. If some kinds of environments disable, then certainly some kinds of environments enable. But what are the exclusionary assumptions in these associations, for both people and environments? Voyles's essay, "The Invalid Sea: Disability Studies and Environmental Justice History," begins to answer this question. Voyles examines the Salton Sea as a lens through which to clarify a variety of contradictions in our understandings of "environment": natural/unnatural, treasure/hazard, wetland/desert. Seen as an "environmental invalid," the Salton Sea was also a place to send people with disabilities. But Voyles also analyzes this rest cure in terms of its gendered history, reinforcing the volume's emphasis on intersectional analysis. In

"La Tierra Pica/The Soil Bites: Hazardous Environments and the Degeneration of Bracero Health, 1942–1964," Mendoza shifts our focus to the Bracero Program, elucidating the haunting story of Adolfo Ramírez Bañuelos to think through the issues in this anthology. With original historical research Mendoza provides new insights about the medicalized racialization at the border. She rejects the dominant narrative that Mexicans coming to the United States to work brought disease with them, and shows how in fact work inside the United States is what disabled Mexican workers. Turning from the Salton Sea and the border to the LA freeway system as a space where the binary of health/disease are once again scrutinized, the last essay in this section is Kim's "Cripping East Los Angeles: Enabling Environmental Justice in Helena María Viramontes's Their Dogs Came with Them." Kim reads Viramontes's novel as offering "a politics and aesthetics of interdependency" that explores how the built environment of East LA is not only disabling but also enabling. The last essay in this section is Sarah Gibbons's "Neurological Diversity and Environmental (In)Justice: The Ecological Other in Popular and Journalist Representations of Autism." Gibbons begins by critiquing how autism is explained by appeals to environmental harms and toxins, but she moves from there to argue that research on autism and environment is framed for the public in ways that turn autistic people into "ecological others"—an extension of the paradigm Ray (2013) proposes in The Ecological Other: Environmental Exclusion in American Culture. Suggesting interesting linkages between neurodiversity and biodiversity, Gibbons concludes, "Concerned environmentalists can first consider whether autistic people are interested in the salvation that research into environmental triggers promises."

The last section, "Interspecies and Interage Identifications," prioritizes a variety of perspectives that do not enjoy the benefits of liberal humanist agency—the child and the animal—supporting resistance from outside the normate position in ways that broaden environmental subjecthood. Two of the essays focus on autism, and so readers might wonder why we did not create a section on autism or neurodiversity, grouping together the essays by David T. Mitchell and Sharon L. Snyder, Robert Melchior Figueroa, and Gibbons. We did consider this possibility in an initial draft, as this is a key contested topic that arises when you bring disability studies and environmental humanities into dialogue. However, we rejected this plan because it would segregate those three pieces on the basis of an identitarian grouping that is not consistent with the thematic arrangement of the rest of the "New Works" section and would therefore potentially limit readers' intellectual engagement with those pieces beyond that cluster, whereas we see each of those pieces contributing to multiple dialogues in the anthology, including but not limited to autism. Further, and perhaps more important, we wanted to avoid reinforcing the mental/physical disability dualism that some of the essays in this volume seek to challenge.

Thinking about the perspectives offered by youth and animals, despite the downside of implying that animals are like children (i.e., naïve) or that children (with or without disabilities) are like animals (i.e., base or less than human), seemed a productive direction for the disability-environment connection compared to the problems created by having a section on neurodiversity and a separate section on animals. We described the former problem earlier; the latter involves implying that people with disabilities, especially children, are more like animals than normate adults. Although other scholars robustly scrutinize this problematic essentializing (see, e.g., Wheeler's essay in this volume), this section's authors make provocative new claims about how a crip epistemology might provide insights into an environmental ethic that includes the more-than-human world. Rather than essentializing children and animals, then, we hope this section amplifies these voices from the margins.

The first essay in this section is by Mitchell and Snyder. "Precarity and Cross-Species Identification: Autism, the Critique of Normative Cognition, and Nonspeciesism" pursues an understanding of disability as an "agential, material, and affective embodiment" to argue that disability studies must allow "ways to meaningfully encounter embodiment." The particular focus of their analysis is the relation between disability and animality and how it plays out in Mark Haddon's novel <u>The Curious Incident of the Dog in the Night-time</u>. Mitchell and Snyder argue that the novel undermines "hierarchical speciesism" and "position[s] autism as an alternative system of devotions to devalued participants." The authors expand the set of approaches of "new materialism" within environmental humanities by showing how it can be applied to produce a more sophisticated disability studies. Figueroa's "Autism and Environmental Identity: Environmental Justice and the Chains of Empathy" further engages with new materialism, adopting a tool from environmental humanities— the affect of "environmental empathy"—to intervene in the familiar discourses around autism. For example, his critical exploration of "autistic environmental trauma" rejects the cordoning-off of therapy solutions because they "[limit] these opportunities in more normate spaces." Wheeler's "Moving Together Side by Side: Human-Animal Comparisons in Picture Books" explores an interspecies "prosthetic community" to exemplify how conversation between fields (in this case animal studies and disability studies) entails enriching interconnections but also contradictions and tensions. Wheeler provides a close reading of two texts, attending to a variety of intersectional dynamics (gender, race, capitalism, culture, postcolonialism). One crucial intervention is her rejection of the way some mergings of animal studies and disability studies fail to challenge humanism and thereby leave people with disabilities essentialized as other than human. Drawing on critical animal studies' preference for the idea of animals as more than human, Wheeler insists that "the richer the prosthetic community, the more humans with disabilities can compare themselves to animals without risking their status as persons." She concludes with a question that encapsulates the shift we hope this volume will make in readers: "How can the vulnerability of disabled people be perceived as part of our shared vulnerability on the planet, and the vulnerability of the planet itself, rather than a unique and separate kind of weakness?"

Intended Audiences and Uses

The intended audiences for this volume include scholars and graduate and undergraduate students in the fields of disability studies and the environmental humanities. In addition it has potential use and appeal to students and researchers in African American studies, animal studies, Asian and Asian American studies, community development, environmental justice, environmental studies, feminist science studies, geography, global studies, Latin@ and Latin American studies, linguistics, literary studies, media studies, medical anthropology, Native American studies, philosophy, and women and gender studies, among other areas. The inclusion of the foundational pieces is intended to make the anthology especially productive for use in undergraduate and graduate courses, either as a full-term textbook in a course on disability and the environmental humanities that will allow students to trace themes from foundational to contemporary works, or as a supplemental text from which instructors can incorporate one or more of the thematic sections or theme-based reading clusters into a more broadly defined course.

Inspirations and Acknowledgments

The editors first conceived this project in 2012 during a conversation at the Association for the Study of Literature and Environment's Off-Year Symposium in Juneau, Alaska. We think it is important to share how we came to this project because that reveals much about the current states and locations of scholarship and activism on disability and environment from which this book emerges.

Sarah writes: As a graduate student in a University of Oregon English seminar, Urban and Social Ecologies in American Literature, my professor and now mentor and colleague Elizabeth A. Wheeler introduced me to disability studies. My training in political ecological approaches to cultural studies already had me attentive to power and the ways nature can become a form of social control, both materially and discursively. I began to think about how nature is a way to exclude people with disabilities from the national body politic. At the same time that I was taking Wheeler's course, I took a course with the environmental historian Mark David Spence (1999), which allowed me to see the ways in which wilderness in America has been constructed to fortify a white, "pure" American citizenry. Simultaneously I was in a graduate seminar, American Empire, with the Wayne Morse Visiting Scholar Neil Smith (2008). These brilliant influences helped me put together big ideas: empire, environment, exclusion, and biopolitics. When I read Donna Haraway's (1989) "Teddy Bear Patriarchy" and Jake Kosek's (2004) "Purity and Pollution," I had a huge revelation: disability, much like Toni Morrison's (1993) "Africanist presence," activated the environmental works I was studying in my literature and environment courses, though disability was never part of this scholarship. I started to see how anxiety about a loss of nature was anxiety about the loss of a certain kind of body and, by extension, national identity. Mapping the social construction of wilderness alongside the social construction of disability became my dissertation and then book project, and since then, with the support of scholars like Rachel Stein, Noël Sturgeon, and Giovanna di Chiro, I have analyzed these connections through environmental justice in much of my work. I organized conference panels for the Association for the Study of Literature and Environment (ASLE) around these themes, started challenging my own ableist assumptions, developed more inclusive pedagogies, and, when I reconnected with Jay in Alaska (years after we had gone to college together), was thrilled to find a kindred spirit with whom I could collaborate to produce a collection like this. Ever since I first encountered disability studies, I have been wanting to bring these fields together more fully and broaden my own understanding of these intersections. In part because of our respective strengths (mine more in environmental humanities and Jay's more in disability studies) and in part because of the chance to rekindle a college friendship, it has been a pleasure to have had these conversations with someone as excited about these connections as I.

Jay writes: I have been engaged with disability studies since 2004, when I first encountered The Disability Studies Reader in an American studies seminar with Rachel Adams at Columbia University. I have lived with disability for much longer. I also got involved in environmental justice activism while living in New York City during the early 2000s but did not discover the relevance of environmental studies to my academic work on disability until late in graduate school. As a doctoral candidate at the University of Southern California I read only a few environmental studies articles and books (Pulido 2000; Tsing 2005) in seminars on American studies, critical race studies, and gender studies. My partner, also a graduate student at USC, had a much deeper background in environmental studies and had just finished her dissertation on the literature of climate change (Sigler Sibara 2012). As I read her work, as well as some of the theorists she engaged, including Rob Nixon (2006–7) on slow violence, I started noticing the environmental concerns in the literary and film texts I was analyzing in my unfinished dissertation on race, disability, and U.S. empire. The primary texts at the center of that project demonstrate that environmental justice concerns have been and continue to be central to many women of color activist movements against racism and imperialism. They also demonstrate the centrality of chronic illness and disability concerns to labor and environmental justice campaigns. When Sarah and her colleague Kevin Maier sent out a call for papers for the ASLE symposium, I noticed in their language an opening for work addressing health and disability concerns. My partner and I each submitted abstracts and with support from USC, were soon headed to the University of Alaska Southeast at Juneau, where Sarah and I reconnected (having first met as undergraduates at Swarthmore College) and forged a new connection based on our shared interest in the intersection of disability and environment. "Let's edit a volume together," Sarah proposed, and the rest is history.

From this point of mutual inspiration, many others have contributed to the enrichment and completion of this project. We would like to thank the two anonymous peer reviewers for their generative critiques, incisive recommendations, and strong support; University of Nebraska Press editors Alicia Christensen, Elizabeth Zaleski, and Marguerite Boyles for enthusiastically shepherding the project from the very beginning; and the professional communities that have helped us develop the concerns of this volume: the Association for the Study of Literature and Environment, the Society for Disability Studies, and the American Studies Association (particularly the Environment and Culture Caucus). For Jay, Colby College has generously supported this project with a Humanities Division Grant as well as with additional funding for a Junior Faculty Writing Group hosted at Colby, for travel to writing residencies where significant work on the anthology was completed, and for travel to conferences to meet in person with the volume's contributors and promote dialogue among interdisciplinary audiences about the anthology's themes and interventions. The Sitka Center for Art and Ecology and Grass Mountain residency programs on the Oregon coast also supported the writing and editing of the project.

Our professors at Swarthmore College nurtured us as undergraduates and sent us out into the world on separate paths, equipped to ask the challenging, interdisciplinary questions that would lead us, serendipitously, to find each other again at the ASLE symposium in 2012. Some individuals have mentored and supported us and the project beyond the call of duty and therefore deserve mention by name here: Elizabeth A. Wheeler, Susan Schweik, Susan Burch, Robert Figueroa, Stacy Alaimo, Kathleen Brian, Mel Y. Chen, Michael Davidson, Janet Fiskio, Julietta Hua, Alison Kafer, Salma Monani, Viet Thanh Nguyen, John Carlos Rowe, Nicole Seymour, Rachel Stein, Julie Sze, Julie A. Minich, and Sarah Wald. It is no exaggeration to say we would never have considered doing this project if it were not for the intellectual work and community building they have done to make ours possible.

Finally, Jay would like to thank family and close friends for support throughout this project, including Josie Sigler Sibara, Anne-Marie Claire, Ron and Cedar Barager, Frank and Jane Boyden, Mindy Chaffin and Taylor Grenfell, Vivian Ducat and Ray Segal, Alexis Lothian and Kathryn Wagner, Emanuel Powell III, Benjamin Shockey, and Miriam Schmidt and Jeremy, Ursula, and Esme Blyth. Sarah would like to thank family for countless forms of emotional, material, and bodily sustenance, not to mention child care: James, Hazel, and Daisy Ray; Jane Jaquette; David

Jaquette; Abraham Lowenthal; and Anette Jaquette. Sarah would also like to honor the memory of one of her most inspiring feminist mentors, her geography professor Susan W. Hardwick, who passed away on November 11, 2015. Susan embodied the ethic of care that is at the heart of this project.

REFERENCES

Alaimo, Stacy. 2010. Bodily Natures: Science, the Environment, and the Material Self. Bloomington: Indiana University Press.

Beck, Ulrich. 1992. The Risk Society: Towards a New Modernity. London: Sage.

Bell, Chris. 2006. "Introducing White Disability Studies: A Modest Proposal." In The Disability Studies Reader, 2d ed., edited by Lennard J. Davis, 275–82. New York: Routledge.

Braun, Bruce. 2003. "'On the Raggedy Edge of Risk': Articulations of Race and Nature after Biology." In Race, Nature, and the Politics of Difference, edited by Donald S. Moore, Jake Kosek, and Anand Pandian, 175–203. Durham NC: Duke University Press.

Chen, Mel Y. 2012. "Lead's Racial Matters." In Animacies: Biopolitics, Racial Mattering, and Queer Affect, 159–88. Durham NC: Duke University Press.

Clare, Eli. 1999. Exile and Pride: Disability, Queerness, and Liberation. Durham NC: Duke University Press.

Davidson, Michael. 2006. "Universal Design: The Work of Disability in an Age of Globalization." In The Disability Studies Reader, 2d ed., edited by Lennard J. Davis, 117–28. New York: Routledge.

Garland-Thomson, Rosemarie. 2013. "Integrating Disability, Transforming Feminist Theory." Feminist Disability Studies 14, no. 3: 1–32.

Gerber, David A. 1994. "Heroes and Misfits: The Troubled Social Reintegration of Disabled Veterans in The Best Years of Our Lives." American Quarterly 46, no. 4: 545–74.

Haraway, Donna J. 1989. "Teddy Bear Patriarchy." In Primate Visions: Gender, Race, and Nature in the World of Modern Science, 20–64. New York: Routledge.

Kafer, Alison. 2013. Feminist, Queer, Crip. Bloomington: Indiana University Press.

Kosek, Jake. 2004. "Purity and Pollution: Racial Degradation and Environmental Anxieties." In Liberation Ecologies: Environment, Development, and Social Movements, 2nd ed., edited by Richard Peet and Michael Watts, 125–59. New York: Routledge.

Meekosha, Helen. 2011. "Decolonising Disability: Thinking and Acting Globally." Disability and Society 26, no. 6: 667–82.

Mitchell, David T., and Susan L. Snyder. 2001. Narrative Prosthesis: Disability and the Dependencies of Discourse. Ann Arbor: University of Michigan Press.

Morrison, Toni. 1993. Playing in the Dark: Whiteness and the Literary Imagination. New York: Vintage.

Nixon, Rob. 2006–7. "Slow Violence, Gender, and the Environmentalism of the Poor." Journal of Commonwealth and Postcolonial Studies 13, no. 2–14, no. 1: 14–37.

Nocella, Anthony J., II, Judy K. C. Bentley, and Janet M. Duncan, eds. 2012. Earth, Animal, and Disability Liberation: The Rise of the Eco-Ability Movement. New York: Peter Lang.

Pulido, Laura. 2000. "Rethinking Environmental Racism: White Privilege and Urban Development in Southern California." Annals of the Association of American Geographers 90, no. 1: 12–40.

Ray, Sarah Jaquette. 2013. The Ecological Other: Environmental Exclusion in American Culture. Tucson: University of Arizona Press.

Rich, Adrienne. 1976. Of Woman Born: Motherhood as Experience and Institution. New York: Norton.

Serlin, David. 2004. Replaceable You: Engineering the Body in Postwar America. Chicago: University of Chicago Press.

Sigler Sibara, Josie Anne. 2012. "Dangerous Climate: Race, Gender, and State Violence in Post-Carbon Fiction." PhD dissertation, University of Southern California.

Smith, Neil. 2008. Uneven Development: Nature, Capitalism, and the Production of Space. Athens: University of Georgia Press.

Spence, Mark David. 1999. Dispossessing the Wilderness: Indian Removal and the Making of the National Parks. Oxford: Oxford University Press.

Tsing, Anna. 2005. Friction: An Ethnography of Global Connection. Princeton NJ: Princeton University Press.

Wheaton, Edward. 2010. Stumbling Blocks before the Blind: Medieval Constructions of a Disability. Ann Arbor: University of Michigan Press.

Part 1
Foundations

1

Risking Bodies in the Wild

The "Corporeal Unconscious" of
American Adventure Culture

Sarah Jaquette Ray

At the heart of outdoor adventure sports is the appeal of personal challenge. The individual—usually male—pits himself against Nature and survives. "Whether climbing, running, jumping or plunging," Bruce Braun (2003, 181) writes, "it is the encounter and the challenge that matter." Not only do adventure sports provide "the consummate image of courage and skill" (181); they also offer transcendence and purification. Adventure culture locates the site of moral purity and connection to nature in the suffering body. As the adventure writer and journalist Jon Krakauer (1997, 136) explains, the appeal of mountaineering is precisely its physical discomfort: "I quickly came to understand that climbing Everest was primarily about enduring pain. And in subjecting ourselves to week after week of toil, tedium and suffering, it struck me that most of us were probably seeking, above all else, something like a state of grace." If getting close to nature is about risking the body in the wild, what kind of environmental ethic is available to the disabled body? How did corporeal risk become an environmentalist practice in the first place?

The appeal of today's adventure sports can be traced to the nineteenth-century enthusiasm for alpine climbing and "wilderness cults" (Nash 1967). Understanding the historical context of wilderness and environmentalism in the Progressive Era illuminates what is at stake in the role of the body in contemporary environmentalism and adventure sports. Environmental historians have shown the modern environmental movement developed in response to various social, economic, and spatial anxieties of the Progressive Era. Environmentalism matured into a movement at a time of turmoil. In part the movement was motivated by the emerging sciences of ecology and evolutionary theory, but the notion of an environmental ethic toward pristine nature was also gaining force, emphasizing a retreat into the wilderness as a palliative for both the individual and the nation.

Wilderness adventure was not just about communing with nature and testing the body; it was a direct response to social instability and nation-building during the Progressive Era. Environmentalism emerged in response to domestic and geopolitical conditions, evolving in tandem with social Darwinism, which portrayed life as a contest for both genetic and national survival. Those who were fit, both individuals and races, "naturally" dominated those who were weaker. Ironically American civilization could be advanced by "going native" (Huhndorf 2001)—practicing wilderness survival exercises, such as hunting, living off the land, and eschewing modernity's conveniences.

The nineteenth-century grandfathers of the modern environmental movement, such as Ernst Haeckel (who coined the term ecology as we use it today) and George Perkins Marsh, promoted an image of the ideal American tested in the wilderness, showcasing self-reliance as achievable through an encounter with "raw nature." The burgeoning movement of environmentalism gained support from many whose interests were potentially in conflict but for whom environmentalism seemed to address their social anxieties: those who were part of the romantic reaction to modernity, such as John Muir; those who wanted to preserve the myth of American exceptionalism, such as Frederick Jackson Turner; and those who feared the loss of white, Protestant dominance and wanted to prepare Americans for the competition ahead, such as Theodore Roosevelt.

But the positive image of environmentalism as protecting nature for "resources" and "refuge" disguised its exclusions and reinforced social norms in ways that helped regenerate the declining power of the Anglo-Protestant elite.[1] Wilderness served as "the theater of American empire" (Cosgrove 1995, 35) and could become a meaningful concept only in the context of environmentalists' racial and social anxieties. It justified the displacement of Native Americans, subsistence farmers, and squatters (Spence 1999; Jacoby 2001) to "conserve" land for white men who came from politically powerful families. The wilderness cults of the Progressive Era promoted wilderness as essential to moral, racial, and national "purity," a focus that reflected American culture's obsession with "social hygiene" in the late nineteenth century (Kosek 2004; Braun 2003).

Similarly scholars have argued that a crisis of white bourgeois identity that drove men into the wilderness was also a "crisis of masculinity," gender, and sexuality. In the Victorian era civilization was thought to be "feminizing" because of unprecedented immigration, which turned the city into a socially unhygienic space. Wilderness parks were a response to a perceived crisis of masculinity at the turn of the century; the appeal of the aesthetics of a sublime, mountaintop transcendence could be appealing (or accessible) to men only in such a context. Krista Comer (1997, 219) thus proposes that a common trope in environmentally themed texts is the "wilderness ideal plot," which defines wilderness as a "space capable of reinvigorating masculine virility while staving off the emasculating tendencies of 'feminine' civilization." Similarly, Adam Rome (2006) contends that urban reform and hygiene in the city was a "domestic" chore for women like Jane Addams, the feminine counterpart to men escaping the unhygienic city to enter a purifying wilderness; both approaches reinforced gender divisions as they helped to build the nation.[2]

Today's "risk culture" enacts many of these racial, gendered, and classist exclusions of the nineteenth-century wilderness movement. Denis Cosgrove (1995) thus observes that environmentalism was riddled with these "hidden attachments" to Manifest Destiny, empire, and whiteness (and, I would add, masculinity). The early wilderness movement's view that the wilderness encounter fosters ideal characteristics in the morally "pure" individual is also central to the appeal of today's adventure culture, as Braun (2003) argues. Adventure culture relies on a "discourse of courage and conquest" to "suture an anxious middle class masculinity" (181). The wilderness encounter continues to give those who participate in adventure sports a sense of moral superiority, but few participants acknowledge the ties between this sense of superiority and white, elite, male identity.

Scholars such as Comer, Rome, Cosgrove, Kosek, Spence, Jacoby, and Braun have thus challenged the race, class, and gender exclusions of early and contemporary environmentalism. They document environmentalism's relationship to patriarchy, Manifest Destiny, and other ideologies of domination, as well as their links to contemporary environmentalism. But no scholarship addresses the extent to which environmentalism, the wilderness movement, and the ideal American identity developed in opposition to a fundamental category of "otherness"—disability. As the passage by Krakauer shows, contemporary adventure culture prizes the "fit" body—able, muscular, young, and male—as a means to transcendence. The role of the body in both the Progressive Era, particularly the wilderness movement, and in contemporary adventure culture calls for an analysis of not just the "racial" but the "corporeal unconscious" of adventure culture and U.S. environmentalism more broadly.[3] To the extent that engaging in adventure culture has become a reflection of environmental sensibility, bodies that do not fit this model are deemed unenvironmental. Extending Progressive Era links between the body, social hygiene, and the wilderness encounter, contemporary adventure culture equates physical fitness with environmental correctness, an equation I challenge in the arguments that follow.

Disability studies perspectives scrutinize the extent to which adventure culture's investments are not just racial, gendered, elitist, or imperialist; they fundamentally hinge on the fit body.[4] Disability studies provides a critique of risk culture's rejection of technology (symbolic of modernity's corrupting force) by challenging its focus on "unmediated" contact between man and nature. Echoing recent work in wilderness studies that probe the "trouble with wilderness,"[5] disability studies theorists contend that everybody's encounter with the physical world is always mediated. They argue that disability is not an ontological category existing outside of a social context; rather social notions of purity and fitness help to construct disability as a social, political, and cultural category and have done so historically.

In this essay I investigate what I call the "corporeal unconscious" of environmental thought and its recreational expression, adventure culture, to broaden what counts as environmentally "good" ways of being in the physical world. Even if the myth of an inaccessible wilderness underpins adventure culture, there is no reason that environmentalism, as an activist and theoretical set of ethical imperatives, must share this attachment to the wilderness myth. Not only does it behoove environmentalism to incorporate an array of corporeal interactions with the physical world, but its failure to do so thus far points to its hidden attachment to the abled body.

Thus the targets of my critique are today's environmental movement, adventure culture, and the historical wilderness movement from which they both emerged. In particular I focus on the mainstream environmental movement, which privileges a myth of the solitary retreat into nature as the primary source of an environmental ethic.[6] I contend that environmentalism is responsible for the ideas of fitness and wilderness that shape risk culture and that risk culture masks its corporeal unconscious behind environmentalism's moral legitimacy. I hope to disentangle the relationship between environmental ethics and adventure and offer a more inclusive model of being in the world.

Locating the Body in Risk Culture

A specific kind of body is associated with the wilderness ideal plot that deserves as much scrutiny as the class, race, and gender politics implied by the plot. As much as the wilderness plot invigorates gendered, racial, and bourgeois identities, today's risk culture codes certain bodies as (already) morally good and pure. In risk culture proving status in challenges and encounters with raw Nature is the best way to attain and display physical fitness, thereby achieving what might be termed the "wilderness body ideal," which promotes a body that risks fitness and the ability to reify it.[7]

The fit body is, figuratively and literally, external evidence of internal qualities. The corporeality implied in the wilderness plot suggests the need for an analysis of the wilderness body ideal, which embodies virtue, select status, and, importantly, genetic superiority. The centrality of the body to the wilderness ideal invokes the historical relationship between social Darwinism and environmentalism on which my argument builds. Braun (2003, 199) hints at these connections: "Climbing the corporate ladder is akin to climbing a mountain . . . [and is] presented as something innate in the person . . . [and] also as a property that belongs to the physically superior specimen whose superiority is deserved." The activities of adventure culture conflate bodily, social, economic, and genetic superiority. In Braun's gloss of this Darwinian argument, the fit body tautologically reflects deserved genetic superiority.

The sports associated with outdoor adventure have taken varying forms since the inception of the appeal of adventure as a recreational activity. Braun explains (2003, 176) that although "adventure has a long history in the United States," it "returned with renewed vigor in the last decades of the twentieth century." He locates adventure culture in "the widespread dissemination of images of 'risk taking' in mainstream media and popular culture" (176),[8] including popular magazines such as Outside and National Geographic Adventurer. Television shows like Survivor, Man vs. Wild, and Survivorman claim to teach viewers how to survive extreme conditions, and the documentary Touching the Void (2003), which dramatized the harrowing mountaineering excursion of two British climbers that nearly killed them both, are examples of the genre.

In the past, alpine clubs and mountaineering appealed because they promised escape and discovery. Today the sport of climbing is about risk taking, not first ascents. Nettlefold and Stratford (1999) contend that the popularity of risk taking suggests a shift away from the sublime view of nature, in which nature is awe inspiring but not dangerous. In the Kantian sublime, nature is simultaneously beautiful and threatening, but the safety of the human figure is always ensured. In contemporary risk culture, by contrast, the "search for jeopardy" is paramount (Williams and Donnelly 1985, 4). Difficulty is central to the appeal and status of climbing.

In Bobos in Paradise: The New Upper Class and How They Got There (2001, 210), David Brooks sardonically observes the importance of jeopardy in adventure sports: "One must put oneself through terrible torment—and this can come either on a cold mountain top or in a malarial rainforest—to experience the spiritually uplifting magnificence of brutal nature. One must mutilate the body for environmental transcendence." Risk culture jeopardizes the very bodies it champions. Ironically bodies "on the raggedy edge of risk," as Braun puts it, are by definition in danger of disablement because risk "mutilates the body," yet environmental transcendence requires this corporeal experience. Just being in the outdoors—gardening or observing nature, for instance—does not offer the same element of risk.

Descriptions of adventure culture frequently emphasize physical fitness but ignore the category of disability against which the risking, adventuring body is defined. They illustrate the logic of what Mitchell and Snyder (1997, 6) call "the double bind" of disability: "While disabled populations are firmly entrenched on the outer margins of social power and cultural value, the disabled body serves as the raw material out of which other socially disempowered communities make themselves visible." In other words, disabled bodies are simultaneously marginalized and invisible, a category of bodily corruption that gives the "normate" body, as Rosemarie Garland-Thomson (2002) calls it, its meaning. The disabled body is made invisible by risk culture's emphasis on fitness, yet risk culture relies on the threat of disability to make the wilderness ideal body meaningful.

Even Braun's (2003) excellent assessment of the racial unconscious of risk culture commits the double bind by overlooking the corporeal implications of his own argument. Note his unconscious emphasis on the fit body, showing how the double bind works to both centralize and erase the disabled body: "Risk culture is seen to have an explicitly ethical dimension, involving a care of self that involves physical and mental tests, and demands an almost ascetic bodily discipline" (179). Risk culture sutures white, male, elite identity, but despite Braun's reference to the importance of bodily discipline and self-care in this passage, he ignores the abled body on which his argument about the white body relies. He thus exemplifies the theory of the double bind: the disabled body is simultaneously the most absent and the most necessary for reifying white bourgeois identity.

The double bind characterizes the corporeal unconscious of risk culture today, depictions of which reveal that the disabled body is necessary to give risk and adventure any meaning, and yet the disabled body must remain invisible. The double bind of risk culture becomes evident because risk in fact threatens disablement. Descriptions of adventure in magazines, survivor shows, and travel literature frequently depict the discomfort, harsh environment, and dangerous challenges the adventurer faces. Advertisements for adventure technologies sometimes even use the prospect of disablement to sell gear. An adventurer who is injured in the wild would become dependent on technological accommodations and support. The imminent possibility of disablement heightens the risk factor of all sports, but particularly outdoor adventure, where there are no trainers, ambulances, or hospitals nearby.

For example, an ACR Electronics advertisement campaign promotes the Global Positioning System (GPS) by presenting images of disabled men alongside their narratives of survival. An analysis of the campaign suggests that disabled bodies signify the absolute opposite of the wilderness body ideal.[9] The ACR personal locator beacon (PLB) advertising campaign turns on the imminence of disability in the outdoors and on the shared assumption that the only place for the disabled body in the wilderness ideal is as an invisible, looming threat—symbolic rather than actual. Although adventure culture valorizes independence and bodily integrity, it simultaneously jeopardizes these very traits. The ads therefore reflect the double bind of disability in risk culture.

The first full-page advertisement includes a full-body image of Dan, standing on artificial legs, alongside text that tells his true story: "Dan got hopelessly lost for five days and eventually lost his legs to frostbite. Sheer willpower helped save his life amid overwhelming odds. It could have been worse. Or it could have been much better if Dan had packed ACR's new TerraFix 406 GPS I/O." Citing "physical prowess and willpower" (qualities Cosgrove [1995] links to fin-de-siècle national character formation), this ad asserts that all that stood between Dan and death was his willpower, but all that stood between him and keeping his legs was a GPS. Avoiding death is testament to the power of will; able-bodiedness is about personal virtue. At the same time the ad exposes the implicit contradiction of adventure culture: the individual is at risk without the GPS, so he is dependent on technological aid to avoid becoming disabled. Technology may help reduce disability, yet relying on technology is itself something like a disability, as it threatens the self-reliance of the adventurer.

To sell this technology ACR must address the problem technology poses for the independent, self-reliant adventurer. A second full-page ad in the ACR campaign exemplifies how ACR glosses this contradiction. Aron Ralston is shown rock climbing with an artificial arm alongside a narrative of his story: "I've been to a place that no one ever wants to visit and I'll never end up there again: Trapped and alone with no way out. With my right arm pinned under a half-ton boulder, I had no way to communicate my position. Five days later I walked out of Utah's Blue John Canyon. I had to leave my arm behind. But I consider it a miracle, not a tragedy: My story has saved lives—it might save yours."[10]

The text continues to describe how important the PLB is for wilderness safety. Aron is quoted in much larger print at the top of the page: "I still climb solo. Unless you count my PLB." This statement allows us to rest assured that his dismemberment did not cause disability, at least in terms of how disability connotes dependence; Aron "still climb[s] solo." We are also assured that the lightweight and "convenient" PLB will not compromise the independence and purity of the wilderness encounter: "I still climb solo, only now I carry a convenient 12-ounce backup by my side. You should too." By taking such care to emphasize Aron's independence despite his reliance on his PLB to avoid further disablement, this ad attests to the double bind of risk culture: dismemberment does not stop Aron, but he is proof that the risks are real. The PLB can help avoid disablement, but the status of the adventurer is preserved by reducing the mediating buffer of such technology. We are reassured that Aron's disability does not get in the way of his independence. But his exceptional recovery proves the rule that disability is feared because it is fundamentally about dependence—on other people and on technology. By foregrounding people with disabilities to promote reliance on technology, this ACR campaign exposes adventure culture's assumption that bodily ability, and the virtue it signifies, must be attained without the aid of technology, "solo."

Like the stories of Erik Weihenmayer, the first blind man to scale Everest, or Rachael Scdoris, the first blind woman to run the Iditarod, Dan's and Aron's narratives are examples of sensationalized "supercrip" stories, as disability theorists call them. Such narratives glorify individual willpower to overcome bodily impairment. Garland-Thomson (2002) argues that supercrip stories are a genre that authorize pity and amazement. Even as they renarrate "tragedy" as "miracle," as in Aron's statement, the corresponding responses are normalization, recovery, or cure. Garland-Thomson suggests that the "visual rhetoric" of images of the disabled simultaneously makes disability "visually conspicuous while politically and socially erased" (56). Because they imply that responsibility for a cure lies in the individual, supercrip narratives express the double bind of disability in risk culture. As

Garland-Thomson adds, "the disabled body exposes the illusion of autonomy, self-government, and self-determination that underpins the fantasy of absolute able-bodiedness" (46). They thus signal risk culture's attachment to the able body. Despite their ostensible aim—to show that people with disabilities can do the same things that people without disabilities can do—supercrip stories reinforce rather than challenge the dominant values of ableism: independence, the role of individual will in self-cure or self-recovery, and bodily self-reliance. Social context is erased.

The prevalence of narratives about supercrips in adventure culture supports my argument that disabled bodies signify not just the opposite of the abled body, but the abled body in the wild. People with disabilities who accomplish extreme outdoor feats capture headlines precisely because disabled bodies are understood as incapable of physically demanding activities. A "disability panic" underpins risk culture. If the wilderness encounter is defined by the fact that it requires more extreme physical fitness than any other activity, then the disabled body literally has no place in the wilderness.[11] In the wilderness myth the body is pure, "solo," left to its own devices, and unmediated by any kind of aid. Its role is to activate jeopardy in the able-bodied as a "disablist presence" that waits just beyond the next extreme thrill.[12] The perpetual threat of disablement is only heightened by the presence of an adventurer who has been disabled by these very activities. However inspiring and heroic, their stories reinforce the audience's attachment to the wilderness body ideal. After all, despite being enabled by technology, Aron "still climb[s] solo."

Risk Culture's Historical Roots

Risk culture's privileging of independence, willpower, bodily fitness, and wilderness borrow much from early environmentalism and from the wilderness movement of the Progressive Era. Examining these roots further exposes the extent to which today's risk culture extends a longer tradition of anxieties about the body, which were directly related to the overlap of social, genetic, spatial, and hygienic concerns of the time. The rapid growth of cities, changing labor relations, an unprecedented influx of immigrants, and concern about the "close of the frontier"—popularized by Turner's 1893 World's Columbian Exposition "frontier thesis" speech—led to a series of perceived crises of masculinity, nature, and national identity. At the same time the emerging theory of social evolution, which saw interactions between racial groups as a struggle for survival, provided a "national" narrative that united "America" (at least white America) against other races and cultures (Bederman 1996; Haraway 1989; Kosek 2004). Because Progressive Era conservationists were beginning to see the environmental costs of modernity, "civilization" could only advance by combining the qualities of progress with man's [sic] primal strengths. In this context returning to "the primitive," "going Native,"[13] and "getting back to nature" rendered wilderness an attractive setting in which to spend leisure time.

The wilderness gained value as a "safety valve," as Turner called it, to replace the role that the frontier had played in defining American identity. When Turner declared the frontier closed, the independent American spirit fostered by lighting out for the territory, popularized in the mainstream by Mark Twain and James Fenimore Cooper, among others, was under threat. If the frontier encounter was necessary for the creation of the ideal American, then the close of the frontier meant no more unique American character. American identity was based on a violent frontier encounter, which converted the wilderness into a "garden," as Henry Nash Smith (1950) famously argued. With the settlement of land once considered frontier, qualities that made Americans unique would have to be artificially produced, which provided the impetus to re-create the frontier in the form of wilderness. Wilderness would allow American identity to be "regenerated through violence," to use Richard Slotkin's (1973) language. Wilderness provided the setting against which the drama of the frontier encounter could be carried out and American identity ensured.

For advocates like Roosevelt, young, virile, American men needed to practice the "savage" arts of war, hunting, and a raw masculinity. The increasing popularity of Darwinian evolutionary theory, which Roosevelt interpreted as legitimizing war and hunting as ways to ensure the survival of the fittest, coincided with various social crises. The result was environmental in two ways, at least: it promoted the preservation of wilderness and naturalized "biologized forms of racism" (Foucault 1978, 149). Along with dramatically increased restrictions on immigration, urban hygiene programs, and the City Beautiful movement, wilderness protection was implemented under the auspices of "social reform." That is, the loss of the frontier and the social hygiene problems associated with urban spaces were in large part responsible for the wilderness movement of the late nineteenth century. As Lawrence Buell (2001, 8) attested, "the first expressions of protectionist sentiment about vanishing woods and wilderness on the part of the dominant settler culture . . . coincided with the first intensive systematic push toward urban 'sanitary' reform." Protecting national health meant enclosing wilderness spaces and honing the fit, white body.[14] Thus Progressive Era wilderness ideology manifested both spatially and corporeally; it spatialized national sentiment through the fortification of U.S. borders, the expansion of territorial boundaries, and the enclosure of land as wilderness against inferior intruders. And the wilderness ideology was internalized in the form of disciplines of the body that merged the health and appearance of individual bodies with the health of the national body politic.

"American nationalism," Jake Kosek (2004, 132) argues, "grows out of persistent connections" between "nation, blood, body, and 'wild' nature in America." Social Darwinism connects these themes, contributing to what Foucault (1978) would argue is a form of nation-building based on "biopower." Turner argued that the confrontation inherent in the frontier encounter—the encounter between civilization and the wild—created a uniquely American character, defined by rugged individualism, good Anglo-Saxon genetic stock, and values of democratic governance. Turner's thesis justified Manifest Destiny on teleological, evolutionary grounds: "It appears then that the universal disposition of Americans to emigrate to the western wilderness, in order to enlarge their dominion over inanimate nature, is the actual result of the expansive power which is inherent in them" (Turner, qtd. in Kosek 2004, 133).

In this logic European Americans possess an "inherent power" to expand and dominate nature, which was perceived as inanimate and uninhabited. This rationale also conveniently justified the domination of Native Americans. Conquest and dominance were about racial survival; not to expand and dominate would mitigate against Anglo instincts and Darwinian necessity, leading to what Roosevelt called "race suicide" (Horsman 1981). With the close of the frontier declared in the early 1890s, Turner worried that the American character, or biopower, was itself endangered. His thesis made wilderness preservation essential to American national and genetic viability.

Environmental determinism backed Darwin and Turner; the success of the Anglo-American "race" required imperial expansion, resting American genetic superiority on territorial appropriation. Progressive Era evolutionists posited evolution not as a matter of natural selection but as a matter of survival of the fittest. This notion revised Darwin's thesis to emphasize dominance over natural selection. Furthermore, in the twisted logic of the survival of the fittest, fitness could be understood on the scale of national identity as opposed to the species, as Darwin had theorized. Thus protected territories were not available for all members of the human species to compete over; they were not even accessible to all members of the American nation.

Eugenics and immigration restriction united race and disability in one project of preserving the American character. The national body politic was taking decidedly genetic form, a fact that made immigration restriction an obvious complement to eugenics in the early twentieth century. That is, eugenicists pushed for immigration restriction to not exclude entire national groups but to deny "entry to individuals and families with poor hereditary history" (Kevles 1985, 47). Immigration restriction based on genetics, as opposed to race, used biological arguments against non-Anglo groups, constructing racial inferiority as disability, as Daniel Kevles notes: "High scientific authority . . . drew upon expert 'evidence' . . . to proclaim that a large proportion of immigrants bordered on or fell into the "feebleminded" category and that their continued entrance into the country made . . . for the 'menace of race deterioration'" (94).

Eugenics pushed racial agendas, to be sure, but it did so in discourses of genetic "flaws"—disabilities. Immigration restriction provided "positive eugenics" (preventing external sources of impurity), and sterilization provided "negative eugenics" (preventing the reproduction of the genetically defective). By the 1920s eugenicist sentiments led to the Immigration Act of 1924 and to forced sterilization of thirty-six thousand white and nonwhite Americans deemed "criminals," "drunkards," "diseased," "feebleminded," and "disabled" from 1907 to 1941 (Kevles 1985, 116). These eugenicist approaches to social reform framed xenophobia as a biological imperative to gain legitimacy.

In such a context it makes sense that eugenics' early proponents called it "biological housecleaning" (Kevles 1985, 114). Ernst Haeckel, the German zoologist considered to be the founder of modern ecology, was engaged in discussions of eugenics as early as 1868, favoring death for the "unfit" long before eugenics gained public support (Pernick 1997, 99). Environmental and eugenics projects reinforced each other: early environmentalists wanted to dictate who belonged on America's precious soil. The purity of American land was linked to the purity of its American genes. The roots of ecology are "tangled up with much of the unsavory racial and eugenic theorizing of the early twentieth century" (Cosgrove 1995, 38).

In her classic essay, "Teddy Bear Patriarchy," Donna Haraway (1989, 57) shows that eugenics and conservation overlapped "in philosophy and personnel." She analyzes the synergy between eugenics and conservation that led to the creation of the Museum of Natural History, which was "dedicated to preserving a threatened manhood." Although "conservation was a policy to preserve resources, not only for industry, but also for moral formation, for the achievement of manhood" (57), natural history was "medical technology, a hygienic intervention" for a "pathology [that] was a potentially fatal organic sickness of the individual and collective body" (55). Haraway argued that Roosevelt understood conquest of the frontier as proof that white men were evolutionarily superior to Indians, which allowed him to see the establishment of wilderness parks in the United States and imperial expansion in the Philippines and Cuba as a two-pronged approach to the same evolutionary imperative.[15] Roosevelt thus spatialized his view of bodily and genetic fitness. He was profoundly influenced by Turner's thesis and developed his conservationist nationalism from its implications.

Some wilderness historians have seen the connections between conservation and eugenics, but the corporeal nature of this connection has received less attention. It is no coincidence that Roosevelt advocated for the purification of the individual body as a justification for preserving wilderness.[16] Gail Bederman (1996) argues that Roosevelt considered outdoor activity—what he called "the strenuous life"—a way to practice a fantasy of raw masculine identity that was endangered by the feminizing work of modern society. Rescuing masculinity involved "wresting the continent from Indians and installing a higher civilization" (182). But as Bryant Simon (2003) attests, it also meant maintaining a fit and healthy body. Once Roosevelt headed west to recover his own masculinity, Simon argues, "national glory, wide-open spaces, and powerful bodies were . . . forever linked" (84).

One of the reasons the body is central to the Progressive Era's response to industrialism is because industrial capitalism's new forms of labor reduced the bodily risks of everyday work for many. City life in particular, Elizabeth Rosen (2007) explains, created conditions that made adventure a preferred form of leisure. She locates the roots of contemporary risk culture in the introduction of technology. "With its urbanity," modern civilization "is so safe compared with life centuries ago. More and more, risk [was] filtered out. . . . Our world is largely explored and there are no nasty surprises waiting over the next hill for us. Our technology erases more and more hardship from our lives" (152). Putting one's body through great discomfort became a prescription for attaining transcendence or virtue because it allowed the privileged to manufacture risk.

Dean MacCannell (1989) adds that the desire to manufacture risk in leisure activities became a feature of bourgeois recreation. Precipitated by the Industrial Revolution, adventure tourism became an example of what MacCannell calls "work displays." The hard physical "work" of outdoor adventure constitutes "leisure" because work itself no longer risks the bourgeois body. "Strangely, we find ourselves in the midst of an age that has turned notions of 'recreation' on its head," Rosen (2007, 147) concludes, "when leisure activities have come to include hard-driving and perilous extreme sports and adventure holidays such as rock climbing, sky surfing, and extreme white water rafting." Work displays correct the moral atrophy associated with bourgeois privilege; they fulfill a Puritan work ethic through bodily toil. And wilderness is the best place to express this ethic, as the environmental historian Paul Sutter (2001, 291) argues: "If virtuous labor in nature was no longer the dominant force of American character, structured leisure in an edifying environment promised to fill the void."

It is within this historical context, in which the purity of the body and the nation led to wilderness, eugenics, and imperialism, that the disabled American body gained meaning. Evolutionary theory was deployed for the purposes of disciplining American bodies as much as for the purposes of imperial expansion and wilderness protection. The relationship between the fit body, national identity, and wilderness that emerged in the Progressive Era ensured that unfit bodies were both a threat to national identity and to Nature itself. In an era increasingly interested in the rationalization of labor and economic models of efficiency, alongside racialized bodies of American Indians, African Americans, women, and the poor, the disabled body had no place.

Disability was defined by the inability to contribute productively to the capitalist system, to the body politic, and therefore to society. "Nowhere is the disabled figure more troubling to American ideology and history," notes Garland-Thomson (2002, 46), "than in relation to the concept of work," which assumes "abstract principles of self-government, autonomy, and progress." The disabled figure could exist only in a context where self-government, autonomy, and progress were prized. The term disability itself implies failure to meet a standard of physical competency, the standards for which were increasingly being defined in the fin-de-siècle industrial capitalist milieu. Only in such a context is it imaginable that a body that cannot perform the actions of "disciplining, optimization of its capabilities, extortion of its forces, parallel increase of its usefulness and its docility, [and] integration into systems of efficient and economic controls" (Rabinow 1984, 261) becomes a liability.

Although historians of disability attribute the construction of disability to the capitalist work ethic, none has made any link between the wilderness movement and disability. By mapping the historical construction of wilderness alongside the historical construction of disability, I contend that there is a material, constitutive relationship between disability and American environmental thought and practice. That is, if the wilderness movement was responsible for imbuing the fit body with values of independence, self-reliance, genetic superiority, and willpower, and if wilderness was the setting in which to rehearse these values and reify the fit and healthy body, then wilderness and disability are constitutively mutually constructed.

The Disabled Body in Environmental Thought

The disabled body has even more symbolic meaning in environmental thought than is evident in the history of eugenics, conservation, and evolution I just described. Perhaps in part because of this history, disability is a dominant symbol of humanity's alienation from nature in literary texts and environmental discourses as well. It is striking that the disablist presence is most evident in texts considered proto-environmentalist, where disability is the category of otherness against which environmentalism is defined. And adventure culture is clearly influenced by environmental thought and literature, for example, in its rejection of modernity as technology. Adventure culture shares with environmental thought the view that humans have been disconnected from a simpler, unmediated, corporeal relationship to the earth. In dominant environmental thought, modernity is a crutch, disconnecting our bodies from nature. In turn, as disability theorists show, ability is about not relying on technology, society, or others' help; independence is understood at the level of the body.

Much of the anxiety about the loss of nature in environmental literature gets expressed as anxiety about the body. The view that the environmental crisis is really a crisis of the body stems from the environmentalist aversion to the machine, which destroyed nature as resource, nature as a space of retreat and regeneration, and nature as an organic system in its own right. Because risk culture borrows environmentalism's aversion to the machine, and because disability so often symbolizes dependence on machines in environmental literature, examining the roots of this aversion is central to a disability critique of risk culture. A disability studies critique of environmental thought best proceeds from an understanding of how values of independence, self-reliance, and environmentalism emerged in opposition to technology.

Some texts that take up environmental themes of the body are central to the American literary canon. Disability literary critics have argued that, for example, Herman Melville's Moby-Dick portrays Ahab's disability as a punishment for his corrupt, instrumental view of nature. Melville captures Ahab's alienation from nature in the sailor's megalomaniacal pursuit of Moby-Dick, the white whale. Ahab's corrupted relationship to nature is symbolized by disability: his lost leg. As the captain of a whaling ship, Ahab symbolizes industrialization's extractive relationship to nature. His bodily incompleteness signals his utilitarian orientation to nature, and justice is served by the ironic use of a whale bone for his prosthesis. Using disability as a metaphor, Ralph Waldo Emerson also invoked the image of the "invalid." For Emerson the invalid was an "icon of bodily vulnerability" against which the self-reliant, ideal man should be defined (qtd. in Garland-Thomson 2002, 42). In Angle of Repose, Wallace Stegner presents his protagonist Lyman Ward's paralysis as symbolic of humanity's malaise, disenchantment, and having been "maimed away from Mother Earth" (Hepworth 1998, 17). These various texts reflected emerging, distinctly modern concerns about the spread of technology, the loss of an Edenic nature, and the impact of these losses on (male) humans. Such losses posed a threat to the notion of a distinct, self-reliant, and yet innocent American national identity. "As modernization proceeded," Garland-Thomson (2002, 47) observes, "the disabled figure shouldered in new ways society's anxiety about its inability to retain the status and old meanings of labor in the face of industrialization and increasing economic and social chaos."

The "disability equals alienation from nature" trope reemerged powerfully in 1968 in a book that is considered canonical to outdoor enthusiasts and environmentalists. In Desert Solitaire: A Season in the Wilderness, Edward Abbey (1968) offers a "polemic against industrial tourism" in which he disparages the machines associated with it: jet skis, motorized boats, RVs, all-terrain vehicles. These machines defeat the purpose of being in the wilderness, making nature too accessible and at the same time distancing humans from the "wilderness experience." Machines disrupt the peace of the outdoors and deaden the human body's ability to perceive and respond to nature. Thus Abbey asks "how to pry the tourists out of their automobiles, out of their back-breaking upholstered mechanized wheelchairs and onto their feet, onto the strange warmth and solidity of Mother Earth again" (64). Elsewhere Abbey explicitly states that disabled people should not be granted the privilege of being in the wilderness if they cannot access it physically. His desire to keep the disabled body out of the wilderness highlights how central physical fitness is to the logic of wilderness in U.S. environmentalism. Modernity as machine has handicapped us by breaking the connection to nature that only our bodies can permit. Getting back to nature requires leaving modern machines behind and stripping the body down to its organic, pure whole.

Abbey's wilderness as a place free of technological interference extends the tradition of the pastoral in environmental literature, a tradition Leo Marx (1964) explores in The Machine in the Garden: Technology and the Pastoral Ideal in America. Marx describes how "the machine" became the antithesis of true "nature": "Industrialization, represented by images of machine technology, provides the counterforce in the American archetype of the pastoral design" (26). The pastoral setting creates a modern Eden, where man can "recover from the fall" (Merchant 2005). The pastoral mode stigmatizes the city as toxic and constructs the garden as morally purifying. These texts hinge on the notion that disability is the best symbol of the machine's corruption of a prelapsarian harmony between body and nature.

Current environmental thought builds on this literary tradition. Like Abbey many contemporary wilderness advocates believe that technologies from automobiles to wristwatches distort the sensual relationship between self and environment. They get in the way of the body's ability to perceive nature. The environmental crisis is portrayed in corporeal terms; an environmental ethic can be achieved only by returning to the intact body. To craft his environmental ethic Paul Adams relies on Abbey's assertion that walking is "the one and only mode of locomotion in which a man proceeds entirely on his own, upright, as a human being should be, fully erect rather than sitting on his rear end" (qtd. in Adams 2001, 195). It is only by "walking through . . . [a natural] environment" that " a kind of rhythmic harmonization" can "produce a heightened sensitivity to the environment, as well as a heightened or special sense of self" (193). Adams's contemporary ethic is deeply indebted to the literary tradition I described earlier: to climb and descend a hill on foot is to establish a kind of dialogue with the earth, a direct imprinting of place on self; this physical dialogue is silent when one moves by merely pressing on a gas pedal. In peripatetic place-experience lies the basis of a special kind of knowledge of the world and one's place in it (188). This suggests that able-bodiedness is necessary for a healthy human life in the natural world, for a "direct imprinting of place on self." For Adams the ideal "multisensory" experience is a "peripatetic place-experience."

Contemporary ecopsychology adopts an environmental ethic of corporeal fitness as well. The ecopsychologist Laura Sewall (1999), for instance, attributes the environmental crisis of our age to a lack of bodily wholeness. Humanity's distance from nature is "muteness" and "cultural blindness." She writes, "The ecological crisis reflects a crisis in perception; we are not truly seeing, hearing, tasting, or consequently feeling where we are. Our blindness has tremendous implications for the quality of relationship between ourselves and the 'more-than-human-world'" (246). Sewall uses blindness as a metaphor to argue that we cannot care about the environment because we do not perceive it correctly, fundamentally a corporeal deficiency. Her uncritical use of disability is another example of the disablist presence in environmental thought: panic about the environment is really panic about the body. For Sewall alienation from nature is (and is like) a disability. She echoes the general move within environmental philosophy to emphasize a corporeal environmental ethic. After all, as the prominent ecophenomenologist David Abrams (1996, x) poses, "direct sensuous reality . . . remains the sole solid touchstone for an experiential world . . . ; only in regular contact with the tangible ground and sky can we learn how to orient and to navigate in the multiple dimensions that now claim us." Only contact with "the tangible ground and sky" and moving away from artificial pleasures and simulacra can bring about the sensuous connection needed for harmony between humans and their environment.[17]

This environmental philosophy based on corporeal experience is being expressed not only in philosophical discussions; it resonates in popular expressions of risk culture as well, further demonstrating its pervasiveness. For instance, Bear Grylls (2007), the star of the television show Man vs. Wild, echoes this environmental philosophy in Born Survivor: Survival Techniques from the Most Dangerous Places on Earth, in which he articulates the fantasy of an unmediated encounter with wilderness available only through the body: "It is only when I return to these so-called 'wilds' of nature that I find my own spirit comes alive. I begin to feel that rhythm within me, my senses become attuned to what is all around; I start to see in the dark, to distinguish the smells of the forest, to discern the east wind from the westerly. I am simply becoming a man again; becoming how nature made us. These 'wildernesses' help me lose all those synthetic robes that society has draped over us" (8). Grylls's emphasis on heightened bodily perception licenses his authenticity. Adventure relieves the body of society's "synthetic robes," which inhibit sensual connection to the world.

But Grylls's use of scare quotes around the words <u>wilds</u> and <u>wilder-nesses</u> exposes a fissure in the wilderness myth; he seems aware of the fact that the very spaces that allow him to shed the robes of society are themselves socially constructed. When these spaces reawaken his senses, however, Grylls becomes "a man again," "how nature made us." Paradoxically, then, only a socially con-structed wilderness can make him feel natural and fully human. His embodied encounter with nature is a form of simulacra; it is more real than "real" nature itself.[18] The encounter substitutes per-formance for the ecological sensitivity that the wilderness encoun-ter claims to cultivate. Thus there is no necessary relationship between the wilderness encounter and an environmental ethic. Grylls's notion of bodily perfection (being manly, as nature made him) is not inherently environmentalist; on the contrary, in risk cul-ture the environment is subsumed by bodily (and other) priorities.

A Disability Studies Critique of the Wilderness Body Ideal

I have argued that the wilderness body ideal is a "hidden attach-ment" of environmental thought and risk culture. The disablist presence in risk culture modernizes the disablist presence of early environmentalism. This view renders some kinds of activities and environments better than others, depending on how well they enhance corporeal connectedness to nature. A disability critique of this position allows, even advocates the centrality of the body as a connection to the physical environment. But it rejects the notion that only certain kinds of physical activities (walking, mountain climbing) and only certain kinds of bodies permit this connection. A disability studies analysis rejects the use of disabil-ity as an overdetermined metaphor for bodily disconnection to the physical environment. Disability studies disrupts risk culture's distinctions between abled and disabled and challenges notions about what are purifying or corrupting forms of technological mediation, distinctions that arbitrarily dictate how a body can connect "correctly" with nature.

A disability studies analysis of risk culture's attachment to the wilderness body ideal helps us see that disability is a social construction, as are the contexts (social, built, and otherwise) in which it exists. Disability theorists demonstrate that "disability is as much a symptom of historical and cultural contingencies as it is a physical and psychological reality" (Mitchell and Snyder 1997, xiv). Historically rooted attitudes toward disability construct it as a negative category, as an overdetermined symbol for an era's fears. This is not to say that disability is entirely a social construction; on the contrary, to acknowledge the ways "disability is a form of disadvantage which is imposed on top of one's impairment" (Tremain 2005, 9) is not to discount the experienced realities of physical impairment. Rather acknowledging the construction of disability allows us to see the extent to which it is "caused by a contemporary social organization that takes little or no account of people with impairments" (9). Susan Wendell (1996, 39) shows how recognizing the construction of disability allows us to look beyond the individual for sources of disablement: "Societies that are physically constructed and socially organized with the unacknowledged assumption that everyone is healthy, non-disabled, young but adult, shaped according to cultural ideals, and, often, male create a great deal of disability through sheer neglect of what most people need in order to participate fully in them." Wendell suggests that neglect constructs disability; disability is not an ontological reality existing prior to society's views of it and, as a reflection of those views, its design.[19]

Wendell (1996) points out that all bodies are in flux, not just those of the disabled. The rigid binary of disabled-nondisabled is a myth: "We are all disabled eventually. Most of us will live

part of our lives with bodies that hurt, that move with difficulty or not at all, that deprive us of activities we once took for
granted or that others take for granted, bodies that make daily
life a physical struggle" (263). Shildrick and Price (1996, 106)
remind the "healthy majority" that "they are merely temporarily able bodies." Disability studies makes us aware that bodies
are abled and disabled at the same time, depending on time,
place, and task at hand (Nussbaum 2006). Ability is relative
to phase of life and to society's structural expectations and
physical designs. Accessibility and design are relative to the
ableism that informs their construction. This relativist view of
disability rejects the notion that disability is a pathology to be
avoided or cured in favor of the view that variation of bodily
form is natural or normal. The "problem" of disability is thus not
located in the individual; rather it lies in social structures and
contexts, not the least of which are built environments, myths
of wilderness, and views of nature.

Gear Fetish or Disability?

Adventure culture's foundational myth is that the value of the
wilderness encounter lies in the fact that the body is going places
and doing things that are inaccessible to those who have not
disciplined their body. Cosgrove (1995, 37) writes, "It is hardly
surprising that [hikers and backpackers on the wilderness trails]
should be young, fit, and well-off: the arduous physical exercise
necessary is unlikely to appeal to the elderly and infirm." Leo
McAvoy (2001, 26) similarly observes that "the very elements that
make outdoor areas and programs attractive are their undevel-
oped nature, their ruggedness, the presence of natural forces at
work, and the challenge to interact with nature on nature's terms
rather than technological human terms," which make "outdoor
recreation and adventure environments" by their very nature

"a challenge for people with disabilities." It would seem that wilderness itself is anathema to disability. As I will continue to show, this is no coincidence.

Inaccessibility is only one aspect of wilderness that creates barriers for people with disabilities. Cosgrove (1995, 37) adds that "the highly elaborated codes of conduct and dress for these [wilderness] areas can be as rigid and exclusive in their moral message" as in their accessibility or expense. Such codes "articulate an individualistic, muscular, and active vision of bodily health" (37). The assumption that people with disabilities do not like wilderness because their body prevents the correct experience of it, an assumption McAvoy's (2001) research demonstrates,[20] fails to recognize risk culture's hidden attachments. Purity, identity, and individualism are associated with independence from technological mediation or the help of others: adventure turns on crossing a great divide between culture and wild nature; it is about physical and moral tests that the encounter with unmediated nature provides. (Hence adventure travel's emphasis on self-propelled transportation is not only a nostalgia for earlier modes of travel; it is also about stripping away the most obvious source of alienation from nature: modern technology [Braun 2003, 194].)

These binaries—culture/wild nature, prelapsarian past/modernity, self-propelled transportation/artificial modes of mobility—are inextricably linked and connect environmentalism's spatial, temporal, and corporeal moral valences. Many scholars challenge the implications of the two former binaries, but what about this question of self-propelled transportation? What happens when we challenge the binary between self-propelled and artificial ways of navigating the physical environment?

The fact that the disabled body often requires technological help to perform adventure activities ignores that able bodies also connect to wilderness in technologically mediated ways. The wilderness ideal body relies on apparatuses of technological support to become "purified" through the wilderness encounter. Braun (2003) calls wilderness a "purification machine" to expose its artificiality. Furthermore, as the ads discussed earlier make clear, technology is central to outdoor adventure culture. Machines are dismissed as impure, but adventure culture relies on, even fetishizes its gear. The success of the adventure equipment industry (REI and Patagonia, for instance) attests to the technological apparatus of risk culture. Such artificial extensions facilitate the wilderness encounter as much as ramps, wheelchairs, walking sticks, Braille signs, and cut curbs—the technologies that are associated with disability. But what distinguishes trekking poles, Camelbacks, GPS units, and crampons—technologies that permit adventurers to encounter wilderness—from the technologies associated with the disabled body? The former is fetishized as "gear," whereas the latter is stigmatized as intrusive or "mediation," as in Abbey's (1968) comparison of a car to a wheelchair.

Adventure activities require "sets of humans, objects, technologies and scripts that contingently produce durability and stability" and "leisure landscapes involving various hybrids that roam the countryside and deploy the kinesthetic sense of movement" (MacNaghten and Urry 2000, 8). The kinds of technologies that would make wilderness accessible to people with disabilities are only qualitatively different from the kinds of technologies that make wilderness available to people without disabilities. All relationships with wilderness are mediated by these objects, technologies, and scripts. The fact that the myth of wilderness obscures the role of culture in its construction and the role of technology in the wilderness encounter allows it to support myths of disability.

Environmental rhetoric claiming that technology corrupted the garden registers disabled figures as unnatural, symbols of the imperfections we must strive to avoid or overcome. A disability critique of risk culture insists that technologies themselves are to be seen not as inherently good or bad but as human constructions: "The social world shapes the meanings of technology" (Gibson 2006, 15). Drawing on the work of Maurice Merleau-Ponty and Gilles Deleuze and Félix Guattari, some disability theorists go further, using phenomenology to argue that all bodies are "becoming." That is, all bodies are in a dynamic state of being between organic and "other," organic and machine. No body is enclosed, static, or purely organic. This insight undermines the notion of the independent, "self-reliant" figure the wilderness body ideal champions. It suggests that all bodies, not just ones designated "disabled" by dominant discourse, are "becoming," dynamic, always in a process of being both abled and disabled relative to context, geography, purpose, or habit. Phenomenology emphasizes that our bodies are not independent objects in the world but are embedded in the world through objects and habits. The relationship between the body and its environment is constitutive. The body's various extensions—clothes, appendages, backpacks, eyeglasses, and chairs, for instance—are technologies that make possible the body's relation to the world.

This argument has important implications for adventure culture. If, as Braun (2003, 179) writes, risk culture is about "refusing the disciplinary regimes of modern society and global capitalism, and about pursuing embodied rather than virtual experiences," then the distinction between embodied and virtual is important to the wilderness encounter. But disability studies challenges risk culture's assumption that the human body is natural, whereas all other objects in the world are unnatural. It suggests instead that the body/world, natural/unnatural distinction is constructed and could therefore be constructed differently. In "Disability, Connectivity, and Transgressing the Autonomous Body" Barbara

Gibson (2006, 188) argues, "The 'non-disabled/disabled' division is actually a false one and . . . all of us inhabit different kinds of bodily differences across a range of experience." Based on her interviews with five people who rely on long-term ventilation machines, Gibson concluded that the relationship between the body and machines ought to be conceived as "becoming." She describes one man's relationship to his wheelchair: Jack's self is uncontained by the material body and spills over into the wheelchair. The chair is more than a symbolic representation of Jack; it is Jack, that is, becoming-Jack, just as the body lying in bed is also becoming-Jack, and the future reuniting of Jack and the wheelchair will also be a reconfigured becoming-Jack (194).

The notion of the body becoming suggests that "selves are distributive," are both "confined to individual bodies and simultaneously connected, overlapping with other bodies, nature, and machines" (Gibson 2006, 189). This challenges "prevailing discourses valorizing independence" (187) and posits the relationship between bodies and machines as "connection," "extension," and testament to the "fluidity of the subject." A becoming body is an "assemblage . . . of multiple bodies, machines, animals, places, and energy ad infinitum" (190). Gibson's use of becoming shifts the valence from dependency to connectivity and accepts as natural the human body's reliance on machines.

Rather than facilitating connection to nature, as adventure culture would have it, the myth of the independent body works against the possibility of an ethic of openness—to other people, to animals, and to nature. The notion of a body becoming rather than being offered by disability theorists reinforces attempts by scholars such as Richard White and Donna Haraway to argue that upholding dichotomies between nature and humans, organic and machine inhibits an ethic of openness not just to nature but to other people as well. A disability approach thus casts in stark relief the hypocrisy of the wilderness body ideal's rejection of technology, because, of course, all persons "employ technologies as extensions of the self" (Gibson 2006, 14). Able bodies do not experience nature any more purely than disabled bodies if we view all technologies as mediating, all bodies as becoming, and all wildernesses as constructed.

Conclusion

An examination of risk culture through the lens of disability studies shows how invested adventure culture and environmentalism are in the fit body. Mainstream environmentalism does indeed have a troubling relationship to disability and should continue to be self-critical about its blanket rejection of technology, often implicit in its use of disability as a metaphor for humanity's alienation from nature and its historical ties to eugenics, national purity, and class and race exclusions. But despite a troubled historical relationship, environmentalists and disability studies theorists share important values, which risk culture's attachment to the fit body unfortunately obscures. Both advocate an increased awareness of place and of various versions of bodies in place. The disability studies theorist Michael Dorn (1998, 183) argues that because the disabled body "remain[s] attentive and responsive to changing environmental conditions," it "exhibits a mature form of environmental sensitivity." Navigating spaces that are constructed by ableist assumptions about the average body can cultivate "geographical maturity." Disability studies does not reject the body as an important site of self- or environmental awareness. It merely challenges the value of the fit and abled body, exposes the constructedness of disability and of environments, and points to the importance of creating both social and physical environments that acknowledge a diversity of bodies.

A common value of many environmentalists and disability studies scholars may point to a connection between their respective notions of an ethical way of being in the world. Like many environmentalists, disability theorists argue that society should be more accommodating to varying "pace of life" abilities. "Pace of life" expectations are in themselves disabling: "expectations of pace can make work, recreational, community, and social activities inaccessible" (Wendell 1996, 38). A slower pace of life can create the conditions for a greater awareness of nature. Even Abbey (1968, 69) was concerned about the environmental consequences of an increased pace of movement: "We could . . . multiply the area of our national parks tenfold or a hundredfold . . . simply by banning the private automobile." To Abbey a slower pace of experiencing nature might lead to a more ethical stance toward it because "a man on foot, on horseback or on a bicycle [which is not unlike a wheelchair, we might note] will see more, feel more, enjoy more in one mile than the motorized tourists can in a hundred miles" (67).

Risk culture sells itself as key to getting back to nature and turns precisely on the threat of disablement. But there is no fundamental relationship between risk and developing a good environmental ethic. Understanding the corporeal unconscious of environmental thought and wilderness preservation reveals that the wilderness body ideal that risk culture performs is a simulacrum of environmentalism at best. The myths of the individual, the genetically superior body, and the wilderness plot all powerfully shape contemporary adventure culture in ways that are at odds with any vision of an inclusive environmental movement. As long as risk culture signifies environmental virtue, its attachment to the abled body will continue to restrict the movement's potential for influence. "After all," the disabled adventurer

Bonnie Lewkowicz (2006, 34) writes, "the more of us there are going out into nature to do these things, the more likely it is that those mountains, rivers, and shorelines will be preserved for all of us for many more years to come."

NOTES

1. Given the scope of this essay I will not elaborate on the debate within environmentalism in the Progressive Era between conservationists (who preferred protecting nature as "resource") and preservationists (who wanted to protect nature for "refuge"). Conservationists such as Gifford Pinchot and Theodore Roosevelt were split from preservationists such as John Muir. See Nash 1967.

2. Susan Schrepfer (2005) records how women were central to wilderness preservation and mountain climbing during many stages of the twentieth-century environmental movement. Although her book contributes an important correction to the notion that the domain of wilderness preservation was strictly male, it fails to question the extent to which wilderness was in itself gendered and therefore a potentially problematic approach for both men and women, not to mention the other hidden attachments of wilderness preservation.

3. I use this term to locate my discussion about disability within Braun's (2003) analysis of race, to highlight the lack of this discussion in similar critical arguments about adventure culture, and to expose the invisibility of this attachment to the fit body. I recognize that the term corporeal unconscious has an established genealogy, arising from Freudian analysis and more recently taken up by cultural studies scholars. Although there may be some overlaps, my use does not directly engage the term's Freudian connotations.

4. Just like critical race studies and feminist theory, the field of disability studies comprises a variety of approaches and political and theoretical agendas. In this essay I draw on the critical theoretical strand of disability studies that historicizes the construction of disability in terms of its relationship to national identity, genetic fitness, and economic productivity. I also draw on geographers of disability who expose the ways disability is both built into and ignored by the

material environment. Finally I engage these strands with critical environmental theories, such as work by Donna Haraway (1989), to identify the relationship between technology and the body in adventure culture and environmentalism, a dialogue that I hope contributes to both environmental theory and disability studies. I want to be careful not to suggest that disability studies is monolithic, and so when I refer to disability studies these are the strands I include.

5. Cronon (1996) famously argued that "wilderness poses a serious threat to responsible environmentalism" because it ignores history, promotes escape from social responsibility, and relies on troubling dualisms of nature/culture, past/present, and natural/artificial.

6. Environmentalism and environmental studies are multifaceted, and when I refer to environmentalism I mean to connote mainstream environmentalism in terms of how it values the fit body and wilderness adventure as constituting the ideal environmental ethic. I locate my project on the corporeal unconscious of adventure culture and mainstream environmentalism within the theoretical and activist subfield known as environmental justice, which eschews any form of environmental protection that fails to consider its relationship to questions of social justice.

7. My attention to risk as a crucial lens through which to understand the relationship between disability and adventure culture supports Ursula Heise's (2008) theorizing of "risk" and "risk society." Following seminal work on risk society by Mary Douglas (1966), Douglas and Aaron Wildavsky (1983), and Ulrich Beck (1992), Heise argues that risk is a fundamental way of understanding, organizing, and describing the modern world, especially as risk increasingly permeates everyday life in ways that are often difficult to corporeally detect and experience. Although she focuses on perceptions of global environmental risk (such as climate change and nuclear fallout), my project supports her thesis that discourses of risk illuminate implications of the environmental agenda. That is, the pursuit of risk in adventure culture can be read as a reflection of the prevalence and perception of risk in modern society that Heise describes.

8. Braun (2003, 178–79) offers the term risk culture to describe "a set of discursive operations around risk and risk taking that help constitute,

and render natural, risk society's racial and class formations." He uses the term "to call attention to the cultural and representational practices that produce risk as culturally meaningful" (178). I use the term interchangeably with <u>adventure culture</u>, although I do want to retain the connotation the term <u>risk</u> implies about the role of risk culture in a "risk society" (Beck 1992).

9. My attempt to obtain copyright permission to reproduce two ACR PLB advertisements in this essay was rejected on the basis that my interpretation of the ads was not what ACR intended. In an email response to my request, ACR's director of marketing explained the rejection: "I cannot provide permission to use these ads for Sarah's article. Our ads are not intended to invoke fear in the minds of outdoor enthusiast[s]. We do not want adventurers to become dependant [<u>sic</u>] on technology. People should not engage in Risky activities without the proper training and preparations to do so. Neither of our spokes persons carries a PLB because they are disabled. The further one treks into the back country, the better the odds that traditional means of communication will not work. PLBs don't save lives. They just provide a means of communication when all means of self-rescue have been exhausted. A PLB would not have saved Aron's arm. It may have saved him the agony of drinking his own urine for 5 days and cutting his own arm off with a dull knife. Our choice of Dan and Aron as spokespersons was driven by the notoriety their stories received amongst backcountry enthusiast[s]. We are using that notoriety to introduce new technology that was not available to that market before July of 2003. Many of the traditional high profile writers and celebrities for the outdoor community tell us that if people need to carry a PLB, than [<u>sic</u>] they don't belong in the back country. We say that even those with the most experience are not immune to accidents." Ironically this response only reinforces my interpretation that the figures of Dan and Aron serve as exceptional "supercrip" narratives that prove the rule that disabled bodies don't belong in the wild, as well as the problem technology poses for adventure culture's attachment to the "pure" encounter between body and Nature.

10. The audience for this ad is expected to know Aron's story, which was famous among outdoor enthusiasts. While rock climbing alone,

Aron's arm was trapped under a boulder in Utah. He cut his arm off after six days to save himself.

11. The tension between disabled access to wilderness and the myth that wilderness should be free of mediating traces of built society is captured in an article titled "Trailblazing in a Wheelchair—An Oxymoron?" by Joe Huber (2005). Huber asks: "Shouldn't minimum impact to the environment and safety of all those involved be balanced equally with one's right to access?" The notion of disabled people "trailblazing" in the wilderness is oxymoronic because of the implicit assumption that access equals impact. But even Huber fails to see the contradiction in his own language. Trailblazing is inherently damaging to the environment; it is only deemed acceptable for abled bodies because of the myth that trailblazing is about independence and escape from technological mediation. But trailblazing with a wheelchair crosses a line because the technology involved is about dependence.

12. I use the term disablist presence as an application of Toni Morrison's (1993) theory of the "Africanist presence" in American literature to suggest that the disablist presence operates in risk culture discourse similarly: just as the "major and championed characteristics of our national literature" are in fact "responses to a dark, abiding, signing Africanist presence" (5), the presence of disability in risk culture and environmental literature and thought "exposes the illusion" (as Garland-Thomson [2002] puts it) of able-bodiedness.

13. Shari Huhndorf (2001) examines this expression in Going Native: Indians in the American Cultural Imagination. Kevin Costner used the expression "going Native" to describe his 1990 box-office hit Dances with Wolves, in which his character returns to the frontier following the Civil War. But few note that he returns to recover from a war injury—disability—a fact that further establishes the relationship between ableism and the wilderness ideal plot.

14. For more on how spending time in the wilderness became understood as a "cure" for psychological and physical maladies, see Harvey Green's (1986) chapter titled "The Sanitation Movement and the Wilderness Cure."

15. For more on Roosevelt and American empire, see Slotkin 1981; Kaplan (1990). Kaplan expands on the role of what Perry Miller

(2009) called America's "errand into the wilderness" in justifying expansion.

16. Roosevelt's focus on the young male body as a site of national integrity was consistent with his historical moment, as Rail and Harvey (1995) argue. At this time "sportization," as they call it, disciplined individual bodies and mobilized the population (171). Sports legitimized a "matrix of bodily surveillance technologies" (172) that helped produce the "deviant body" (173). Again we see that the construction of the fit body at this moment coincided with the construction of disability as the deviant body.

17. This move in environmental philosophy echoes early ecofeminist calls to challenge the dualism between mind/body and sacred/profane that corresponds to the split between nature/culture. Some ecofeminists argue that modern society's mistreatment and exploitation of nature is parallel to its exploitation of women. Getting back to nature is understood therefore as also a feminist move and requires reconnecting to the body's natural cycles and functions. Other feminists also ground theories of liberation in the body by challenging how patriarchy privileges the public sphere and cerebral projects over the private sphere of the body. And then there are feminists such as Haraway (1989), who reject these binaries entirely. The feminist intervention that my argument provides is perhaps most in line with Haraway's, although I am also sensitive to some of the tensions between some disability studies theorists and what is often perceived as Haraway's rejection of the body.

18. The show demonstrated further simulacra in a 2007 controversy surrounding its authenticity; when it was released that the show staged many of its "wild" encounters and Grylls was often aided behind the scenes (given indoor accommodation, assistance building rafts, for instance), the premise of the show was threatened. The Discovery Channel managed the controversy by including a statement about these interventions at the beginning of every show.

19. Disability theorists have analyzed the way built environments create "design apartheid" that constructs disability (see, e.g., Gleeson 1999; Hall and Imrie 1999).

20. McAvoy's (2001) article debunks myths about people with disabilities and outdoor recreation. The first myth he debunks is "that people

with disabilities do not prefer the same kind of outdoor environments as do people without disabilities" (26). Although his research attests to the prevalence of myths about people with disabilities and expectations of outdoor recreation, McAvoy does not critique the root of these myths: the "corporeal unconscious" assumed in the wilderness encounter to begin with.

REFERENCES

Abbey, Edward. 1968. Desert Solitaire: A Season in the Wilderness. New York: Ballantine.

Abrams, David. 1996. The Spell of the Sensuous: Perception and Language in a More-Than-Human World. New York: Vintage.

Adams, Paul C. 2001. "Peripatetic Imagery and Peripatetic Sense of Place." In Textures of Place: Exploring Humanist Geographies, edited by P. C. Adams, S. Hoelscher, and K. E. Till, 186–206. Minneapolis: University of Minnesota Press.

Beck, Ulrich. 1992. Risk Society: Towards a New Modernity. London: Sage.

Bederman, Gail. 1996. Manliness and Civilization: A Cultural History of Gender and Race in the U.S., 1880–1917. Chicago: University of Chicago Press.

Braun, Bruce. 2003. "On the Raggedy Edge of Risk: Articulations of Race and Nature after Biology." In Race, Nature, and the Politics of Difference, edited by D. Moore, J. Kosek, and A. Pandian, 175–203. Durham NC: Duke University Press.

Brooks, David. 2000. Bobos in Paradise: The New Upper Class and How They Got There. New York: Touchstone.

Buell, Lawrence. 2001. Writing for an Endangered World: Literature, Culture, and the Environment in the U.S. and Beyond. Cambridge MA: Belknap Press of Harvard University Press.

Comer, Krista. 1997. "Sidestepping Environmental Justice: Natural Landscapes and the Wilderness Plot." In Breaking Boundaries: New Perspectives on Women's Regional Writing, edited by S. A. Inness and D. Royer, 216–36. Iowa City: University of Iowa Press.

Cosgrove, Denis. 1995. "Habitable Earth: Wilderness, Empire, and Race in America." In Wild Ideas, edited by D. Rothenberg, 27–41. Minneapolis: University of Minnesota Press.

Cronon, W. 1996. "The Trouble with Wilderness; or, Getting Back to the Wrong Nature." In Uncommon Ground: Rethinking the Human Place in Nature, edited by W. Cronon, 7–28. New York: Norton.

Dorn, Michael. 1998. "Beyond Nomadism: The Travel Narratives of a Cripple." In Places through the Body, edited by H. Nast and S. Pile, 183–206. New York: Routledge.

Douglas, Mary. 1966. Purity and Danger: An Analysis of the Concept of Pollution and Taboo. London: Routledge.

Douglas, Mary, and Aaron Wildavsky. 1983. Risk and Culture: An Essay on the Selection of Technological and Environmental Dangers. Berkeley: University of California Press.

Foucault, Michel. 1978. History of Sexuality. New York: Pantheon.

Garland-Thomson, Rosemarie. 2002. "The Politics of Staring: Visual Rhetorics of Disability in Popular Photography." In Disability Studies: Enabling the Humanities, edited by S. L. Snyder, B. J. Brueggemann, and R. Garland-Thomson, 56–75. New York: Modern Language Association.

Gibson, Barbara E. 2006. "Disability, Connectivity, and Transgressing the Autonomous Body." Journal of Medical Humanities 27: 187–96.

Gleeson, Brendan. 1999. Geographies of Disability. New York: Routledge.

Green, Harvey. 1986. Fit for America: Health, Fitness, Sport, and American Society. New York: Pantheon.

Grylls, Bear. 2007. Born Survivor: Survival Techniques from the Most Dangerous Places on Earth. London: Transworld.

Hall, P., and R. Imrie. 1999. "Architectural Practices and Disabling Design in the Built Environment." Environment and Planning B: Planning and Design 26: 409–25.

Haraway, Donna. 1989. Primate Visions: Gender, Race, and Nature in the World of Modern Science. New York: Routledge.

Heise, Ursula. 2008. Sense of Place and Sense of Planet: The Environmental Imagination of the Global. New York: Oxford University Press.

Hepworth, J. R. 1998. Stealing Glances: Three Interviews with Wallace Stegner. Albuquerque: University of New Mexico Press.

Horsman, Reginald. 1981. Race and Manifest Destiny: The Origins of American Racial Anglo-Saxonism. Cambridge MA: Harvard University Press.

Huber, Joe. 2005. "Trailblazing in a Wheelchair—An Oxymoron?" Palaestra, July 28, 52.

Huhndorf, Shari. 2001. Going Native: Indians in the American Cultural Imagination. Ithaca NY: Cornell University Press.

Jacoby, Karl. 2001. Crimes against Nature: Squatters, Poachers, Thieves, and the Hidden History of American Conservation. Berkeley: University of California Press.

Kaplan, Amy. 1990. "Romancing the Empire: The Embodiment of American Masculinity in the Popular Historical Novel of the 1890s." American Literary History 2: 659–90.

Kevles, Daniel. 1985. In the Name of Eugenics: Genetics and the Uses of Human Heredity. New York: Knopf.

Kosek, Jake. 2004. "Purity and Pollution: Racial Degradation and Environmental Anxieties." In Liberation Ecologies: Environment, Development, Social Movements, edited by M. Peet and R. Watts, 125–65. New York: Routledge.

Krakauer, Jon. 1997. Into Thin Air. New York: Anchor.

Lewkowicz, Bonnie. 2006. "Accessible Outdoors: Opening the Door to Nature for People with Disabilities." Bay Nature Magazine, October–December, 21–34.

MacCannell, Dean. 1989. The Tourist: A New Theory of the Leisure Class. Revised ed. New York: Schocken.

MacNaghten, P., and J. Urry. (2000). "Bodies of Nature: Introduction." Body & Society 6, nos. 3–4: 1–11.

Marx, Leo. 1964. The Machine in the Garden: Technology and the Pastoral Ideal in America. New York: Oxford University Press.

McAvoy, Leo. 2001. "Outdoors for Everyone: Opportunities That Include People with Disabilities." Parks and Recreation 36, no. 8: 24–36.

Merchant, Carolyn. 2005. Reinventing Eden: The Fate of Nature in Western Culture. New York: Routledge.

Miller Perry. 2009. Errand into the Wilderness. Cambridge MA: Harvard University Press.

Mitchell, D., and Sharon L. Snyder. 1997. The Body and Physical Difference: Discourses of Disability. Ann Arbor: University of Michigan Press.

Morrison, Toni. 1993. Playing in the Dark: Whiteness and the Literary Imagination. New York: Vintage.

Nash, Roderick. 1967. Wilderness and the American Mind. New Haven CT: Yale University Press.

Nettlefold, P. A., and E. Stratford. 1999. "The Production of Climbing Landscapes-as Texts." Australian Geographical Studies 37, no. 2: 130–41.

Nussbaum, Martha. 2006. Frontiers of Justice: Disability, Nationality, and Species Membership. Cambridge MA: Belknap Press of Harvard University Press.

Pernick, M. S. 1997. "Eugenics and Public Health in American History." American Journal of Public Health 87: 1767–72.

Rabinow, Paul. 1984. The Foucault Reader. New York: Pantheon.

Rail, G., and J. Harvey. 1995. "Body at Work: Michel Foucault and the Sociology of Sport." Sociology of Sport Journal 12: 164–79.

Rome, Adam. 2006). "Political Hermaphrodites: Gender and Environmental Reform in Progressive America." Environmental History 11 (July): 440–63.

Rosen, Elizabeth. 2007. "Somalis Don't Climb Mountains: The Commercialization of Mount Everest." Journal of Popular Culture 40: 147–68.

Schrepfer, S. 2005. Nature's Altars: Mountains, Gender, and American Environmentalism. Lawrence: University of Kansas Press.

Sewall, Laura. 1999. Sight and Sensibility: The Eco-Psychology of Perception. New York: Jeremy P. Tarcher/Putnam.

Shildrick, M., and J. Price. 1996. "Breaking the Boundaries of the Broken Body." Body & Society 2, no. 4: 93–113.

Simon, Bryant. 2003. "New Men in Body and Soul: The Civilian Conservation Corps and the Transformation of Male Bodies and the Body Politic." In Seeing Nature through Gender, edited by V. Scharff. Lawrence: University of Kansas Press.

Slotkin, Richard. 1973. Regeneration through Violence: The Mythology of the American Frontier, 1600–1860. Middletown CT: Wesleyan University Press.

———. 1981. "Nostalgia and Progress: Theodore Roosevelt's Myth of the Frontier." American Quarterly 33: 608–37.

Smith, Henry Nash. 1950. Virgin Land: The American West as Symbol and Myth. Cambridge MA: Harvard University Press.

Spence, Mark. 1999. Dispossessing the Wilderness: Indian Removal and the Making of the National Parks. New York: Oxford University Press.

Sutter, Paul. 2001. "Terra Incognita: The Neglected History of Interwar Environmental Thought and Politics." Reviews in American History 29: 289–98.

Touching the Void. 2003. Directed by Kevin Macdonald. London: FilmFour Productions.

Tremain, Shelly. 1997. Extraordinary Bodies: Figuring Physical Disability in American Culture and Literature. New York: Columbia University Press.

———, ed. 2005. Foucault and the Government of Disability. Ann Arbor: University of Michigan Press.

Wendell, Susan. 1996. "The Social Construction of Disability." In The Rejected Body: Feminist Reflections on Disability, edited by S. Wendell, 35–56. New York: Routledge.

White, Richard. 1995. The Organic Machine. New York: Hill and Wang.

Williams, T., and P. Donnelly. 1985. "Subcultural Production, Reproduction, and Transformation in Climbing." International Review of the Sociology of Sport 20, no. 1: 3–15.

2

Bringing Together Feminist Disability Studies and Environmental Justice

Valerie Ann Johnson

Writing this essay has been like falling down Alice's proverbial rabbit hole into Wonderland.[1] The more I reflect on feminist disability studies and environmental justice, the more connections between the two I find. And the more connections I find, the more complexity there seems to be. To paraphrase Alice, it gets curiouser and curiouser. Still it is a complexity worth exploring. This essay represents an initial venture into what I believe to be a fruitful area of scholarship and activism. I bring together ideas from several social justice perspectives in order to connect environmental justice and feminist disability studies in a way that provides a coherent framework to address activist work for women and girls.

Two ideas should be kept in mind as this essay unfolds. The first is that feminist disability studies frames disability as a representational system that is socially constructed and of interest as an intellectual concern across a broad spectrum of inquiry; it is not just the intellectual concern of those in areas designed to "fix" the "problem" (e.g., medicine, social work, rehabilitation [Garland-Thomson 2001]). The second is that environmental justice generally is defined as "the pursuit of equal justice and equal protection under the law for all environmental statu[t]es and regulations, without discrimination based on race, ethnicity, and/or socioeconomic status" (Johnson 2004, 82). Absent from that definition are both gender and ableness, which is why feminist disability studies provides such a compelling framework from which to discuss this gap in environmental justice consciousness.

It is also worth noting that both feminist disability studies and environmental justice are grounded in social justice. In the introduction to Cultural Bodies: Ethnography and Theory, editors Helen Thomas and Jamilah Ahmed (2004) observe that in the radical social and cultural climate of the latter years of the twentieth century, when the nature-culture debate was seriously challenged, we inherited from the social movements of that time the "awakening consciousness of the body as 'an instrument of power'" (quoting Bordo 1993, 4). Feminists are concerned with the environment, as reflected in ecofeminism and feminist environmental studies. Although social injustice is addressed in both these perspectives, disability is rarely in the foreground.[2] And it is important to note that environmental justice also is not the same as environmentalism. The Earth Charter (Earth Charter Initiative 2001) is a document created by an independent global organization after the Earth Summit in 1992 in order to codify a global consensus around sustainability; it outlines sixteen principles. Principle 12 states:

> Uphold the right of all, without discrimination, to a natural and social environment supportive of human dignity, bodily health, and spiritual well-being, with special attention to the rights of indigenous peoples and minorities.
>
> a. Eliminate discrimination in all its forms, such as that based on race, color, sex, sexual orientation, religion, language, and national, ethnic or social origin.
>
> b. Affirm the right of indigenous peoples to their spirituality, knowledge, lands and resources and to their related practice of sustainable livelihoods.

c. Honor and support the young people of our communities, enabling them to fulfill their essential role in creating sustainable societies.

d. Protect and restore outstanding places of cultural and spiritual significance.

It is significant to me that, while many forms of possible discrimination are listed, the category of ability or ableness is absent. This omission is troubling because it means that disability is subsumed under one of the other categories, and such sublimation can mask or obscure the issues that need to be attended to when considering sustainability as it relates to mental and physical ability. Without explicitly naming ability or ableness as a category where discrimination can occur, we cannot be sure that sustainability (for example) in relation to persons with disabilities will in fact be addressed.

My thinking about the nexus between disability and environmental justice began in earnest as a result of my daughters' participation in the 11th Annual North Carolina Environmental Justice Summit in Whitakers, at Franklinton Center at Bricks.[3] My older daughter is classified as "special needs" so that, though her chronological age was twelve years at the time, developmentally she tested around six or seven. I maintained a watchful eye and ear from afar, reluctant to be too intrusive as she participated in the Youth Summit (with the help of her one year younger sister), at which young people addressed environmental issues separately from the larger summit.

For the most part her experience was positive, although some of the concepts discussed were hard for her to understand at the moment she heard them. I knew, however, that in her own time she would figure out what the organizers were trying to convey. Although my daughter contributed to the discussion on recycling and helped with the tree planting and other activities, I wondered whether her ideas were fully embraced or just tolerated. And I started thinking then, in a more deliberate manner, about whether the environmental justice community is one of true inclusivity when it comes to those deemed disabled.

In fact one participant at the Summit, Dr. Della McQueen, reminded us that reliable transportation for those with impaired sight was just as much an environmental justice issue as access to clean air and water.[4] In a private conversation with Lynice Williams, executive director of North Carolina Fair Share and a member of the Summit organizing committee, we agreed that the subject of disability and environmental justice had not been formally addressed at the Summit but needed to be.[5] Williams felt that a discussion of disability as it relates to environmental justice would draw more (and different) people to these meetings. And as one of the Summit organizers, I know that this has been an unintentional oversight. In that moment, between witnessing my daughter's participation and hearing the comments from my sister activists, I realized that though we talk about "all peoples' needs" in the environmental justice movement, rarely do we directly address the issues affecting persons with disabilities. And more subtly, we tend to conflate disability, disease, and environmental injustice. We need to disaggregate the possible results of environmental injustice (e.g., exposure to toxic substances emanating from landfills or hog operations that injure the body) from the person, however they are embodied.

As an activist and scholar within the environmental justice movement, I have noted, beyond my local and statewide activist community, the absent voices and perspectives from those who self-identify or are identified as disabled. It is especially troubling that the disabled women and girls who contribute to the environmental justice movement as advocates and policymakers are rendered invisible. Even when movement activists rail against the adverse health effects of environmental policies and practices (e.g., placement of landfills, hazardous waste sites, bus depots) the complexities of disability are seldom part of the discussion.

What is not seen is the implicit assumption that we want healthy environments so that we do not end up damaged (i.e., disabled). This is especially true when we consider what can happen to women and girls, who so often are marginalized. Though we may discuss at length the harms created by bad environmental policies and practices, often with special emphasis on what happens to women and girls, we seldom question our underlying biases and prejudices regarding what is "normal." How can we call for justice and equity without inviting everyone to the table?

The need for a more visible connection between environmental justice and feminist disability studies was brought into even sharper relief for me in December 2009 as I watched news clips from the UN Climate Change Conference in Copenhagen, searching in vain for any coverage from the perspective of disabled activists. I even telephoned one of the national activist groups for disability rights to see if they had any representatives at the conference. They did not, and they said that climate change was beyond their mission. Who, then, represents the concerns of persons with disabilities with regard to climate change?

As I participate in the environmental movement in my various capacities (activist, scholar, community member) I now pay more attention to the connection between environmental justice activism and disability rights activism. This is not just an academic exercise for me. As a parent of a teenage girl with developmental delay I see where we miss opportunities to be more holistic in addressing environmental challenges.

Defining Feminist Disability Studies

Feminist disability studies represents the merging of feminism and disability activism. I accept the broadest definition of feminism, which says it is a movement to end sexism, sexist exploitation, and oppression (hooks 2000). The framework provided by Rosemarie Garland-Thomson's (2001) paper on feminist disability studies is the lens through which I discuss how the environmental justice movement is enriched by the work in feminist disability studies. First, it is worthwhile to unpack a cultural notion of disability. The first definition of <u>disability</u> on Dictionary.com is "lack of adequate power, strength or physical or mental ability; incapacity." The second is "a physical or mental handicap, especially one that prevents a person from living a full, normal life or from holding a gainful job."[6] Using the feminist disability studies analytical framework allows us to see how such a definition is socially constructed. It denies agency for the person given this appellation. In fact this definition could easily describe what it means to be female.

If disability is defined in large part as a lack of power, then we should consider the flip side of this coin. Hyperability is the excess of power, strength, or physical or mental ability, and for the select few who participate at the highest level in sports, that unusual ability (such as the unusual height required of the best basketball players) is richly rewarded. But a girl reaching seven feet or more in height is considered especially "odd" or "unusual" in a negative sense unless she plays professional, semiprofessional, or collegiate basketball or volleyball. She is conferred a "social" disability because this enhanced physical ability has limited application as defined by our society. We celebrate and desire the "abnormal" athletic body that, outside of athletics, puts the person at a disadvantage. Instead we accommodate the extra large sizes, the need for more space in all types of conditions (travel, seating, amount of food consumed, etc.), admiring hyperable persons when they are performers, entertainers, or athletes.

We learn from feminist disability studies that we shape normalcy and in doing so place at the margins those who do not fit our ideas of "the normal." Feminist disability politics upholds the right of women to define for themselves their physical difference and their femininity rather than conform to received interpretations (Garland-Thomson 2001). Our society, however, creates the parameters in which people are stigmatized. I remember when Warrior Marks (Walker and Parmar 1993) first came out Alice Walker was criticized for equating the loss of her eye with female genital circumcision. How could she, a Western woman, understand the meaning of female circumcision as well as women and girls who had undergone the operation? How dare she depict these operations as mutilation? Yet Walker defined for herself the meaning of her eye loss and translated disability into a "warrior mark."

We should also consider that "the concept of disability unites a heterogeneous group of people whose only commonality is being considered abnormal," and "as the norm becomes neutral in an environment created to accommodate it, disability becomes intense, extravagant, and problematic" (Garland-Thomson 2001, 1, 2). As an analytic concept and framework, disability studies is a system for interpreting bodily variations, a relationship between bodies and their environments, a set of practices that produce both the able-bodied and the disabled, and a way of describing the inherent instability of the embodied self (Garland-Thomson 2001). The overlap with feminism illuminates the sexist ways disability injustice differentially impacts women and men.

Merging Feminist Disability Studies and Environmental Justice

The civil rights movement has largely shaped the ideology of the environmental justice movement. Race, ethnicity, and socioeconomic considerations have been the major ways social justice has been envisioned within this movement. Bullard (2001, 9) outlines five principles that should be considered when addressing environmental justice concerns: the right to environmental protection, prevention of harm before it occurs, shifting the burden of proof to the polluters, obviating proof of intent to discriminate, and targeting resources to redress inequities. However, the population affected by the application of these principles is usually depicted solely in racial and class terms. Gender is largely absent when environmental justice is defined and outlined. Even the prominent role black women played and continue to play in the environmental movement is not regularly highlighted.

In an earlier essay (Johnson 2004) I wrote about black women's involvement in the environmental justice movement as framed by a concept of ethical consciousness reflected in black womanist and feminist ideology and spiritual authority and as linked to black feminist activity, demonstrated in my recounting of the stories of individual black women in North Carolina involved in the environmental justice movement. Though disability justice is an important social justice movement, it is not explicitly referenced in the context of the environmental justice movement.

We are more accustomed to depicting environmental justice in racialized ways (see, e.g., Westra and Lawson 2001). Even in the otherwise important collection, New Perspectives on Environmental Justice (Stein 2004), that brought attention to diverse feminist voices in environmental justice work there was little discussion or consideration of disability or the possibility of merging feminist disability studies with feminist environmental justice. In an otherwise excellent collection of work on the many issues affecting environmental justice, this gap was apparent to me (as a contributor) only after much later reflection.[7]

Merging feminist disability studies and environmental justice forces us to confront the power dynamics that reinforce a narrow view of "normal," one that privileges a particular sense of the human body that is constrictive, not expansive.

Feminist disability studies can be integrated into the praxis of environmental justice by utilizing Garland-Thomson's (2001, 20) four aspects of disability: "as a category of analysis, as a historical community, as a set of material practices, and as a representational system." The community of persons with disabilities is a heterogeneous group unified by their common depiction as "abnormal" (2). This makes it easier to overlook disabled persons collectively and instead see individuals with disabilities as unique or exceptional. One way environmental justice activists can consider disability, therefore, is in terms of exceptionalism.

Exceptionalism

One way to frame the particularities of gender, ableness, race, ethnicity, socioeconomic status, and other "identities" as they shape our lives is to look at the concept of exceptionalism, which I define a little differently than is common.[8] In brief, exceptionalism is when a person is assigned to a class because of bodily appearance or phenotype and held to be marginal to what is considered mainstream or dominant in our society. This designation can carry either positive or negative connotations depending on the context.

Exceptionalism can also be thought of as another facet of the Du Boisian concept of double consciousness. A twofold concept, exceptionalism describes the labeling that occurs when an individual (1) is thought to be different, unique, and unlike other people of his or her "class" (e.g., disabled, female, or of a particular racial or ethnic identity) because he or she has achieved some measure of success as defined by extant normative cultural standards; and (2) transcends his or her singular identity and is subsumed into a corporate identity of nonsuccess as defined by these same cultural standards, which, in both instances, relegate the "exception" to a marginal space outside of the "normal" ideal. Each aspect of exceptionality relies on the assumption that identity can be essentialized and used as an emblematic category. For example, one could look at the success of the skier Bonnie St. John, held out as an individual who overcame her disability by medaling in the 1984 Winter Paralympics and who therefore is exceptional (i.e., rising above her disability).[9] At the same time nonathletic disabled persons are characterized as part of a corporate disabled identity that is pathological (remember the popular definition quoted earlier) and therefore an exception to "normal" society (the dominant culture).

For another example, speak with a group of black college students about their experiences in the educational system, and overwhelmingly they will describe how they were treated as "different" (meaning "better") than other blacks because of their successful academic accomplishments. Exceptionalism does more than describe; it is also an explanatory model. Conceptual use of what is considered exceptional identifies that part of the abnormal that will not be assimilated into the normal and therefore can help us see more clearly how individuals placed in the exceptional category move in our society.

Disability is also defined by one's inability to fit comfortably in society. I cannot help but quote Sontag (1977, 82) here: "The people who have the real disease are also hardly helped by hearing their disease's name constantly being dropped as the epitome of evil." We need to ask ourselves what it means for disabled persons when we use the fear of possible disability in confronting environmental injustice and advocating for changes in policy regarding the environment. Constant reference to environmental causes of disability renders those who are disabled passive recipients of harm and implies their inability to be full participants in environmental justice work. It removes agency from those identified as disabled, especially when those working for disability rights are not part of the environmental justice conversation.

Implicit in environmental justice concerns is that we work to ensure that people are not exposed to those environmental assaults that lead to the creation of "the disabled" or "disability." Here is the challenge to those of us in the environmental justice movement, to do as Mia Mingus (2010) outlines: "Creating Collective Access (CCA) was about re-thinking how we, as disabled and chronically ill people, engage in movement spaces. This was about imagining something more and knowing that we had to do it for ourselves because it is so rare for movement spaces to ever consider disability and access in ways that go beyond logistics; in ways that challenge the ableist culture of our work. This was about being very clear that we wanted to shift the individualized and independent understanding of access and queer it and color it interdependent. This was about building crip solidarity." If we treat disability as an add-on or second thought, we continue a practice of marginalization that does not advance social justice. Who has standing to speak on the environmental issues impacting persons with disabilities? If ableism is not seen as equally destructive as the other isms (racism, sexism), then we do what Audre Lorde admonished us not to do: create a hierarchy of oppression. This serves to mask as well as marginalize those environmental justice issues that are salient to people with disabilities.

In environmental justice work a good portion of our activity is spent on identifying the problems and advocating for remedies. We do not have the luxury to theorize when lives are at stake. Yet when race, for example, is the focal point for our activities, then other categories, such as ableness, are obscured, thus hampering our ability to fully identify and critique the underlying values that drive various environmental policies and practices. One of the positive aspects of environmental justice activism is that those most impacted by environmental injustices compose our environmental justice leadership. Often these are the people who are ignored. But the merger between environmental justice and feminist disability studies could illuminate those environmental justice leaders who are disabled women and girls.

Those of us in the environmental justice movement cannot back away from our privileged ideas of ableness. Nor can we ignore how women and girls face different sets of issues regarding ability than do men and boys. Using perspectives from feminist disability studies allows us to better identify quality-of-life issues with respect to ableness. If we advocate for an improved quality of life, then we must be prepared to be truly inclusive by making sure the perspectives from disabled activists are centered in our activities.

What does this mean for someone who is differently abled? In practical terms, as we advocate for improved living conditions in various communities we also must include in our consideration what that means for those with developmental, emotional, and physical challenges. For example, after Hurricanes Katrina and Rita much of the public discussion revolved around how unprepared government disaster relief agencies were and the slowness of the response when called to action. One remedy has been to engage the public in disaster preparedness training. Is there a systematic effort, across all communities, to make sure that the disaster relief kits are accessible to people who are sight-impaired, who have limited cognitive skills or impaired dexterity? Are there kits available or designed to be accessible to those who use prostheses?

A further concern is the need for postdisaster trauma counseling. According to a study by Madrid et al. (2009), even after all the recent national disasters (going back to the Oklahoma City terrorist bombing more than sixteen years ago and up to the recent Gulf oil spill), the U.S. government is still not adequately prepared to respond to the next natural or human-created disaster.

Inadequate preparation and response also leads to "needless creation of psychiatric disability" (Madrid et al. 2009, 12). Madrid et al. also found that one of the most enduring effects of Hurricane Katrina has proven to be psychological distress (12). And we know that women are disproportionately the caregivers in their families and communities. What is needed are community-based mental health services that are "adequately available, readily accessible," and remain in place as long as the need is there (12).[10]

Of course harm is a major concern in environmental justice activism, and environmental injustice creates profound harm in communities of color. These harms include exposure to unsafe emissions from hazardous waste facilities, concentrated animal feeding operations, and bus depots and contamination of the water table from diverse toxic leakages. The warming of our climate has set in motion various natural disasters (such as drought and flooding) that disproportionately hurt women and children.[11] But when harm occurs, do the people harmed become disabled in a way that renders them less capable of active participation in the movement work? Are they stigmatized? How do we talk about girls of color so injured by toxins in their community that they become sterile or struck with various uterine-related cancers? Is this disability? An injury? An assault?

If unable to bear children, are women and girls less woman, less girl, de-feminized?[12] What are the rights of disabled women to reproduce, and how should we address those who question those rights? How should we address concerns regarding possible limitations on physical and intellectual ability? Some people are still concerned that those identified as disabled pass on deleterious genes. Here is where the convergence of social justice activity by environmental justice activists, disability rights activists, and reproductive rights activists could be quite powerful in promoting more humane and woman-centered reproductive health policies (locally, nationally, and internationally).

Applying Environmental Justice and Feminist Disability Studies to a Current Issue

Ableism, sexism, and environmental injustice are interconnected systems of exclusion and oppression that also depend on the other oppressive systems (racism, classism, religious intolerance, etc.) to support unequal treatment of people based on category. We, as a society, construct these inequalities; they are not natural or inherent. In order to better understand disability as socially constructed we can use representation, the body, identity, and activism (concepts identified by Garland-Thomson 2001) as our analytical categories and filter these categories through an environmental justice perspective.

One of our current national debates involves defining obesity as a disability. Popular culture encourages us to view obesity as a disability. Witness the proliferation of so-called reality shows regarding weight reduction. In a recent study of a nationally representative sample of 2,290 American adults Puhl (2010) and fellow researchers found that not only was weight discrimination common, but the rate of such discrimination was relatively close to the prevalence of race and age discrimination. However, there is no consensus regarding how we define obesity as a disability. There is variability across racial and ethnic identities. Not all "fat" is fat equally. Do we use a legal definition that can be used in litigation?

Medical definitions of disability regarding obesity may differ considerably from legal definitions of obesity. Do insurance companies use a definition of disability that includes obesity? Or do we accept the popular presentation of "normal" that still idealizes the thinner beauty standard? These questions and others suggest how complex a matter it is to define a concept that has such strong objective and subjective criteria attached to it. We need to be in conversation with those disability rights activists who have a feminist perspective so that together we can develop a clear critique and understanding of the issues involved in defining obesity as a disability. Even our first lady's anti-obesity campaign, an admirable and worthy endeavor, can be misconstrued if we focus too much on the biomedical depiction of obesity as evidenced in the report from the White House Task Force on Childhood Obesity (2011).[13]

Another approach to addressing obesity as an environmental justice issue involves the issue of food deserts, which, according to the Centers for Disease Control and Prevention (2011), are areas that lack access to affordable fruits, vegetables, whole grains, low-fat milk, and other foods that make up the full range of a healthy diet. To lift a community out of a food desert, we would need to identify the structural reasons for the existence of such a desert, learn how the community defines fatness as well as healthiness, formulate descriptions of daily food consumption patterns, and work with community activists on the food issues they feel are important. While food deserts can be found in urban,

semirural, and rural communities, in many urban areas the proliferation of fast-food restaurants that serve high-fat, high-sodium,
high-cholesterol foods, coupled with the lack of clean and safe
play areas, are structural concerns that impede people's ability
to engage in lifestyles that encourage wellness.

We also should recognize that when a woman is identified as
obese there are implicit and explicit, usually negative assumptions regarding her moral values. So when environmental justice
activities identify an environmental concern, we need to also be
aware of the social and cultural dimensions, beyond race and
class, of the identified problem. In this case today's obesity discourse comes out of an earlier antifat bias from the early twentieth century, a sentiment that came about in part through the
interaction of several social factors: industrialization, allowing
more people access to more foods; promotion of the ethic of self-
denial; and control of undesirable populations through eugenics
(Sherwood 2009). Not recognizing the genesis of our ideas about
the body allows us to fall into the trap of prescribing remedies
to help people, as if they need rescuing and are not capable of
generating their own solutions.

Those of us in the environmental justice community are not
immune to our society's standards of health, beauty, and normality, and until we formally confront those values we will replicate
the oppressive structures we seek to overturn. One of the positive effects of preparing this essay has been my own increased
consideration of the interconnections between environmental
justice and feminist disability studies. With this newly heightened
awareness, I noted with increased interest the announcement of
an upcoming event sponsored by the Environmental Protection
Agency (Region 9), the 2011 Disability Employment Opportunities
Job Fair. The advertisement read in part, "The U.S. Environmental

Protection Agency is seeking talented people with disabilities who have an interest in human health, environmental protection, and environmental justice. They specifically seek people who have degrees in Engineering, Physical Science, Biology, Chemistry, Environmental Management/Science, and Environmental Studies, who would like an opportunity to gain professional workforce experience in the San Francisco, California Regional Office." I want to know more about this job fair. Are the people the EPA seeks to recruit, who hold the degrees listed in the announcement, really prepared to address environmental justice issues? Will they see the connections between disability, feminism, and environmental justice? We need to hold the EPA and other employers responsible for the way they interact with the environmental justice community and the disability rights community. Asking these and other questions, pushing for the answers, and standing at the ready to act as needed are just a few ways to foster the accountability we need from EPA and other employers.

The ideas put forth in this essay are part of a work in progress. I am setting the parameters for further investigation. To be responsible as a scholar and activist as I merge environmental justice and feminist disability studies means that I must work collaboratively with women and girls in the environmental justice movement who identify themselves as having disabilities. Such a collaboration allows us to discover the appropriate questions to ask and to challenge unjust environmental policies so that the communities where we live, play, pray, and become educated are safe, clean, and fruitful.

NOTES

My appreciation goes to my family for their support and Leslie Wolfe for her patience. I thank God for Her Wisdom in guiding my thoughts.

1. This essay was previously published under the surname Kaalund.
2. For a thorough critique of ecofeminism and feminist environmentalism see Agarwal 2001.
3. A yearly meeting usually held in one of the more rural areas of North Carolina that brings together grassroots and community activists with academics and government representatives to discuss pertinent environmental justice issues.
4. Comment made by Dr. McQueen during one of the discussion sessions at the 11th Annual NCEJN Summit in which I participated.
5. North Carolina Fair Share was founded in 1987 to help North Carolinians, particularly those with low income, work for a fairer share of economic and political power (http://ncfairshare.org/).
6. The other aspects of this definition are "anything that disables or puts one at a disadvantage; the state or condition of being disabled; and legal incapacity, legal disqualification" (www.dictionary.com).
7. Another collection on environmental justice that outlines the diverse issues affecting grassroots communities is Adamson et al. 2002.
8. I have written more extensively on this concept in an unpublished paper, "Deciding to Be 'Blacknificent': Transforming Bioethics through Black/Africana Studies."
9. Bonnie St. John, an amputee, became the first African American to win Olympic medals (silver and bronze) in ski racing. More information can be found at her website: http://www.bonniestjohn.com/.
10. See Madrid et al. (2008) for another perspective on the effects of disaster on mental health.
11. The environmental activists Vandana Shiva, working primarily in India, and Wangari Maathi, working primarily in Kenya, have elevated to international consciousness the challenges of severe environmental degradation faced by women and children.
12. Andrea Simpson (2002) wrote about the environmental justice activist Doris Bradshaw from Memphis, Tennessee, who became particularly concerned with the occurrences of reproductive organ cancers among women in her community. I met Doris (and her husband, Ken)

at one of the first North Carolina Environmental Justice Summits (in 1998), where they presented their concerns regarding the level of toxicity in their community due to the Memphis Defense Depot. The EPA has since conducted clean-up activities at the site, according to the Memphis Defense Depot website: EPA Superfund Program: Memphis Defense Depot (DLA), Memphis TN, https://cumulis.epa.gov/supercpad/cursites/csitinfo.cfm?id=0404159.

13. First Lady Michelle Obama's Let's Move campaign is outlined in detail at Let's Move, http://www.letsmove.gov.

REFERENCES

Adamson, Joni, Mei Mei Evans, and Rachel Stein, eds. 2002. The Environmental Justice Reader: Politics, Poetics and Pedagogy. Tucson: University of Arizona Press.

Agarwal, Bina. 2001. "Environmental Management, Equity, and Ecofeminism." In Feminism and Race, edited by KumKum Bhavnani, 410–55. New York: Oxford University Press.

Bhavnani, KumKum. 2001. Feminism and Race. New York: Oxford University Press.

Bordo, Susan. 1993. Unbearable Weight: Feminism, Western Culture and the Body. Berkeley: University of California Press.

Bullard, Robert D. 2001. "Decision-Making." In Faces of Environmental Racism: Confronting Issues of Global Justice, 2d ed., edited by Laura Westra and Bill E. Lawson, 3–28. Lanham MD: Rowman & Littlefield.

Carroll, Lewis. 2008. Alice's Adventures in Wonderland. London: Puffin Books.

Centers for Disease Control and Prevention. 2011. "A Look inside Food Deserts." http://www.cdc.gov/Features/FoodDeserts/.

Earth Charter Initiative. 2001. "The Earth Charter." file:///C:/Users/user/Downloads/echarter_english.pdf.

Garland-Thomson, Rosemarie. 2001. "Re-shaping, Re-thinking, Re-defining: Feminist Disability Studies." Barbara Waxman Fiduccia Papers on Women and Girls with Disabilities. Washington DC: Center for Women Policy Studies. www.centerwomenpolicy.org/pdfs/dis2.pdf.

hooks, bell. 2000. Feminism Is for Everybody: Passionate Politics. Boston: South End Press.

Johnson, Valerie A. 2004. "Witness to Truth: Black Women Heeding the Call for Environmental Justice." In New Perspectives on Environmental Justice: Gender, Sexuality, and Activism, ed. Rachel Stein, 78–92. New Brunswick NJ: Rutgers University Press.

Madrid, Paula, Richard Garfield, Parham Jaberi, Maureen Daly, Georgina Richard, and Roy Grant. 2008. "Mental Health Services in Louisiana School-Based Health Centers Post-Hurricanes Katrina and Rita." Professional Psychology: Research and Practice 39, no. 1: 45–51.

Madrid, Paula, Roy Grant, and Rachel Rosen. 2009. "Creating Mental Health Disability through Inadequate Disaster Response: Lessons from Hurricane Katrina." In Disabilities: Insights from across Fields and around the World. vol. 2: The Context: Environmental, Social and Cultural Considerations, ed. by Catherine A. Marshall, Elizabeth Kendall, Martha E. Banks, and Reva Mariah S. Gover, 1–16. Westport CT: Praeger.

Mingus, Mia. 2010. "Reflections on an Opening: Disability Justice and Creating Collective Access in Detroit." Incite, August. http://inciteblog.wordpress.com/2010/08/23/reflections-from-detroit-reflections-on-an-opening-disability-justice-and-creating-collective-access-in-detroit/.

Puhl, Rebecca. 2010. "Weight Discrimination: A Socially Acceptable Injustice." Obesity Action Coalition. http://www.obesityaction.org/wp-content/uploads/Obesity-Discrimination.pdf.

Sherwood, Jessica Holden. 2009. "Weighing In." Review of The Fat Studies Reader, ed. by Esther Rothblum and Sondra Solovay (New York: NYU Press). Ms. Magazine, Fall, 57–58.

Simpson, Andrea. 2002. "Who Hears Their Cry? African-American Women and the Fight for Environmental Justice in Memphis, Tennessee." In The Environmental Justice Reader: Politics, Poetics and Pedagogy, edited by Joni Adamson, Mei Mei Evans, and Rachel Stein, 82–104. Tucson: University of Arizona Press.

Sontag, Susan. 1977. Illness as Metaphor. New York: Vintage Books.

Stein, Rachel, ed. 2004. New Perspectives on Environmental Justice: Gender, Sexuality, and Activism. New Brunswick NJ: Rutgers University Press.

Thomas, Helen, and Jamilah Ahmed, eds. 2004. Cultural Bodies: Ethnography and Theory. Malden MA: Blackwell.

Walker, Alice, and Pratibha Parmar. 1993. Warrior Marks: Female Genital Mutilation and the Sexual Blinding of Women. New York: Harcourt, Brace.

Westra, Laura, and Bill E. Lawson, eds. 2001. Faces of Environmental Racism: Confronting Issues of Global Justice. (2d ed. Lanham MD: Rowman & Littlefield.

White House Task Force on Childhood Obesity. 2011. "One Year Progress Report." February. http://www.letsmove.gov/sites/letsmove.gov/files /Obesity_update_report.pdf.

3

Lead's Racial Matters

Mel Y. Chen

If animality is coarticulated with humanity in ways that are soundly implicated in regimes of race, nation, and gender, disrupting clear divisions and categories that have profound implications, ramifying from the linguistic to the biopolitical, here I pluck an object from the lowest end of the animacy hierarchy: lead metal, a chemical element, an exemplar of inanimate matter. I bring animacy theory to bear on metals by looking at recent racialized discourses around lead and by focusing on mercury toxicity to discuss the vulnerability of human subjects in the face of ostensibly inanimate particles. These particles are critically mobile, and their status as toxins derives from their potential threat to valued human integrities. They further threaten to overrun what an animacy hierarchy would wish to lock in place.

Toys Off Track

This essay considers the case of "lead panic" in the United States in 2007 regarding potentially toxic toys associated with Chinese manufacture. I label this recent lead case a panic to suggest a disproportionate relationship between its purportedly unique threat to children's health and the relative paucity of evidence at its onset that the contaminated toys themselves had already caused severe health consequences.[1] I measure this panic against other domestic public health lead concerns, including spectacles of contagion, to investigate lead's role in the complex play of domestic security and sovereign fantasy (defined here as the national or imperial project of absolute rule and authority). I suggest that an inanimate but migrant entity such as industrial lead can become racialized, even as it can only lie in a notionally peripheral relationship to biological life. Rather than focus exclusively on the concrete dangers to living bodies of environmental lead, which are significant and well documented, I consider lead as a cultural phenomenon over and above its material and physiomedical character.

In the summer of 2007 in the United States a spate of specific recalls and generalized warnings about preschool toys, pet food, seafood, lunchboxes, and other items began to appear in national and local newspapers and on television and radio news.[2] In this geopolitical and cultural moment the most urgent warnings were issued for toys. Lead's identity as a neurotoxic heavy metal was attributed to a set of toys whose decomposable surfaces when touched yielded up the lead for transit into the bloodstreams of young children, giving it a means for its circulatory march toward the vulnerable developing brain. Nancy A. Nord, acting chair of the Consumer Product Safety Commission, issued a statement that declared, "These recalled toys have accessible lead in the paint, and parents should not hesitate in taking them away from children."[3]

Descriptions of the items recalled tended to have three common characteristics. First, they pointed to the dangers of lead intoxication as opposed to other toxins. Second, they emphasized the vulnerability of American children to this toxin. Third, they had a common point of origination: China, for decades a major supplier of consumer products to the United States and responsible for various stages in the production stream: "As more toys are recalled, trail ends in China," reported the New York Times in June 2007.[4] These alerts arose out of direct testing of the toys rather than from medical reports of children's intoxication by lead content in the indicated toys; one Consumer Reports article said, "Our latest tests find the toxic metal in more products."[5] In other words, no children had yet fallen demonstrably ill from playing with these specific toys. One image for a lead testing kit, the Abotex Lead Inspector, shown on the company's website, shows a smiling white baby seated next to a plush toy flower. The baby's right sleeve appears to have been pushed up its arm so that its prominent skin contact with the toy can visibly indicate the intimate bodily contact between toys and children in the course of everyday play (figure 3.1).

The toy's obviously facial front naturalizes its status as a primary interlocutor for the infant. Its anthropomorphization reifies parents' fantasy that the toy must be a familiar and safe substitute for a person. If the toy flower presents a friendly face to the socializing infant, the testing kit suggests that this idealized scene of interactivity has a threatening undercurrent. The logo features a silhouette of a man's face and a magnifying glass, a deliberate anachronism that makes it seem as if this kit will turn a parent into Sherlock Holmes, able to hunt down clues, searching for visible traces of lead as if looking for fingerprints.

The Abotex Lead Inspector can investigate for a consumer which toys and other personal effects have toxic levels of lead. Its color-coded test strips can be bought in quantities of eight to one hundred. The diagnostic reference colors range from a "faint yellowish tint" (the least toxic range) to "medium brown" to "black" (most toxic; figure 3.2). Critical race scholars have usefully parsed the distinctions between "colorism" and "racism," investigating how regionally and culturally specific discourses (including legal ones) regarding tones, shades, and colors may or may not synch up with relevant discussions on race.[6] Yet the graded valuation of color, the higher valuation of light shades and lower valuation of darker shades, remains a popular habit

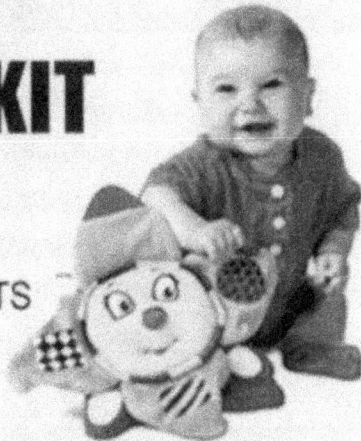

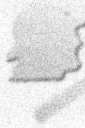

ABOTEX Lead INSPECTOR® Lead Test Kit

PREMIUM

LEAD TEST KIT

EASY TO USE

IMMEDIATE TEST RESULTS

ECONOMICAL

The only PREMIUM Lead Test Kit on the market that will test surfaces for lead, as well as water, and tell you the approximate lead release in the sample!

QUICKLY AND EASILY TEST:

Baby Bibs	Mexican Candles	Mini-Blinds	Plastic Parts
Ceramic Tile	Folk Remedies	Paint	Play Sand
Lunch Boxes	Lipstick/Make-up	Pet Toys	Pottery / Dishes
Electronics	Food Can Seams	Jewelry	Sidewalk Chalk
Plumbing	Soil/Dust	Toys	Water

Fig. 3.1. "Easy to use, immediate test results, economical." Abotex Lead Inspector Lead Test Kit. From the promotional website, 2007.

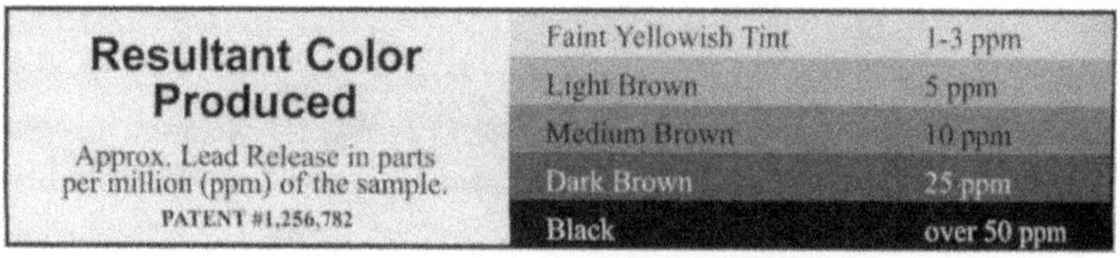

Resultant Color Produced	Faint Yellowish Tint	1-3 ppm
	Light Brown	5 ppm
	Medium Brown	10 ppm
Approx. Lead Release in parts per million (ppm) of the sample. PATENT #1,256,782	Dark Brown	25 ppm
	Black	over 50 ppm

Fig. 3.2. Abotex lead color chart. From the promotional website, 2007.

of mainstream colorism in the United States, and the Abotex reference chart complies with this chromatic logic.

At the height of the lead toy scare, media outlets paraded images of plastic and painted children's toys as possibly lead-tainted and hence possible hosts of an invisible threat; guest doctors repeated caveats about the dangers of "brain damage," "lowered IQs," and "developmental delay," directing their comments to concerned parents of vulnerable children. Toy testing centers were set up across the country, and sales of inexpensive lead test kits like the Abotex Lead Inspector rose as concerned parents were urged to test their toys in time for the holiday season in 2007, in effect privatizing and individualizing responsibility for toxicity in the face of the faltering dysfunction of the Food and Drug Administration and Environmental Protection Agency, whose apparent failure to regulate these objects was thrown into sharp relief.

One of the more prominent visual symbols of this recall debacle was the toy train, generally smiling, in different colors and identities. In a photograph accompanying an article on the toy recall in 2007 in the New York Times an anthropomorphized engine is graphically headed off the tracks (figure 3.3). The photograph affiliates the toy panic with one particular toy, Thomas the Tank Engine, the eponymous head of the Thomas & Friends series. Originally a creation of the British author Wilbert Awdry in a book

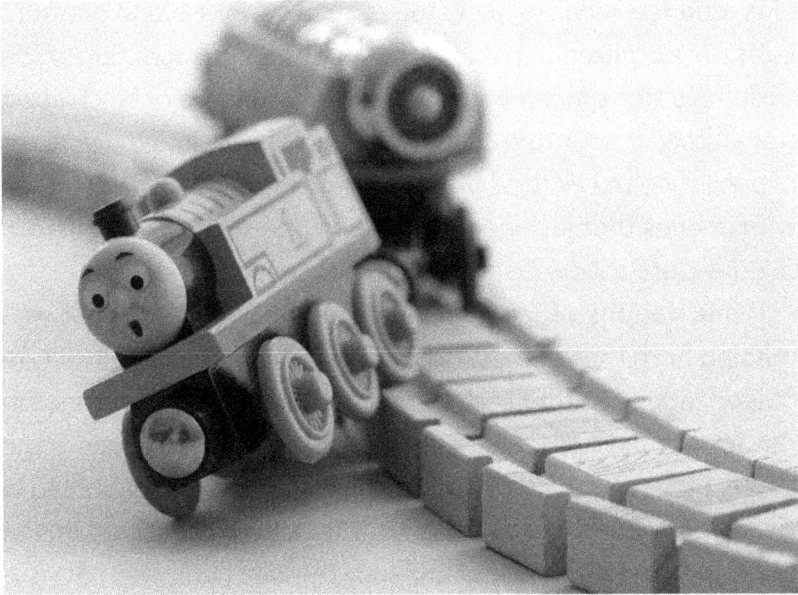

Fig. 3.3. Thomas the Tank Engine headed off the tracks. Photo by Lars Klove, from David Barboza and Louise Story, "RC2's Train Wreck," <u>New York Times</u>, June 19, 2007.

published in 1946, Thomas the Tank Engine has spawned an entertainment industry that today spans the globe; its central significance to the toy panic is discussed later. In this photograph Thomas's open mouth and raised eyebrows suggest surprise at his derailing as the wooden tracks under his wheels gently curve away. The maker of Thomas & Friends toys, the U.S. company RC2 (whose manufacturing is outsourced to China), also produces Bob the Builder and John Deere toys, model kits, and the Lamaze Infant Development System; the prevalence of toys related to construction and industrial transportation reflects a slant toward fostering young masculinities.[7]

Other media images specific to lead-tainted toys abounded: stuffed animals, plastic charms, necklaces and bracelets, teething aids, and toy medical accessories such as fake blood pressure cuffs. (Medicalized playthings were particularly ironic since the toxic toys transposed expected subjects and objects: children were turned from future doctors and nurses back into the patients of public health.) Pictures of the decontextualized toys alternated with images that included overwhelmingly white and generally middle-class children playing with the suspect toys.

While notions of lead circulated prolifically, lead itself was missing from these renderings. Neither the molecular structure of lead, nor its naturally occurring colors, nor its appearance in raw form or industrial bulk were illustrated. Rather images of the suspect toys and the children playing with them predominated in visual representations of the toxic threat. Even the feared image of a sick American child that underlay the lead panic was not visually shown, only discussed in the text as a threatening possibility. Together the associative panoply of images, the nursery-school primary-color toys associated with domestic, childlike innocence and security, served as a contrastive indictment. The lead toxicity of painted and plastic toys became the newest addition to the mainstream U.S. parental (in)security map.

The ensemble of images seemed to accelerate the explosive construction of a "master toxicity narrative" about Chinese products in general, one that had been quietly simmering since the recalls in 2005 of soft Chinese-made lunchboxes tainted with dangerous levels of lead. Journalists, government officials, and parents soon drew alarming connections between Chinese-made products and environmental toxins. Their lists now included heparin in Chinese-made medicines, industrial melamine in pet food, even Chinese smog, which had become unleashed from its geographic borders and was migrating to other territories. The visual representations of Chinese toxicities not related to lead that flourished in 2007 included rare-earth magnets haphazardly arrayed in the intestines of a child's X-rayed body; medicine vials; toothpaste tubes; cans of dog food; lipstick tubes; dogs lying on veterinary tables; and Chinese female workers in factory rows, in what Laura Hyun Yi Kang has called "one of the emblematic images of the global assembly line."[8] If RC2 shared legal responsibility for the lead found in Thomas the Tank engine, this fact seemed lost on the news media; it was the Chinese site of assembly (and the U.S. child as the site of contact or ingestion) that received the lion's share of attention.[9]

A generalized narrative about the inherent health risk of Chinese products to U.S. denizens thus crystallized. But this narrative is a highly selective one dependent on a resiliently exceptionalist victimization of the United States. Chinese residents are continually affected by the factories called their own, through the pollution of water, air, food, and soil. A growing awareness of the regular failure of local and national governments to strengthen protections for residents and workers from industrial toxins has led to a dramatic rise in community protests, lawsuits, and organized activist movements.[10] These industries are deeply bound up with transnational industrialization, in which China has been a major participant for decades, as well as the vulnerabilities it generates. According to David Harvey, the governments of industrializing nations are tempted to "race to the bottom" in their striving for participation in systems of transnational capital. In the process they are more than willing to overlook unjust labor remunerations or benefits and the lack of protection from adverse labor conditions. As a result local populations and industry workers, because they are deeply tied to the very environments in which these industries are animated, must forcibly consume (literally) the byproducts of those industries.[11]

In the United States in 2007 mass media stories pitched Chinese environmental threats neither as harmful to actual Chinese people or landscapes nor as products of a global industrialization that the United States itself eagerly promotes but as invasive dangers to the U.S. territory from other national territories. These environmental toxins were supposed to be "there" but were found "here." Other countries, including Mexico, were named in relation to manufacturing hazards, yet, perhaps in proportion to its predominance in world markets, China remained the focus of concern for the vulnerability of the United States to consumer product toxicities. It seems no coincidence that just before this year, in 2006, China overtook the United States in global exports, a fact documented by the World Trade Organization and widely reported throughout 2006 and 2007.[12] This rise in manufacturing led to fears about the trade deficit, fears hardly contained, and in fact in some sense paradoxically fueled, by Commerce Secretary Carlos Gutierrez's proclamation that the swelling Chinese output was "not a threat."[13]

Alarm about the safety of Chinese products entered all forms of discourse, from casual conversations to talk shows and news reports. In what might be called a new, shrewd form of unofficial protectionism, U.S. citizens were urged to avoid buying Chinese products in general, even though such products are essentially ubiquitous given the longtime entrenchment of trade relations between the United States and China. That an estimated 80 percent of all toys bought in the United States are made in China is the sign of such entrenchment. An investigative reporter recounted that attempting to avoid anything made in China for one week was all but futile. He wrote, "Poisoned pet food. Seafood laced with potentially dangerous antibiotics. Toothpaste tainted with an ingredient in antifreeze. Tires missing a key safety component. U.S. shoppers may be forgiven if they are becoming leery of Chinese-made goods and are trying to fill their shopping carts with products free of ingredients from that country.

The trouble is, that may be almost impossible."[14] One lesson of this panic was that inanimate pollutants could now "invade" all kinds of consumer products, and other pollutants could always climb on board.

The Chinese toy panic in 2007 was a twist on an earlier theme in recent U.S. history regarding the toxicity of lead. Since 1978, the year the U.S. Consumer Product Safety Commission banned residential paint containing lead, there have been public-awareness campaigns and legislation regarding exposure from house paint. Lead-based paint is present in many buildings constructed before 1978, though public-awareness campaigns and municipal abatement programs have been quite successful in reducing the threat of residential lead to the middle and upper classes. More recently, however, environmental justice activists from polluted neighborhoods and public health advocates have insisted that lead toxicity remains a problem for children in impoverished neighborhoods. Lead poisoning among black children was thus figured as an epidemiological crisis linked to the pollution of neighborhoods populated largely by people of color, including older buildings whose once widespread lead paint had not been remediated and where lead-polluting industrial centers were located. But in 2007 news media coverage of this kind of lead toxicity began to fade, overtaken by the heightened transnational significance of lead. Toys from China quickly became the primary source of threat, displacing this previous concern.[15]

I thus argue that a new material-semiotic form of lead emerged in 2007. This new lead, despite its physiological identity to the old lead, was taking on a new meaning and political character and becoming animated in novel ways. Why were painted trains and beaming middle-class white children chosen to represent the lead toxicity this time? If the spread of transnational commodities reached into all classes and privileges, how did middle-class white children morph into the primary victims of this environmental lead, when poor black children had previously been represented as subject to the dangers of domestic lead? Why could only China, or occasionally a few other industrial sites not in the United States, such as Mexico and India, be imagined as lead's source? Ultimately what, or who, had this new lead become?

Animate Contaminants

At first glance lead is not integral to the biological or social body. In the biomythography of the United States, lead is "dead." Rather than being imagined as integral to life, and despite its occurrence in both inorganic and organic forms, lead notionally lies in marginal, exterior and instrumental, and impactful relation to biological life units, such as organic bodies of value. The concept of animacy suggests there can be gradations of lifeliness. If viruses, also nonliving, nevertheless seem "closer" to life because they require living cells for their own continued existence, lead seems more uncontroversially dead and is imagined as more molecular than cellular. The metarubric of animacy theory proves useful here, as lead appears to undo the purported mapping of lifelines, deadliness scales onto an animate hierarchy. Not only can dead lead appear and feel alive; it can fix itself atop the hierarchy, sitting cozily amid healthy white subjects.

Furthermore lead deterritorializes, emphasizing its mobility through and against imperialistic spatializations of "here" and "there." The lead that constitutes today's health and security panic in the United States is figured as all around us, in our toys, our dog food, and the air we breathe, streaming in as if uncontrollably from elsewhere. Lead is not supposed to, in other words, belong here. Even popular reports of the export of electronics waste to developing countries for resource mining still locate the toxicity of lead, mercury, and cadmium away from here; their disassembled state is where the health hazard is located, and disassembly happens elsewhere.[16] Now, however, the new lead is here, having perversely returned in the form of toxic toys. Lead's seeming return to the middle and upper classes exemplifies the "boomerang effect" of what the sociologist Ulrich Beck calls a "risk society": "Risks of modernization sooner or later also strike those who profit from them. . . . Even the rich and the powerful are not safe from them."[17] The new lead thus represents a kind of "involuntary environmental justice," if we read justice as not the extension of remedy but a kind of revenge.[18]

While the new lead fears indicate an apparent progressive development of the interrelations of threat, biology, race, geographic specificity, and sovereign symbolization, lead's present-day embodiment may not be such an unusual admixture. It is instructive to trace lead's imbrication in the rhetorics of political sovereignty and globalized capital, remaining attentive to what is present and what is absent. If lead is at the present moment imagined to come from places <u>outside</u> the geographic West, in spite of the longtime complexity of transnational relations, and to threaten definitive U.S. citizenry, then how might we assess its status against a history of race rendered as biological threat and a present that intensifies the possibilities of biological terrorism? How might we contextualize the panic around lead as a hyperstimulated war machine in which the U.S. government perceives and surveils increasing numbers and types of "terrorist" bodies? And how does a context of an increasingly fragile U.S. global economic power texture and condition this panic, one that sits adjacent to discussions of contamination and contagion?

While lead has long worn an identity as a pollutant, associated with industry and targeted in environmentalist efforts, today's lead might first suggest a new development in the domain of contagion discourse. Contagion can be invoked precisely because the touching and ingestion of lead represents, for children, a primary route of exposure, just as with living biological agents. Yet there may be still further structural forces at play. Priscilla Wald, writing about complex narratives of biological contagion, has shown how epidemiology itself can be informed by circulating "myths," understood as stories that are authoritative and serve to buttress communitarian identity.[19] One could argue that the black children who disappeared from the lead representations did so precisely because the new lead was tied to ideas of vulnerable sovereignty and xenophobia, ideas that demanded an elsewhere (or at least not interior North America) as their ground. However, as I argue later, black children did not quite disappear. In the United States the genuine challenge of representing the microcosmic toxicity of lead and a human group's vulnerability to it defers to a logic of panics, falling back on simplified, racially coded narratives. Such narratives, by offering ready objects, doubly conceal the deeper transnational, generational, and economic complexity of the life of lead.

The behavior of lead as a contaminating, but not technically contagious, toxin (but, again, not necessarily as a pollutant in wall paint or as an airborne dust) contains many of the elements of Wald's "outbreak narrative," a contemporary trope of disease emergence involving multiple discourses (including popular and scientific) that has been present since the late 1980s. Wald asserts that the specific form of the outbreak narrative represented a shift in epidemiological panics because it invoked tales that reflected the global and transnational character of the emerging infection and involved the use of popular epidemiological discourses to track the success of actions against the disease. Lead, however, is not a microbe, not an infectious agent; it does not involve human carriers like those profiled in Wald's examples of outbreak narratives. The lead panic depends not on human communicability but on the toxicity of inanimate objects, so it is technically not the stuff of contagion. What it does clearly and by necessity involve, however, is transnational narratives of the movement of contaminants in the epidemiology of human sickness. In migration (the Pacific Rim) and source (China) the lead story significantly resembles the SARS epidemiological and journalistic trajectories of 2002, when the "outbreak" occurred. Finally, lead's major route of contamination is by ingestion, and it is epidemiologically mappable; when lead is attached to human producers, even if transnationally located far away, a kind of disease vectoring still can happen, even if its condition is not (even transitively) communicable.

Yellow Terrors

There is in fact very little that is new about the lead panic in 2007 in the United States. At least we can say that it is not sufficient to turn to popular and scientific epidemiology's overapplied cry that contemporary ailments bear the mark of this globalizing world's heightened interconnectivities (a cry that says, for instance, that lead travels more than it used to, which would require us to accept, somehow, that lead came only from China). In fact anxieties about intoxications, mixings, and Chinese agents have steadily accompanied U.S. cultural productions and echo the Yellow Peril fears articulated earlier in the twentieth century. That lead was subject to an outbreak narrative works synergistically with these anxieties, and these narratives may indeed have been partially incited or facilitated by them. One wonders in particular about the haunted vulnerability of Western sites that Elizabeth Povinelli incisively describes as ghoul health:

> Ghoul health refers to the global organization of the biomedical establishment, and its imaginary, around the idea that the big

scary bug, the new plague, is the real threat that haunts the contemporary global division, distribution, and circulation of health, that it will decisively render the distribution of jus vitae ac necris and that this big scary bug will track empire back to its source in an end-game of geophysical bad faith. Ghoul health plays on the real fear that the material distribution of life and death arising from the structural impoverishment of postcolonial and settler colonial worlds may have accidentally or purposefully brewed an unstoppable bio-virulence from the bad faith of liberal capital and its multiple geo-physical tactics and partners.[20]

Povinelli traces a kind of looming materialization, in the form of threatened health, of the latent affects of imperialist "just deserts."

The recent lead panic echoes, yet is a variation of, the turn-of-the-century Orientalized threat to white domesticity, as detailed by Nayan Shah in relation to San Francisco's Chinatown in the late nineteenth century and early twentieth.[21] Shah describes local investments in white domesticity in this period and its connection to nationalism and citizenship. Two perceived threats to white domesticity came in the form of activities believed to reside exclusively in Chinatown: prostitution and opium dens. Significant among concerned white residents' and policymakers' fears at the time was the contractibility of syphilis and leprosy, which was imagined to happen in direct contact with the Chinese, whether this contact was sexual or sensual in nature. Notably they also worried that the passing of opium pipes "from lip to lip" was a major route of disease transmission; this image resonates with the licking scene of contamination of the lead-covered toys, a scene to which I return later.[22] This indirect mode of imagined transmission resonates with the nature of the lead panic, for the relation contamination in the case of both the opium pipes (disease contagion) and the new lead (pollution, poisoning) is one of transitivity. While the imagined disease transmission mediated by an opium pipe was more or less immediate and depended on proximity, if not direct contact, between human bodies, the new lead is imagined to be associated with national or human culprits somewhere far away.

Since the current reference to lead produces an urgent appeal to reject Chinese-made products, and since mentions of China arouse fantasies of toxins such as lead, heparin, and so on, then in effect so has lead at this moment become just slightly Chinese (without being personified as such). That is to say, on top of the racialization of those involved, including whites and Chinese, lead itself takes on the tinge of racialization. This is particularly so because lead's racialization, I suggest, is intensified by the non-proximity of the Chinese who are understood as responsible for putting the lead in the toys; that is, lead's presence in the absence of the Chinese, in a contested space of U.S. self-preservation, effectively forces lead to bear its own toxic racialization. As toys become threatening health risks, they are rhetorically constructed as racialized threats. This racialization of lead and other substances both replicates a fear of racialized immigration into the vulnerable national body at a time when its economic sovereignty is in question and inherits a racialization of disease assisted by a history of public health discourse.

The corrupted Chinatown arguably still lives, albeit now understood as an entire nature covered in irresponsible factories that spread their poisons far and wide. In the twenty-first-century lead panic, exogenous (i.e., "unassimilated") mainland Chinese still face the old accusations of poor hygiene and moral defect. Thus today's images of toy-painting laborers too readily attract narratives of moral contagion: they demonstrate irresponsibility toward "our" consumers and blithe ignorance of the consequences of their work, properties that effectively reinforce their unfitness for U.S. citizenship. This is a moral standard that has already been increasingly imposed on the working class by legal and social expressions of U.S. neoliberalism.

Chinese lead panics are sticky; they are generated by and further borrow from many already interlaced narratives. The spread of war discourse within the West and of the imaginary fount of bioterrorist plotting, dramatized by the U.S. government in its second Gulf war, was a convenient additive to narrations about toxins.[23] Bioterrorism involves the intentional use of toxic agents that are biologically active, even if not live themselves, against populations. They often cannot be perceived by the naked eye. While bioterrorist intentionality cannot be attached to the lead narrative (the China case might more aptly be called "bioterrorist negligence"), it is nevertheless fairly easy to read the discourses on lead as a biosecurity threat, conflating the safety of individual bodies with the safety of national concerns.[24] Other biosecurity threats have also been recruited as Asian, in the case of contagious diseases such as SARS and bird flu. Consultants and safety advocates deemed red and yellow colors, precisely those colors used to indicate heightened levels of security threat in U.S. airports, to have particularly dangerous levels of lead and suggested color as an effective criterion ("profile") by which toys should be identified and returned.[25]

Thus lead was an invisible threat whose material loci and physical provenance, much like a terrorist sleeper cell, needed to be presumed in advance and mapped not only geographically but sensorily, sometimes through visual coding schemes like color itself (recall the Abotex lead test color chart which codes faint yellow the least toxic, black the most).[26] Popular responses in the United States and in other countries affected by the China toy recall bore this out; one blog entry's title, for instance, was the indignant "Why Is China Poisoning Our Babies?"[27] News about heparin contamination in pharmaceuticals originating from China became particularly explosive when it was thought to be deliberate, highlighting the sense of insidious invasion in the same way that bioterrorism does.[28] Given the apparent blithe disregard or dysfunction of both the Chinese and U.S. governmental safety controls along the way, the sign of biosecurity and protection falls on the head of a young child who wishes to play with a toy and, by implication, that child's parents. Indeed the body of the young white child playing with a toy train is not signified innocently of its larger symbolic value at the level of the nation; its specific popularity suggests this metonymic connection.

The past few decades have seen a strengthening of affects around terrorism, associating it with radical extranationality as well as nonstate agentivity. Jasbir Puar has incisively examined the escalating agitation around purported terrorism, particularly its potential to consolidate national interests (including white and neoliberal homonationalisms) in the face of such a perceived threat.[29] Nonstatehood, while always potentially unstable, has come into a mature relationship with the imagined possibility of terrorism. This is evidenced, for example, by the fact that in 2010 Senator Joe Lieberman proposed that Congress revoke the citizenship of those who demonstrate financial support or other forms of allegiance to organizations deemed terrorist by the United States. Under these conditions the invisible threat of cognitive and social degradation in the case of lead meant that the abiding, relatively more methodical, and diversified work of environmental justice activists on lead toxicity was here transformed into something that looked less environmental and increasingly like another figure in the war on terror, a war that marked the diffuseness, unpredictability, and sleeper-cell provenance of enemy material and its biological vectors.[30]

This war on terror was doubly pitched as a neomissionary insistence on the dissemination of the American way, including its habits of free choice and its access to a free market at its core, defined by the proliferation of consumer products. The very title of a New York Times article by Leslie Wayne published in 2009 about corrosive drywall for new homebuilding sourced from China, "The Enemy at Home," betrays toxic drywall's coding as a biological threat metaphorized as war (itself not at great notional distance from biological warfare).[31] The idea of this "enemy at home" makes lead into a symptomatic signifier of a war of capital flows, particularly the struggle over trade protectionism and the Chinese resistance to allow the Chinese yuan to float against the dollar, a resistance that has only recently seen a measured lessening as of this writing (2011). Lead is animated to become simultaneously an instrument of heightened domestic panic, drawing from and recycling languages of terror, and a rhetorical weapon in the rehearsal of the economic sovereignty of the United States. A story by the financial interest magazine Forbes at the height of the toy recall made these slippages baldly evident; its title was "Chinese Toy Terror."[32]

What are blended in this collapse of narratives, and what are of particular interest for animacy, are precisely the subjects and objects, recipients and perpetrators, terrorists and innocents of lead toxicity. In other words, the fused stories about lead displace the normal agents of the contagion narratives and scramble the normal pairings between protector and protected and self and other. As such they cannot rhetorically function as effectively as they might strive to. This easily recognizable failure of boundaries may be the sole rehabilitative counterthrust of the new lead panic.

Lead's Labors

The image of the vulnerable white child is relentlessly promoted over and against an enduring and blatant background (i.e., unacknowledged) condition of labor and of racism: the ongoing exposure of immigrants and people of color to risk that sets them up for conditions of bodily work and residence that dramatize the body burden that projects of white nationalism can hardly refuse to perceive. Blithely overlooked, or steadfastly ignored, are the toxic conditions of labor and of manufacture, such as inattention to harmful transnational labor and industrial practices that poison, in many cases, badly protected or unprotected workers.[33] Other persistent conditions include the invisibility within the United States of the working, destitute, or agrarian poor in favor of idealized consumers who are white and middle or upper middle class; electronic wastes as extravagant and unattended exports of the United States to countries willing to take the cash to mine it; the dumping of toxic wastes and high-polluting industries into poorer neighborhoods within municipalities; and the common practice in the United States of exporting products of greater toxicity than is permitted within its own borders.[34] Here the cynical calculus of risk, race, and international trade continually reproduces a specific configuration of toxic expulsion to othered lands or peoples. As Cheri Lucas Jennings and Bruce H. Jennings report, the international economic director of the World Bank suggested that Third World countries might be better off trading for the toxic waste of First World countries, since "poverty or imminent starvation" was a greater threat to life expectancy than the toxicity of the waste they would receive.[35] These authors point to the greater access in the United States to less persistent toxins (such as pesticides) by those with economic privilege, leading to a bifurcated distribution of greater and lesser toxic infusion along lines of class and race.

The contemporary fears in the United States about lead contamination and mental degradation are complexly interwoven with race, class, and cognitive ability, both as they externally manifest (i.e., the racialization of imports from China) and as they dovetail with internal registers of classism and regional stereotyping. Take, for example, one toy, Hillbilly Teeth, made in China and distributed by the company Funtastic (of Houston, Texas), which was recalled due to concerns about lead in 2008 (figure 3.4). The recall notice of this product issued by the U.S. Consumer Product Safety Commission singled out the gray paint on the teeth as the source of lead.[36] Though it was coded as threatening or harmful due to its potentially tainted plastic (which would by design be placed in the child's mouth), one could equally find alarm in its perpetration of classed, ableist, and ruralized violence in its identity as a toy.

The package's cardboard backing depicts a smiling, presumably "nonhillbilly" white male child wearing the denture insert, and the discolored, out of proportion, and otherwise imperfect teeth are designated "yucky," "gross," and "scary." An inset fake frame, labeled "My Name's Bubba," has a cartoon speech bubble ("Yain't I purdy?") that uses a distorted caricature of rural or southern accents. The prefatory and framing "Let's Get Goofy!" resembles the youthful refrain "Let's Get Retarded!" and signifies a willful and temporary loss of rationality and cognitive measure. The extant class coding of the "bad teeth" further builds on the myth of rural and working-class degradation by hinting at the acute dental issues that often accompany addiction to methamphetamines (aka "meth mouth"). Methamphetamines are the most recognized drug problem in "hillbilly country," that is, the rural South and Midwest. The juxtaposition of Hillbilly and Teeth

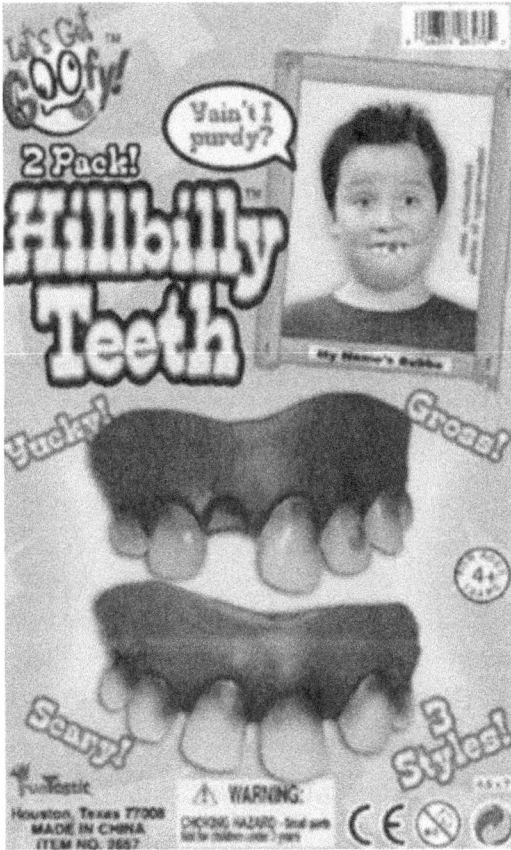

Fig. 3.4. Funtastic's "Let's Get Goofy" Hillbilly Teeth, made in China, recalled in 2008.

reminds us that both the urban gentrified center and the pastoral myths of the United States have their own white undersides.[37] Against such a consolidated scenario the leaden gray-tinted tooth paint seems even more intent on the protection of a limited few, the urban kids who have the voluntary luxury, every year on Halloween, of assuming the mask of fallen class and intellectual ability, only to snap it off later.

A different toy, however, sat at the center of the lead panic in 2007: the expensive toy series Thomas the Tank Engine, seen earlier. Thomas and his "friends" are immensely popular objects and are accompanied by a range of lucrative tie-ins, including a television show, games, activity books, candy, and other merchandise bearing Thomas's characteristic blue "body" and round gray and black face. These are not meant for children only. The series is marketed to middle-class parents who insist on high-status "quality" products, which in this case are tuned toward boys and quite explicitly direct their proper masculine development. An article in the New York Times in 2007 explicitly associated the toys' high prices with their presumed quality and safety. The article bears one visual image, a photograph of the James Engine from the Thomas series, and a description of one member of the vulnerable population (identified as children), a white four-year-old boy whose mother points to the expectation of quality for these toys and whose class membership appears to be middle to upper middle class: "The affected Thomas toys were manufactured in China. . . . 'These are not cheap, plastic McDonald's toys,' said Marian Goldstein of Maplewood, N.J., who spent more than $1000 on her son's Thomas collection, for toys that can cost $10 to $70 apiece. 'But these are what is supposed to be a high-quality children's toy.'"[38] Presumably the "cheap," working-class McDonald's toys are the toxic ground on which the nontoxic quality toys are to be built and compared.

Goldstein may have a point about the train's symbolic privilege at least. Trains occupy an iconic place in the mythology and economic actuality of the creation of the American West. Symbolically and materially trains are intrinsically connected to commerce and the circulation of economic goods as well as, in the United States, a hidden history of Chinese labor. Both the extension of railroad systems to the American West and the development of the Sacramento River Delta in California heavily depended on imported Chinese labor that was rendered invisible in certain interested histories of labor.[39] Narratives about lead toxicity in toys from China largely obscure the conditions of Chinese labor in the production of these toy trains.[40] Nevertheless these narratives deploy the fact of labor obliquely, in an explication of the pathway of toxicity. (Lead must be painted on.) How to explain the incipient visibility?

An accusatory narrative in which Chinese are the criminal painters of the toy Thomas trains sets things up differently from the story of the Chinese laborers who extended the railroads to the American West: while the latter were made invisible in the interest of the white ownership of land, property, and history, for the toy painters the conditions of labor needed to be made just visible enough to facilitate the territorial, state, and racial assignation of blame, but not enough to generally extend the ring of sympathetic concern around the workers themselves.[41] I found very few instances among concerned parents or journalists in the United States in which lead was also understood to be a source of toxicity for the immigrant or transnational laboring subjects who take part in the manufacture of the product.

So the story of lead, a story of toxicity, security, and nationality, is also necessarily about labor: when it is registered, when it is hidden, and who pays what kind of attention to whose labor. The regular erasure or continued invisibility in the lead narratives of the textile sweatshops, device assemblers, and toy painters, who are largely young women who have migrated into the Chinese cities from rural satellites, renders quite ironic the care work that is so poignantly provided by the toys, and transitively by the women who make them. The transitive criminalization of Chinese toy assemblers is all the more ironic when we consider the routinization of child care inside the United States by African Americans and immigrants from Central and South America, the Philippines, South Asia, the Caribbean, and elsewhere, for middle-class parents of all ethnicities.[42] In some respects the economy itself and changing kinship structures have increasingly meant that parents hire help while they work away from home, a creep of the care crisis into higher echelons of society, as the feminist labor scholar Evelyn Nakano Glenn notes.[43] From the 1980s middle-class mothers increasingly joined the labor force as neoliberalism took hold in the racialized sphere of the care of children; as they increasingly left the house and their children, mothers had to accomplish more intimate care in less time, suggesting that care work be taken up by others in their place.[44] The racial mapping of the desirable subjects in the United States thus occurs in the context of the erasure of its disposable ones; I refer here to Grace Chang's notion of (immigrant female) "disposable domestics."[45]

Just as lead particles travel, so too does Thomas the Tank Engine. It is a mobile vehicle, not only symbolically but also materially, one that has journeyed from England to the United States and to China and back again. A trip I took to China in 2010 revealed many knock-offs of Thomas, who is just as popular there as he is in the United States. These packaged toys, puzzle books, and candies were immediately recognizable but had slightly incorrect English spellings of his name, such as "Tromas" or "Tomas," as if to match the impossibility of perfect translation (figure 3.5). These "illegal" copies show that, like the lead he allegedly carries with him on his back, Thomas is not containable within a given trajectory of movement and desire. The global spread of this commodity complicates the one-way vector of contamination from China to the United States, indicating a multidirectional flow. And yet little is known within the United States about how these toys may or may not harm Chinese children or the Chinese workers who produce them.

I referred earlier to a mode of transmission, from contaminated toy to child, as one of transitivity. For the late capitalist,

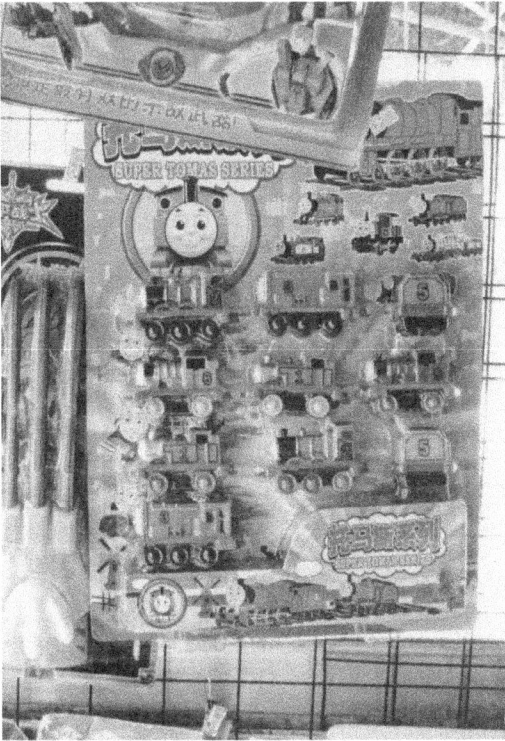

Fig. 3.5. Super Thomas Series toy train set, outdoor market, Guilin, China, 2010. At lower right, the first three Chinese characters are to-ma-sz, a phonetic spelling of Thomas. Photographed by the author.

high-consumption, and highly networked sectors of the world, transitivity has arguably become a default mode not only of representation but of world-relating. The asymmetry of this world relation is no barrier to the toxic effectivity of simmering racial panics. The sphere of the world that is well rehearsed in the flow of transnational commodities, services, and communications has become the perfect host for such transitivity, or at least the collapsing of transitive relations into conceptualizations of immediate contact. Patricia Clough, in her theorization of the complex, even nonhuman agencies and affects participating in television and computer-consuming information societies, aptly writes that "even as the transnational or the global become visible, proposing themselves as far-flung extensions of social structure, they are ungrounded by that upon which they depend: the speed of the exchange of information, capital, bodies, and abstract knowledge and the vulnerability of exposure to media event-ness."[46]

An advertisement on the airport trolleys in Shanghai Pudong Airport in June 2010 demonstrates this relentlessly productive metonymic and economic transitivity in stark white letters on a red background: "Your Eyes in the Factory! Book and Manage your Quality Control on www.Asiainspection.com." Below the website is an icon of inspection, the magnifying glass. In an inset picture a male worker, possibly an inspector, possibly an assembler, handles a product (figure 3.6). The transitivity here is not between the Chinese workers and the toys they have assembled but rather of participants in production monitoring. It exists between the eyes of international corporate managers, the advertisement's English-reading addressees, and another set of eyes that is ambiguously either that of local Chinese inspectors or that of remote cameras that focus on Chinese workers. The ad further represents the interest in surveillance, glossed here as more benign "quality control," that arose after the toxicity of Chinese products illuminated Chinese production as a troubled site.[47]

Blackened Lead

Some years ago, as I indicated earlier, before the domestic narrative largely disappeared in favor of the Chinese narrative, the greater public was invited to consider the vulnerability of black children to lead intoxication. What happened to this association? Did it simply disappear, as I hinted? Or did it meaningfully recede? I turn here to take a closer look at the medicalization of lead. Lead toxicity is medically characterized as at least partly neutral; that is, it involves the nerve system, most notably comprising the brain and nerve pathways throughout the body. Medical accounts of lead toxicity, including those invoked in the toy lead

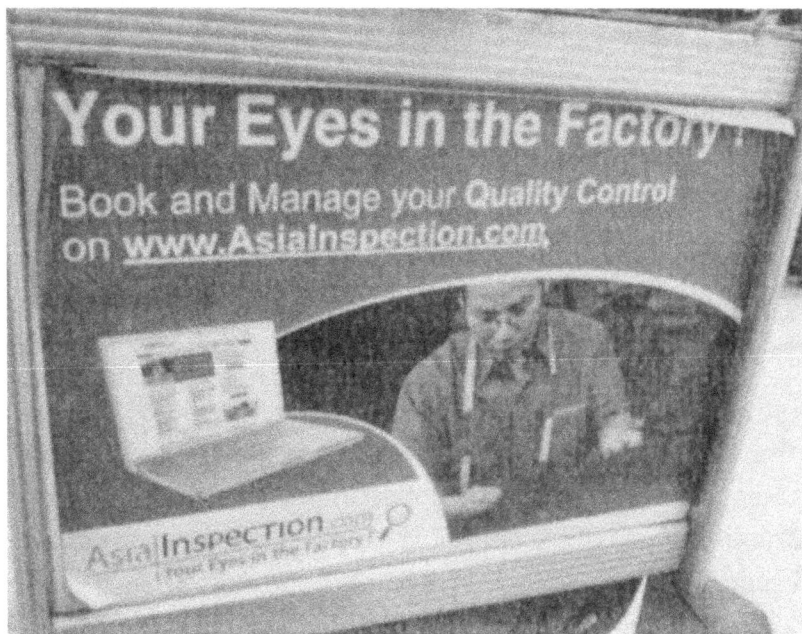

Fig. 3.6. Airport trolley ad for Asianspection, June 26, 2010.
Photographed by the author.

panic of 2007, invoke its ability to lower the intelligence quotient
of a child. The IQ measure bears a distinctly eugenicist history
and remains the subject of controversy regarding whether it has
adequately shed its originary racial and socioeconomic biases.[48]
To what extent might we imagine that lead-induced IQ loss not
only threatens the promise of success in an information economy
but also involves subtle racial movement away from whiteness,
where the greatest horror is not death but disablement, that is,
mental alteration and the loss of rational control?

Julian B. Carter's study of neurasthenia, or "nervous exhaustion," and its characterization in the 1880s by the neurologist
George Beard as a specific property of genteel, sensitive, intelligent, well-bred whiteness (rather than, it was assumed, a prop-

erty of the working or peasant classes) gives us a more specific backdrop against which to consider neurotoxicity and its connection to the new lead's poster boy, the white middle-class child. Carter argues that the very vulnerability expressed by neurasthenia as a property cultivated primarily in privileged whites, both men and women, is what legitimated their claim to power in modernity, even as industrialization was blamed as a cause of the condition.[49]

Within the United States blackness has its own specific history with regard to rhetorics of contamination, not least the "one drop of blood" policies against racial mixing and miscegenation. Later policies of racial segregation in the Jim Crow South were also linked to white fears of contamination. Referring to the debates in Plessy v. Ferguson, Saidiya Hartman writes of white concerns about the "integrity of bodily boundaries and racial self-certainty": "As Plessy evinced, sitting next to a black person on a train, sleeping in a hotel bed formerly used by a black patron, or dining with a black party seated at a nearby table not only diminished white enjoyment but also incited fears of engulfment and contamination."[50]

Lead contamination in the United States continues to be scrutinized for its racial bias, albeit unevenly. One recent contested conjunction of African American populations and lead was a study led by the Kennedy Krieger Institute. This study, conducted between 1993 and 1995, tracked lead levels in the children of Baltimore public housing occupants (primarily African Americans) who were exposed to various degrees of lead toxicity in residential paint, without adequate warning of the dangers of that lead. A storm of debate erupted around this study, in which healthy families were recruited to live in lead-contaminated houses. (This experiment harked back to the notorious Tuskegee Institute study, conducted between 1932 and 1972, which monitored poor black men who had syphilis but neither treated nor informed them in any way about the disease.)[51]

I have claimed that the year 2007 represented a year of transition, as a new and imaginatively more dominant, exogenous Chinese lead was entering the public domain. In this very same year National Public Radio symptomatically both remembered and forgot received knowledge about domestic lead toxicity. First, a National Public Radio (NPR) show called Living on Earth updated its coverage of a longitudinal study on the urban poor and lead toxicity. That same year another NPR show noted the higher levels of lead toxicity among African American children and pronounced these statistics "puzzling," leaving it at that.[52] "Puzzling": this illogic or failure of deduction occurred despite all kinds of widely available evidence pointing to increased urban regional pollution, lower access to information, and lower financial capacity to remediate or conceal lead paint. This easy disregard explains how black children in representations of toxic lead largely disappear and are replaced by white children: the national security project of the United States is less interested in profiling African American children as victims of lead poisoning, especially when the novel lead is situated as an externally derived attack.

Even the remembering of urban toxicity in the NPR Living on Earth show in 2007 is of a certain kind. This show updated its audience on an acclaimed longitudinal study on lead's effects on children that was begun in the 1970s, led by Kim Dietrich of the University of Cincinnati, and revisited over the years by NPR. Dietrich reported that early exposure to lead toxicity can be linked to later criminal behavior. By design the study was focused on "inner-city" children, according to Dietrich, "who are largely minority."[53] In the NPR update in 2007, which functions as a symptomatic piling up of racial constructs, Dietrich actively legitimated the interviewer's prompts, gathering a stunning assemblage: poverty, proximity of weapons, violence, lead, and poor nutrition as collective determining factors for inner-city criminality:

> GELLERMAN (interviewer): So if you look at inner cities, if you look at the poor, if you look at their exposure to weapons, you look at their exposure to violence, you look at their exposure to lead, and their poor nutrition. Is this sort of the perfect combination of factors for crime?

> DIETRICH: Yes, it's in a sense, the perfect storm. Uh, the environment provides a lot of incentives for crime. The child is in a community where he or she sees violence—the availability of guns, the availability of illicit drugs. So I would say that the inner-city environment provides the weapon, lead pulls the trigger.

"Lead pulls the trigger." This metaphor of weaponry is used to characterize a latent violent criminality domestic to the United States, naturalized to an urban underclass of color, using a co-construction of guns, "ghettoes," and racialized pathology. In some sense it is an old story: to pump people full of lead is to kill them. But the form and objects of death have become molecular, intentionality has shifted to neglect, and a fragile self-identification rather than potency reshapes the threat into the other person, conflated with the lead that afflicts them.

Contrast this metaphor of weaponry to the title of the New York Times article on toxic Chinese drywall, "The Enemy at Home," which partakes of a war metaphor not because of some naturalizing co-construction of guns, "ghetto," and racialized pathology but in relation to a transnational (i.e., extradomestic) exchange that simultaneously seems to threaten representative individual bodies and criminalize Chinese trade participation. This enemy, that is, should not be at "home," with this word understood both as a generalized national body and as the domicile of family units (who are in a position to afford the construction of new homes).

One wonders to what degree any newfound alarmism about the vulnerability of black children to environmental lead can succeed, given the abiding construction of affinities between racist constructions of blackness and those of lead, long integral to the American racial and gendered corporeal imaginary.[54] A racial construction of blacks as already unruly, violent, contaminated, and mentally deficient lies inherent in the current neoliberal economy, which not only positions people of color in a labor hierarchy that matches them with literally disabling forms of manual labor but is also conditioned and supported by a growing and incredibly powerful prison industrial complex structured according to race, class, and gender.[55] If lead exposure itself is associated with cognitive delay, enhanced aggressivity, impulsivity, convulsions, and mental lethargy, then we might read such characterizations of blackness as attributions or intimations of disability, as much as we already understand them as damaging racial profiles. Eric Lott's study of blackface minstrelsy relates the suturing of impulsivity or sudden bodily displacement to fears about black masculinity in this performance culture in the United States. Lott reads Charles Dickens's account of the dancing in a New York blackface performance as stunned by its spasticity: "The whole passage reads as if Dickens did not really know what to do with such energy, where to put it."[56] Would lead toxicity, hence overdetermined with legacies of the negative characteristics of blackness, succeed quite so successfully as an imagined property of other racialized bodies, such as the Mexican braceros of the Second World War and modern-day maquiladora workers, both of whom have suffered from lead toxicity?[57] If disability can be read into constructs of blackness, disability itself is also a critically important axis of difference. Scholars such as Nirmala Erevelles and Andrea Minear point out the dangers of being both black and disabled; the authors suggest that within critical race feminism, while disability is sometimes recognized, it can often analytically function for scholars as a "nuance" of intensity rather than its own structural difference, leading to a loss of complexity in the reading: "The omission of disability as a critical category in discussions of intersectionality has disastrous and sometimes deadly consequences for disabled people of color caught at the interstices of multiple differences."[58] These are just some ways criminality, race, and disability can be mutually produced and reproduced.

Thus it is not necessarily correct to say that African American youth are no longer viewed as vulnerable to lead. Rather it is easier to imagine that in this pointedly transnational struggle between major economic powers, black children are now the less urgent population under threat. It is instead as if black children are constructed as more proximate to lead itself, as naturalized to lead; they serve as ground to the newest figure.

In the case of the Thomas trains, lead toxicity is racialized not only because the threatened future has the color of a white boy but also because that boy must not change color. The boy can change color in two ways: First, lead lurks as a dirty toxin, as a pollutant, and it is persistently racialized as anything but white. Second, black children are assumed to be toxic, and lead's threat to white children is not only that they risk becoming dull and cognitively defective but precisely that they lose their class-elaborated white racial cerebrality and that they become suited racially to living in ghettoes.[59]

Queer Licking

Let me return to the visual symbolic of media coverage of lead toxicity. The florid palette of toy-panic images yielded two prominent and repeating icons: the vulnerable child, more frequently a young, white, middle-class boy, and the dangerous party, Thomas the Tank Engine. The iconic white boy's lead toxicity must be avoided: he should not be mentally deficient, delayed, or lethargic. His intellectual capabilities must be assured to consolidate a futurity of heteronormative (white) masculinity; that is to say he must not be queer. This is not only because one of lead's toxicities reported by the Centers for Disease Control and Prevention is reproductive disability and infertility; I suggest that one aspect of the threat of lead toxicity is its origin in a forbidden sexuality, for the frightening originary scene of intoxication is one of a queer licking. Here again is the example of the white boy, who in the threatening and frightening scene is precisely licking the painted train, a train whose name is Thomas, a train that is also one of the West's preeminent Freudian phallic icons.[60] This image of a boy licking the train, though clearly the feared scene of contamination, never appears literally, or at least I have not found it; rather, if a boy and a train are present, the boy and the train are depicted proximately, and that is enough to represent the threat. (The licking boy would be too much, would too directly represent the forbidden.) But suggestions are sometimes loaded onto the proximities. In one representative image from a website alerting its readers to RC2's recall of Thomas trains, we see the head and chest of a blond boy lying alongside a train that is in the foreground. The boy's moist lips are parted and smiling, his eyes intent and alert; he grasps a dark-hued train car with his right hand, gazing slightly upward at it. The other cars, receding toward the camera, fall out of focus. The scene is, at the very least, physically and emotionally intimate, pleasurable, and desirous.

On its website the Centers for Disease Control and Prevention issued a fact sheet about lead, including the following statement under the heading "How Your Child May Be Exposed": "Lead is invisible to the naked eye and has no smell. Children may be exposed to it from consumer products through normal hand-to-mouth activity, which is part of their normal development. They often place toys, fingers, and other objects in their mouth, exposing themselves to lead paint or dust."[61] The language here, which means to reassure anxious parents, twice uses the word normal in describing children's orality: their hand-to-mouth activity is "normal . . . part of their normal development." This redundancy betrays a nervousness about children, with its language of proper development and its delineation of what is or is not permissible in normal play.

Returning to that fantasy that images could only approximate: What precisely is wrong with the boy licking the train? The boy licking Thomas the Tank Engine is playing improperly with the phallic toy, not thrusting it forward along the floor but putting it into his mouth. Such late-exhibited orality bears the sheen of that "retarded" stage of development known as homosexuality. I am invoking the impossible juncture between the queernesses naturally afforded to children and the fear of a truly queer child.[62] I recently had a conversation with a British man in his seventies about the lead panic in the United States. With a twinkle in his eye, he said, "We had that lead in toys when I was young! Perhaps we just didn't suck them?" His comment highlights the limitations on some kinds of national memory, the invested forgetting that is necessary for such a lead panic to become so enlivened.

Given that lead's very threat is that it produces cognitive disabilities, the scene of the child licking his toxic train slides further into queerness, as queer and disabled bodies alike trouble the capitalist marriage of domesticity, heterosexuality, and ability. The queer disability theorist Robert McRuer writes of the development of domesticity within capitalism that the ideological reconsolidation of the home as a site of intimacy and heterosexuality was also the reconsolidation of the home as a site for the development of able-bodied identities, practices, and relations.[63] Exhibiting telltale signs of homosexuality and lead toxicity simultaneously alerts a protected, domestic sphere to the threat of disability. One could say that lead itself is queered here as a microcosmic pollutant that, almost of its own accord, invades the body through plenitudes of microcosmic holes (a child's skin), sites the state cannot afford to acknowledge for the queer vulnerabilities they portend.

Animacy theory embraces the ramified sites and traces of shifting being. It claims first that the tropes by which lead threatens to contaminate "healthy" privileged subjects rely fundamentally on animacy hierarchies. Lead can drag vulnerable people down, through variously lesser positions of animateness, into the realms of the "vegetable" or the nonsentient. At the same time it has already weighed on some bodies more than others. The strength of anxieties about lead toxicity microcosmically, and very compactly, demonstrates that race, class, sexuality, and ability are unstable. These are not assured categories or properties that could operate intersectionally in a binary analysis but are variably "mattering participants" in dominant ontologies that cannot therefore securely attach to anybody. Animacy theory objectifies animate hierarchies, assessing their diverse truth effects against the mobilities and slippages that too easily occur within them, and asks what paths the slippages trace.

Notwithstanding my claims about lead's racialization in relation to a context, lead is of course not always specific to China.

Rather, like any toxin, perhaps especially because it is not alive, it can be detached and reattached to diverse cultural and biological forms. This means that it is readily racialized, but with a set of preferences provided by the discursive structures it inhabits. Lead as a toxin, more generally, has already become in this global context racialized in excess as nonwhite; for instance, Mexican lead-tinged candy also received much media attention in 2007.[64] Yet lead's attachment preferences are perhaps not so flighty as one might think; the yellow hue of today's lead seems to swirl in with the brown and black layers of lead's naturalized image.

I have suggested that the mediation of lead in and around categories of life undoes lead's deadness by reanimating it. In other words, lead has the capacity to poison definitively animate beings, and as such achieves its own animacy as agents of harm. By examining the signifying economies of health, imperialism, and degradation that paint race onto different bodies, and by directing attention to the multiplicity of "contact zones" of those engaging lead, from working on the assembly line and using the new products that contain them to the downstream use of the products and the recycling and mining of them, we witness the inherent brokenness of races, geographies, and bodies as systems of segregation, even as they remain numbingly effective in informing discourses of combat, health, and privilege. An environmental history of toxic objects must minimally register the gendered, laboring, and chronically toxically exposed bodies of globalized capital, which systematically bear less frequent mention in narratives of toxicity than the cautionary warnings from the seat of U.S. empire. With this registration lead's spectacle remains connected to the possible forging of justice.

NOTES

1. I do not wish to fully privilege available medical evidence when I note that, to the degree that lead toxicity was medicalized, there were no known reports of poisoning from the specific toys recalled. It is the relationship between the high levels of panic and low levels of documented poisoning that points to a disproportionate response. I caution, however, that medically documented poisoning can often be an unreliable criterion, since documentation levels for testing may be calibrated to detect acute rather than chronic levels of poisoning.
2. See, for example, "Mattel Issues New Massive China Toy Recall."
3. Story, "Lead Paint Prompts Mattel to Recall 967,000 Toys."
4. Lipton and Barboza, "As More Toys Are Recalled, Trail Ends in China."
5. "New Worries over Lead."
6. See the essays in the excellent book edited by Evelyn Nakano Glenn, Shades of Difference, for a variety of approaches to the complex mappings between colorism and racism.
7. On April 29, 2011, the Illinois company RC2 was acquired by the Japanese toy-making corporation Tomy Company, Ltd.
8. Kang, "Si(gh)ting Asian/American Women as Transnational Labor," 403. Kang's essay focuses on the Asian female body's appropriation and decontextualized uptake for symbolic representation of transnational working bodies.
9. See Jain, Injury, for a discussion of injury law and "American injury culture" from cultural anthropology and legal studies perspectives.
10. Lei, Environmental Activism in China; Tilt, The Struggle for Sustainability in Rural China.
11. Harvey, A Brief History of Neoliberalism, 168.
12. "WTO: China Overtakes U.S. in Exports."
13. Lague, "China Output Not a Threat, Officials Say."
14. Lammers, "What to Do When Everything Is 'Made in China'?"
15. Such extravagant and rapid displacements in mainstream media do not, however, reflect the continued attention to this issue among environmental justice activists. The activist and artist Mel Chin has embarked on a campaign to raise awareness about lead level in lower-income, historically black neighborhoods in post-Katrina New Orleans; for more on his "Operation Paydirt" project, see Brookhardt,

"Mel Chin's Operation Paydirt Aims to Get the Lead Out of New Orleans' Inner City Neighborhoods."

16. However, many scholars are taking more sensitive views on the permeability of national borders when it comes to industrial pollutants, including environmental studies such as Pulido, Environmentalism and Economic Justice.

17. Beck, Risk Society, 23.

18. For this phrasing I am indebted to Gabriele Schwab, who was responding to my talk at the University of California, Irvine, on this topic on October 30, 2009.

19. Wald, Contagious. In the case of SARS, for instance, Gwen D'Arcangelis writes that microbial modes of transmission were explained by way of animals, linking these to U.S. imperialism in relation to China ("Chinese Chickens, Ducks, Pigs and Humans, and the Technoscientific Discourses of Global U.S. Empire").

20. Povinelli, The Empire of Love, 77.

21. Shah, Contagious Divides.

22. A phrase from Williams, The Demon of the Orient and His Satellite Fiends of the Joint, quoted in Shah, Contagious Divides, 54.

23. The Bioterrorism Act was enacted in 2002. According to Andrew Lakoff, concerns about bioterrorism merged with existing disease outbreaks in national security discourses in the late 1990s ("National Security and the Changing Object of Public Health").

24. A somewhat different argument is made by Marion Nestle in Safe Food, who writes about concerns over food safety and links them to rhetoric about bioterrorism.

25. Austen, "Lead in Children's Toys Exceeds Limit, Magazine Says."

26. I am reminded here of Jake Kosek's articulation of another invisible threat, radiation near nuclear sites, and the fungibility it portends, precisely because it must be imagined: "Radiation is a strange beast. It is undetectable by our very senses. . . . Living next to a deeply secretive, historically deceptive nuclear research complex that produces a highly volatile, mobile, odorless, tasteless, invisible substance that is unimaginably enduring and deadly in its toxicity blurs the traditional boundaries between material and imaginary. The very essence of an object changes meanings: a dust cloud from the east, smoke from Los Alamos, firewood, drinking water, an elk

steak, all become haunted by possibilities of what is not perceptively present but always a threat. What makes sense in a context where senses are useless?" (Understories, 258–59).

27. Harris, "Why Is China Poisoning Our Babies?" This blog is by an Australian writer. Other ambiguous and not so ambiguous titles included the conservative website Americans Working Together, which posted an article titled "Greed, China Poisoning Our Children with Lead."

28. Harris, "Heparin Contamination May Have Been Deliberate, F.D.A. Says."

29. Puar, Terrorist Assemblages.

30. For more accounts of the rhetorical strategies of environmental justice activism, see Sze, Noxious New York; Calpotura and Sen, "PUEBLO Fights Lead Poisoning." For general approaches to environmental justice, see Bullard, The Quest for Environmental Justice.

31. Wayne, "The Enemy at Home." This is the print title; the online version is titled "Thousands of Homeowners Cite Drywall for Ills."

32. Chen, "Chinese Toy Terror." See also Cottle, "Toy Terror."

33. See, for example, Nash, "Fruits of Ill-Health," and the film Maquilopolis, which refers to the poisoning of the environment in which maquiladoras are located as well as of the maquiladora workers' bodies themselves.

34. Pediatric mercury-laden vaccines are one example of such practices. The Food and Drug Administration and the Centers for Disease Control and Prevention bought up surpluses of thimerosal-preserved children's vaccines banned in the United States, then oversaw their exportation to other countries. On October 15, 2008, President George W. Bush signed into law the Mercury Export Ban, prohibiting the export of elemental mercury from the United States by 2013. The United States has been a top source of mercury distribution throughout the world, particularly by selling its stores of surplus mercury to industrializing countries. The ban does not, however, address the continuing export of electronic wastes (which contain lead, mercury, cadmium, and other toxic chemicals) to industrializing countries for resource mining, which results in highly toxic exposures.

35. Jennings and Jennings critique the shallow, still racist remedies inherent in "organic" and "sustainable" agricultural practice and policy developments ("Green Fields/Brown Skin," 180).

36. U.S. Consumer Product Safety Commission, recall release 08-247, April 10, 2008.

37. For more on the opposition between rural and metropolis and this divide's organizations based on class and sex, see Herring, Another Country.

38. Jennings, "Thomas the Tank Engine Toys Recalled Because of Lead Hazard."

39. In Racial Castration David Eng discusses a photograph commemorating the construction of Western railroads that, through omission, performs the erasure of Chinese labor in the building of the railroads. He uses Walter Benjamin's considerations of history, temporality, and the photograph to perform a literary analysis of the rhetorical invisibilization of Asian American presence, building an argument about "racial melancholia" in the United States.

40. There has been some popular attention to the conditions of Chinese labor; for example, Chang, Factory Girls, and the documentary directed by Micha Peled, China Blue, on the exploitative living and working conditions of young female Chinese workers who have come to the city to make blue jeans.

41. There are some exceptions. Among individual public responses to either professional journalism or blogged expressions of the toxicity of lead toys and the toxicity of Chinese products, one can find alerts to the more complex, sometimes imperial relationships between U.S. and transnational corporate interests, U.S. consumer interests, the Chinese government, and Chinese transnationalized labor. To my knowledge, however, for all the complexity it might have included in its coverage, no mainstream publication has not also symptomatically either assisted in retreating to occasional gestures of alarmism or conflations of biosecurity threats with the catch-all nomination of China.

42. For a study of situations in which the employers of child care are themselves people of color, see Qayum and Ray, "Traveling Cultures of Servitude."

43. Glenn, Forced to Care, 2. Glenn's book historicizes the long-standing racialization, gendering, and class structuring of all kinds of care work within the United States.

44. Briggs, "Foreign and Domestic."

45. Chang, Disposable Domestics.
46. Clough, Autoaffection, 3.
47. See also Chun, Control and Freedom.
48. The first IQ measure in the United States was broadly and inaccurately adapted from the French Simon-Binet scale by H. H. Goddard. Goddard believed that intelligence was inborn and could not be altered environmentally; the IQ measure factored prominently in his and others' eugenicist efforts. Since then several biases inherent in the test have been recognized, including the fact that IQ can dramatically change in relation to one's environment.
49. See Carter, The Heart of Whiteness. Carter discusses neurasthenia diagnoses of men and their associations with weakness and white vulnerability in general. In The Ugly Laws Susan Schweik notes that neurasthenia was gendered as female and "turns out to be high-class mendicancy," illustrating the ease of alteration between one's vulnerability to disability and being disabled.
50. Hartman, Scenes of Subjection, 206.
51. See Roig-Franzia, "Probe Opens on Study Tied to Johns Hopkins."
52. I heard this story when it aired in 2007 and inadequately understood it as a symptom of willful forgetting in light of "Chinese lead." However, I am unable to find the exact citation since not all NPR programs are transcribed and archived.
53. "The Living Legacy of Lead."
54. Paul Gilroy implicitly arouses the specter of such a "savage" body when he critiques the naïvely rehabilitative reading of the contained and fluid image of the black athlete in Leni Riefenstahl's filming of Jesse Owens: "Her superficially benign recognition of black excellence in physicality need not be any repudiation of raciological theory. In this world of overdetermined racial signs, an outstandingly good but temperamental natural athlete is exactly what we would expect a savage African to become" (Against Race, 173).
55. Davis, "Masked Racism."
56. Lott, Love and Theft, 116.
57. In a chapter called "Animatedness," Sianne Ngai suggests the legacy of blackface minstrelsy haunts modern-day animation shows centering on black life, such as The PJs; what Lott reads as Dickens's textual "jump-cuts" in describing minstrel dance might be found

in the bodily displacements and exaggerations of the stop-motion sequencing of the PJs characters (<u>Ugly Feelings</u>, 89–125).

58. Erevelles and Minear, "Unspeakable Offenses," 128.

59. "A mind is a terrible thing to waste" is the slogan of the United Negro College Fund's campaign to further African Americans' access to education. Dan Quayle's perversion of this slogan, "What a terrible thing it is to lose one's mind," suggests what fantasies about blackness might underlie benevolent white liberal representations.

60. I thank Don Romesburg for first getting me to indulge in this sensory fantasy.

61. See the Centers for Disease Control and Prevention's webpage on lead and toys, "Toys," October 15, 2013, http://www.cdc.gov/nceh/lead/tips/toys.htm.

62. See Bruhm and Hurley, <u>Curiouser</u>; Stockton, <u>The Queer Child</u>.

63. McRuer, <u>Crip Theory</u>, 88–89.

64. See, for instance, the website Lead in Mexican Candy, www.leadinmexicancandy.com. (In a possible reflection of both policy changes and political sensitivity, on October 21, 2016, this address redirected to a topical coverage of lead-free candy by the Environmental Health Coalition with minimization of the provenance of the lead).

BIBLIOGRAPHY

Americans Working Together. "Greed, China Poisoning Our Children with Lead." 2008. www.americans-working-together.com.

Austen, Ian. "Lead in Children's Toys Exceeds Limit, Magazine Says." <u>New York Times</u>, October 19, 2007.

Beck, Ulrich. <u>Risk Society: Towards a New Modernity</u>. Translated by Mark Ritter. London: Sage, 1992.

Briggs, Laura. "Foreign and Domestic: Adoption, Immigration, and Privatization." In <u>Intimate Labors</u>, edited by Eileen Boris and Rhacel Parreñas, 49–62. Stanford: Stanford University Press, 2010.

Brookhardt, D. Eric. "Mel Chin's <u>Operation Paydirt</u> Aims to Get the Lead Out of New Orleans' Inner City Neighborhoods." <u>Art Papers</u>, January–February 2009.

Bruhm, Steven, and Natasha Hurley, eds. <u>Curiouser: On the Queerness of Children</u>. Minneapolis: University of Minnesota Press, 2004.

Bullard, Robert, ed. The Quest for Environmental Justice: Human Rights and the Politics of Pollution. San Francisco: Sierra Club Books, 2005.

Calpotura, Francis, and Rinku Sen. "PUEBLO Fights Lead Poisoning." In Unequal Protection: Environmental Justice and Communities of Color, edited by Robert Bullard, 234–55. San Francisco: Sierra Club Books, 1994.

Carter, Julian B. The Heart of Whiteness: Normal Sexuality and Race in America, 1800–1940. Durham NC: Duke University Press, 2007.

Chang, Grace. Disposable Domestics: Women Workers in the Global Economy. Cambridge MA: South End Press, 1999.

Chang, Leslie. Factory Girls: From Village to City in a Changing China. New York: Spiegel and Grau, 2008.

Chen, Shu-Ching Jean. "Chinese Toy Terror." Forbes, August 2, 2007.

China Blue. Directed by Micha Peled. San Francisco: Teddy Bear Films and Independent Television Service, 2005.

Chun, Wendy Hui Kyong. Control and Freedom: Power and Paranoia in the Age of Fiber Optics. Cambridge MA: MIT Press, 2006.

Clough, Patricia Ticineto. Autoaffection: Unconscious Thought in the Age of Teletechnology. Minneapolis: University of Minnesota Press, 2000.

Cottle, Michelle. "Toy Terror." New Republic, August 13, 2007.

D'Arcangelis, Gwen. "Chinese Chickens, Ducks, Pigs and Humans, and the Technoscientific Discourses of Global U.S. Empire." In Tactical Biopolitics: Art, Activism, and Technoscience, edited by Beatriz da Costa and Kavita Philip, 429–42. Cambridge MA: MIT Press, 2008.

Davis, Angela. "Masked Racism: Reflections on the Prison Industrial Complex." Color Lines, September 10, 1998, 12–17.

Eng, David. Racial Castration: Managing Masculinity in Asian America. Durham NC: Duke University Press, 2010.

Erevelles, Nirmala, and Andrea Minear. "Unspeakable Offenses: Untangling Race and Disability in Discourses of Intersectionality." Journal of Literary and Cultural Studies 4, no. 2 (2010): 127–45.

Gilroy, Paul. Against Race: Imagining Political Culture beyond the Color Line. Cambridge MA: Harvard University Press, 2002.

Glenn, Evelyn Nakano. Forced to Care: Coercion and Caregiving in America. Cambridge MA: Harvard University Press, 2010.

———. Shades of Difference: Why Skin Color Matters. Stanford: Stanford University Press, 2009.

Harris, Gardiner. "Heparin Contamination May Have Been Deliberate, F.D.A. Says." New York Times, April 30, 2008.

Harris, Samela. "Why Is China Poisoning Our Babies?" Adelaide Now, November 9, 2007.

Hartman, Saidiya. Scenes of Subjection: Terror, Slavery, and Self-Making in Nineteenth-Century America. Oxford: Oxford University Press, 2007.

Harvey, David. A Brief History of Neoliberalism. Oxford: Oxford University Press, 2007.

Herring, Scott. Another Country: Queer Anti-Urbanism. New York: New York University Press, 2010.

Jain, S. Lochlann. Injury: The Politics of Product Design and Safety Law in the United States. Princeton NJ: Princeton University Press, 2006.

Jennings, Angel. "Thomas the Tank Engine Toys Recalled Because of Lead Hazard." New York Times, June 15, 2007.

Jennings, Cheri Lucas, and Bruce H. Jennings. "Green Fields/Brown Skin: Posting as a Sign of Recognition." In The Nature of Things: Language, Politics, and the Environment, edited by Jane Bennett and William Chaloupka, 173–94. Minneapolis: University of Minnesota Press, 1993.

Kang, Laura Hyun Yi. "Si(gh)ting Asian/American Women as Transnational Labor." positions: East Asia Cultures Critique 5, no. 2 (1997): 403–37.

Kosek, Jake. Understories: The Political Life of Forests in Northern New Mexico. Durham NC: Duke University Press, 2006.

Lague, David. "China Output Not a Threat, Officials Say." New York Times, April 1, 2006.

Lakoff, Andrew. "National Security and the Changing Object of Public Health." In Biosecurity Interventions: Global Health and Security in Question, edited by Andrew Lakoff and Stephen J. Coller, 33–60. New York: Columbia University Press, 2008.

Lammers, Dirk. "What to Do When Everything Is 'Made in China'?" MSNBC.com, June 29, 2007.

Lei, Xie. Environmental Activism in China. London: Routledge, 2009.

Lipton, Eric S., and David Barboza. "As More Toys Are Recalled, Trail Ends in China." New York Times, June 19, 2007.

"The Living Legacy of Lead." Living on Earth, National Public Radio, November 2, 2007.

Lott, Eric. Love and Theft: Blackface Minstrelsy and the American Working Class. New York: Oxford University Press, 1993.

Maquilopolis: City of Factories. Produced by Vicky Funari ad Sergio de la Torre. Distributed by California Newsreel, 2006.

"Mattel Issues New Massive China Toy Recall." MSNBC.com, August 14, 2007.

McRuer, Robert. Crip Theory: Cultural Signs of Queerness and Disability. New York: New York University Press, 2006.

Nash, Linda. "Fruits of Ill-Health: Pesticides and Workers' Bodies in Post–World War II California." In Landscapes of Exposure: Knowledge and Illness in Modern Environments, edited by Greg Mitman, Michelle Murphy, and Christopher Sellers, 203–19. Chicago: University of Chicago Press 2004.

Nestle, Marion. Safe Food: Bacteria, Biotechnology, and Bioterrorism. Berkeley: University of California Press, 2003.

"New Worries over Lead." Consumer Reports, December 2007.

Ngai, Sianne. Ugly Feelings. Cambridge MA: Harvard University Press, 2005.

Povinelli, Elizabeth. The Empire of Love: Toward a Theory of Intimacy, Genealogy, and Carnality. Durham NC: Duke University Press, 2006.

Puar, Jasbir K. Terrorist Assemblages: Homonationalism in Queer Times. Durham NC: Duke University Press, 2007.

Pulido, Laura. Environmentalism and Economic Justice: Two Chicano Studies in the Southwest. Tucson: University of Arizona Press, 1996.

Qayum, Seemin, and Raka Ray. "Traveling Cultures of Servitude." In Intimate Labors: Cultures, Technologies, and the Politics of Care, edited by Eileen Boris and Rhacel Parreñas, 101–16. Stanford: Stanford University Press, 2010.

Roig-Franzia, Manuel. "Probe Opens on Study Tied to Johns Hopkins." Washington Post, August 23, 2001.

Schweik, Susan M. The Ugly Laws: Disability in Public. New York: New York University Press, 2009.

Shah, Nayan. Contagious Divides: Epidemics and Race in San Francisco's Chinatown. Berkeley: University of California Press, 2001.

Stockton, Kathryn Bond. The Queer Child: Or Growing Sideways in the Twentieth Century. Durham NC: Duke University Press, 2009.

Story, Louise. "Lead Paint Prompts Mattel to Recall 967,000 Toys." New York Times, August 2, 2007.

Sze, Julie. Noxious New York: The Racial Politics of Urban Health and Environmental Justice. Cambridge MA: MIT Press, 2007.

Tilt, Bryan. The Struggle for Sustainability in Rural China: Environmental Values and Civil Society. New York: Columbia University Press, 2010.

Wald, Priscilla. Contagious: Cultures, Carriers, and the Outbreak Narrative. Durham NC: Duke University Press, 2007.

Wayne, Leslie. "The Enemy at Home." New York Times, October 8, 2009.

Williams, Allen S. The Demon of the Orient and His Satellite Fiends of the Joint: Our Opium Smokers As They Are in Tartar Hells and American Paradises. New York: Allen S. Williams, 1883.

"WTO: China Overtakes U.S. in Exports. Asian Nation Set to Become the World's Biggest Exporter by 2008." MSNBC.com, April 12, 2007.

4

Defining Eco-ability

Social Justice and the Intersectionality of Disability, Nonhuman Animals, and Ecology

Anthony J. Nocella II

Earth, Animal, and Disability Liberation: The Rise of the Eco-ability Movement (Nocella et al. 2012) is the first book to connect ecology, disability, and animal advocacy, couched in terms of interlocking social constructions and the interwoven web of interdependent global life.[1] Both the natural world and disability will be viewed as socially constructed entities. I suggest that for the current global ecological crisis to transform into a more sustainable global community, including nonhuman animals, the field of environmental studies needs to engage in a discussion of colonization and domination of the environment. I explain and deconstruct the meaning of disability while critically examining environmentalism and environmental studies from an anti-oppression perspective. Finally, I demonstrate how disability studies can take a position on the current ecological crisis, showing that disability theory, animal advocacy, and ecology can be brought together in a philosophy of eco-ability. Eco-ability combines the concepts of interdependency, inclusion, and respect for difference within a community; and this includes all life, sentient and nonsentient.

Crisis of Ecological Domination and Normalcy

"Voice for the voiceless" is a saying that has been used repeatedly by disability rights activists, environmentalists, and animal advocates. These traditionally oppressed groups—nonhuman animals, people with disabilities, and the ecological world—have much in common and have arguably been marginalized more than any other segment of society. In today's colonized and capitalist-driven world, one of the worst things is to be considered or called an "animal," "wild," or a "freak" (Snyder and Mitchell 2006). If one is not recognized as human by "normal society," one is either an animal or disabled, as was the case for women and people of color less than fifty years ago, who were also once identified by law as property. Between the seventeenth and early twentieth century the predominantly white patriarchal scientists, using the racist, sexist, and ableist theory of eugenics, claimed that women and people of color had smaller brains, were "by Nature" less intelligent, psychiatrically inferior to men (labels such as "hysterical" were applied), and less than human. As Snyder and Mitchell explain, "American eugenics laid bare the social and national goals newly claimed for medical practices. It promised an empirically sound, cross-disciplinary arena for identifying 'defectives' viewed as a threat to the purity of a modern nation-state. Turn-of-the-century diagnosticians came to rely on the value of bureaucratic surveillance tools, such as census data, medical catalogues, and intelligence testing" (74).

With this mind-set established, from the early 1870s onward the rise of strategic, repressive, and pathological medical categorization of those with mental disabilities or perceived inferior physical attributes (especially among the poor) permitted new immigration officials to deny any person with an assumed mental disability entrance into the United States. Next came the incarceration and institutionalization of those within the country, and finally the testing, medical experimentation, and killing of them in the name of purification (Snyder and Mitchell 2006). The institutionalization of and Nazi experimentation on those with disabilities was a little-known mass genocide in the name of genetic purity and perceived normalcy promoted by the medical field (Snyder and Mitchell 2006). Striving for a genetically and psychologically pure society was the taken-for-granted, popular view of scientists at the turn of the twentieth century (Dowbiggin 2003). The rise of intelligence testing by Binet (Binet and Simon 1973) gave scientists the tool to officially determine a person's competence.

In contrast, while Western colonial science constructs a "perfect norm," some theories of ecology argue that everyone and everything is interdependent and diverse and that there exists no "norm" or "normal." The inherent philosophy within the natural world is that the environment strives to be in harmony and balance. The ecological world, or biosphere, is itself an argument for respecting differing abilities and the uniqueness of all living beings. Moreover humans as a species are a part of the "animal kingdom" and nature rather than separate and dominant. Ecofeminists, environmental justice scholars and activists, and environmental revolutionaries represent the antithesis of genocidal thought. They foster an appreciation and love of difference and mutual aid rather than a fetishization of sameness and individualism (Best and Nocella 2006).

Eco-ability, a concept I developed, is a philosophy that respects differences in abilities while promoting values appropriate to the stewardship of ecosystems. Eco-ability is in its infancy as a concept, and I encourage further dialogue and discussion of its implications. At this point a basic understanding will suffice.

Disability studies as a discipline also praises difference, uniqueness, and interdependency. Disability studies suggests that every being has differing abilities. Each being plays an important role in the global community and is valuable within the larger ecological context. Eco-ability respects differences while challenging the concepts of equality, sameness, and normalcy. These concepts are social constructions that fail to respect the uniqueness of individual abilities and differences, which, as the ecological and disability communities realize, are interdependent. Further, nature, nonhuman animals, and people with disabilities have been institutionalized, tortured, and murdered not because they have committed a crime or for profit but for being recognized as different and as a commodity. "Difference" is a threat to the advancement of normalcy, which is the philosophical foundation of social control and discipline (Pfohl 2009).

The label different is important to eco-ability because it becomes an assumed descriptor within societal institutions, as do the seven Ds of stigmatization: demonic, deviant, delinquent, disabled, debtor, disorder, and dissenter. If you are not labeled normal by society, you are inherently viewed as abnormal, a threat that must be controlled, disciplined, and punished. Repressing people with disabilities has always been a complex system of stigmatization of those who are different. Even to this day some counselors, doctors, and religious leaders state that if an individual has committed a highly controversial act that challenges socioeconomic or political norms, that person is deemed to be evil and is demonized in the news and official reports. Critical criminology shows that there is a slippery slope when one is stigmatized as deviant by teachers or counselors. Police and judges can more easily stigmatize an individual as delinquent when he or she is arrested. After the individual is convicted and institutionalized, he or she is put through rigorous examinations by doctors and psychologists who are determined to finally and permanently label the individual as someone having a disability.

How Did All This Begin with Western Society?

In Western civilization the marginalization of those who are different was first fostered and reinforced by the concept of civilization and its divide between nature and humans. (This divide arguably began when human beings first began cultivating the land ten thousand years ago.) Those considered wild, savage, or primitive were situated on one side, and those considered civilized, privileged, and normal on the other. This corresponded to the ideological policy of foreign relations that Kees van der Pijl (2007, 24) calls "empire-nomad relations." In time, civilization took the further step of establishing state borders in what we know today as Europe, amid the project of global conquest, which today we call "colonization." In addition to establishing an elitist, antinatural culture at home (i.e., civilization), the predominant goal of empires was to conquer, assimilate, or destroy every non-colonial-influenced culture. For example, non-Christian religious sites were destroyed in the New World, and Christian churches were built on top of them. Every popular religion attempted to assimilate others through religious domination (forced conversions) in addition to economic and cultural usurpation.

With European colonialism spreading across the world, an economic system that upheld the values of capitalism was created, placing a value on everything and everyone. For example, whites were more valuable than people of color, birds, trees, water, and even land. All of nature was viewed as a natural resource, a commodity, and typically marked as property—something owned by someone—to be used any which way its owners saw fit. Over time everything, including people (such as slaves), had an inherent worth and was viewed as a commodity.

The concept of ownership of property, critiqued by anarchists (Amster et al. 2009), created the haves and the have-nots. Societal classes were split between the owners and the working classes. With the establishment of natural resources as a commodity and ownership of goods, the producer-consumer relationship was forged. This symbiotic relationship was the foundation of the industrialized world that became dominant in nineteenth-century Europe and North America. The primary economic system was supported by institutions, ostensibly developed to care for others and keep the public safe and the culture orderly. Similarly "scientific" treatments to benefit the common good were developed and hailed as improvements in a society eager to become "modern" and civilized. Institutions such as colleges, prisons, hospitals, and religious centers worked closely with political and educational systems to justify their existence. Violent acts such as experimentation, dissection, and vivisection using people with disabilities, nonhuman animals, plants, water, and other elements were condoned as the foundation of modern advancements in science and knowledge.

From Personal to Political

Beating, killing, imprisonment, surveillance, raids, and framing have been taking place since the creation of a class, race, and state divide established by the elite and reinforced by governments (Bodley 2005). Faced with dark times, survival is often the only hope for victims, both humans and nonhumans, of repressive and controlling authoritarian structures. The oppressed typically do not think of speaking out, fighting back, writing their stories, or uniting to share their experiences (Harding 2003). They simply want to move on, endure, and live!

It took me four years to watch a video of myself being arrested. It was too emotional to relive. I was arrested and searched by the chief of police in Corpus Christi, Texas, for an act of civil disobedience in protecting dolphins from captivity (which I argue is a prison). I was subsequently framed for felony charges of possession of crack cocaine with the intent to sell. The framing was strategic. I was the lead organizer of a political campaign to keep dolphins out of a nonprofit entertainment and educational facility similar to Sea World. The facility was bringing in a lot of money to the city from tourists. Law enforcement needed to figure out how to stigmatize me and other activists, as arresting us was only bringing us more sympathy from the public and the media. They needed to stigmatize me and the campaign with something that would make people disregard our efforts. Marijuana, PCP, LSD, heroin, and other drugs, although vilified, do not have the universally negative image of crack cocaine, a drug stigmatized because of its political history. Crack cocaine was strategically placed into the black community in the 1970s by government agencies, including the CIA, to destroy those communities (Schou 2006; Scott and Marshall 1998; Webb 1999). It is an interesting coincidence, or a strategic act by law enforcement, that I was framed for crack cocaine for protesting dolphins in captivity in Texas, and crack cocaine was used to destroy the black community. Since its inception crack cocaine has been a powerful tool to destroy and repress political and social groups by U.S. law enforcement.

After my release from jail I did not speak much to my friends about the incident; neither did I speak to the media or make buttons or stickers about my case. Rather I kept fighting for the dolphins. Yes, people knew about my case, but they were mainly one of two types of people: activists who supported me or the media and law enforcement personnel who portrayed me as a crack-selling, vegan dissenter needing to be silenced. I remember making one flyer relating the imprisonment of dolphins to my possible imprisonment, but I produced only a hundred copies. It was then that I understood a prisoner is a prisoner is a prisoner, no matter if the prisoner is an elephant in a zoo, a human in Attica, a bird in a cage, or a dolphin in an aquarium.

No one spoke up to write my story; if someone had done so I would have told him or her to focus on the dolphins. Now, upon further reflection, I realize that my case tells another story. It tells how everything is connected and that when one fights against systems of domination and oppressive institutions, one will be repressed. Many others in the animal rights movement have been arrested on trumped-up charges, receiving ridiculous prison sentences and fines.

I, a Quaker and straightedge practitioner (someone who does not engage in illegal drugs, alcohol, or promiscuous sex), was among the first in this group to be framed for something I did not do. As a result I later received numerous calls from activists wondering what to do about being targeted by police. I provided them with this advice: stick with your community and protect each other, and tell your story, as I am doing now. It is through our shared experiences and knowledge that we build a stronger understanding of political repression and oppression from systems of domination.

The Stigmatization of Disability, the Inclusion of People with Disabilities in Society, and Animal Rights Rhetoric

At a very young age (before first grade) I was diagnosed as having severe mental disabilities.[2] This diagnosis resulted in my being directed to special education classes from first to fourth grade. It was a nightmare for me. I could neither read nor speak well. I shook all the time, and I had difficulty focusing my energy, both in the classroom and in general. At times I would be held down or kicked out of class. The only wonderful relationship I had in those years was with my cat, Sparkle, who was my best friend and someone I was able to communicate with emotionally in a humane manner. While I was still a child Sparkle was killed by three dogs. It was that death that later inspired me to become highly involved in the animal rights movement. From fifth to twelfth grade I went to a school for students with mental and learning disabilities. Both the classes in the "normal" school and those in the disability school represent segregation.

It is important to connect the social construction of ableism and speciesism. Ableism, a term created by activists with disabilities, is discrimination against people with disabilities by promoting normalcy carried out through structural barriers, personal actions, and theories (Davis 2002). Speciesism is discrimination against nonhuman animal species by arguing that humans are more important and superior to nonhuman animals (Dunayer 2004). Both speciesism and ableism are social constructions interwoven into society, promoting civilization, normalcy, and intellectualism grounded in modernity, which arose out of the European Enlightenment. Modernity is "a progressive force promising to liberate humankind from ignorance and irrationality" (Rosenau 1992, 5). Therefore the intellectual movement's goal was to create theory after theory to divide adherents from everything that was savage and what they would soon deem abnormal and deviant, that is, nature, nonhuman animals, women, and people with disabilities. Snyder and Mitchell (2006, 31) explain how the narrative of modernity was "key" to constructing disability as deviant and undesirable:

> Modernity gives birth to the culture of technology that promises more data from less input. This unique historical terrain is characterized by Bauman [2001, 12] as "the morally elevating story of humanity emerging from pre-social barbarity." This progressive narrative is key to the development of disability as a concept of deviant variation. In a culture that endlessly assures itself that it is on the verge of conquering Nature once and for all, along with its own "primitive" instincts and the persistent domain of the have-nots, disability is referenced with respect

to these idealized visions. As a vector of human variability, disabled bodies both represent a throwback to human prehistory and serve as the barometer of a future without "deviancy."

In other words, for modernity, the eradication of disability represented a scourge and a promise: its presence signaled a debauched present of cultural degeneration that was tending to regress toward a prior state of primitivism, while at the same time it seemed to promise that its absence would mark the completion of modernity as a cultural project.

To challenge this movement of domination over nature, nonhuman animals, and disability, I united the three groups to create the field of study called eco-ability. Eco-ability is the theory that nature, nonhuman animals, and people with disabilities promote collaboration, not competition; interdependency, not independence; and respect for difference and diversity, not sameness and normalcy.

Dr. Liat Ben-Moshe (personal communication, January 20, 2011) states that the value of people with disabilities sometimes falls between humans and nonhumans, but, depending on their physical or mental disability, they may also be viewed as less than nonhuman. Many of us in the United States are familiar with the demeaning comments directed toward humans that are exploitative of nonhuman animals: "You are such a pig"; "What are you, an animal?"; "Stop acting like a bitch"; "You are such a dog"; and "You are as fat as a whale." Similarly people with disabilities are stigmatized and marginalized when those without disabilities are faced with insults such as the following: "You are so retarded," suggesting a person is not being cool; "You are such a freak," suggesting a person has uncommon sexual behaviors; "Why are you acting so lame?," suggesting a person is boring;

and "You are acting crazy," suggesting a person is not in control of his or her actions (Snyder and Mitchell 2006).

In U.S. culture, and even within social movements, we are used to homophobic, racist, classist, and sexist language. While those acts of oppression are important to address, this eco-ability focuses on addressing the stigmatization of nonhuman animals as property, activists as terrorists, and people with disabilities as abnormal or less than human.

For example, a connection between ableism and speciesism has recently become manifest in the animal advocacy movement with the concept of being a "vegan freak." The term was first coined by Bob Torres and Jenna Torres (2010), authors of Vegan Freak: Being Vegan in a Non-Vegan World. Dedicated animal advocates and vegans, Torres and Torres developed the title and term ironically to spotlight the social deviance of veganism as marginalized and "abnormal" behavior. They write, "So, regardless of how 'normal' you are, in a world where consuming animal products is the norm, you're always going to be seen as the freak if you obviously and clearly refuse to take part in an act of consumption that is central to our everyday lives, our cultures, and even our very own personal identities" (8).

Torres and Torres (2010) are social justice scholar-activists who, like most animal advocates who challenge the norm that veganism is an oddity, do not critically address the use of the term freak or other ableist language. In their book a possible example connecting animal advocacy and disability is the reference to Bob's disorganization when trying to plan ahead for navigating vegan cookery: "If you're like Bob, planning ahead is something for organized people without ADHD, so it may strike you as incredibly dull" (33). This sentence, which was not critically unraveled in the book, suggests that people like Bob Torres who have ADHD are disorganized and that being disorganized is some-how exciting. Further, because this sentence is not examined, it is not clear if Bob has ADHD or if the authors are simply making a common ableist "joke."

Freak is a term historically associated with those with disabilities. As defined by Robert Bogdan (1988, 6) in Freak Show, freak can refer to either those living in a "non-Western world then in progress," when Western explorers brought back uncommon and unfamiliar descriptions of people and cultural traditions of indigenous groups, or "'monsters,' the medical term for people born with a demonstrable difference" (i.e., "freak of nature"). Bogdan provides a summary of the attitude toward people with physical disabilities (i.e., freaks, which he is critical of, but he uses the term to examine its historical and social construction): "Our reaction to freaks is not a function of some deep-seated fear or some 'energy' that they give off; it is, rather, the result of our socialization, and of the way our social institutions managed these people's identities. Freak shows are not about isolated individuals, either on platforms or in an audience. They are about organizations and patterned relationships between them and us. 'Freak' is not a quality that belongs to the person on display. It is something that we created: a perspective, a set of practices—a social construction" (x–xi).

Therefore, from an ableist perspective, there can be only two reasons that justify and explain someone being vegan: veganism is a behavior that people with disabilities adopt, or people become disabled when they adopt a vegan diet. Being a "vegan freak," however, is not the only ableist term in the animal advocacy movement, for we also have moral schizophrenia to consider. Introduced by Gary Francione (2000), a law professor at Rutgers University, in his book, Introduction to Animal Rights: Your Child or the Dog?, moral schizophrenia is the action of caring for nonhuman animals such as dogs and cats but also exploiting them for food, product testing, clothes, and entertainment. In short, moral schizophrenia is hypocrisy: saying one thing but doing the complete opposite. Francione used the term schizophrenia not in a medical sense but to stigmatize those who do not support animal liberation. While most members of the animal advocacy movement agree with the term and the argument, there are a few who do not agree with the term but do agree with the argument. After a number of writers criticized Francione's use of the term schizophrenia as ableist, he published a defense on his blog: "Some people accuse me of confusing moral schizophrenia with multiple/split personality. When I talk about moral schizophrenia, I am seeking to describe the delusional and confused way that we think about animals as a social/moral matter. . . . Our moral schizophrenia, which involves our deluding ourselves about animal sentience and the similarities between humans and other animals . . . is a phenomenon that is quite complicated and has many different aspects" (Francione 2009).

Francione (2009) begins his argument by stating that schizophrenia is a "personality," with which people in the field of disability studies would agree, but he quickly changes his description of schizophrenia to a "condition," as seen in the following section. He then apologizes to those people who are offended by his using the term in a stigmatizing manner while continuing to defend his rationale: "Some people think that by using the term, I am stigmatizing those who have clinical schizophrenia because it implies that they are immoral people. I am sincerely sorry . . . if anyone has interpreted the term in that way. . . . Schizophrenia is a recognized condition that is characterized by confused and delusional thinking." Now, instead of identifying schizophrenia as a personality, he identifies it as a "condition," which quickly snowballs into a condition that people "suffer" from and that is not a "desirable" condition, as he states in the following passage from that same blog post: "To say that we are delusional and confused when it comes to moral issues is not to say that those who suffer from clinical schizophrenia are immoral. It is only to say that many of us think about important moral matters in a completely confused, delusional, and incoherent way. I am certainly not saying that those who suffer from clinical schizophrenia are immoral!" Francione goes on to provide some additional responses to the criticisms he had received on the original blog posting. He notes:

> When it comes to nonhuman animals, our views are profoundly delusional and I am using that term literally as indicative of what might be called a social form of schizophrenia. . . . Some critics claim that it is sufficient to use "delusional." But delusion is what characterizes the clinical form of schizophrenia and anyone who objected to the use of schizophrenia as ableist would have the same, and in my view groundless, objection to "delusional." . . . In any event, if "moral schizophrenia" is ableist, then so is the expression "drugs are a cancer on society" or "our policies in the Middle East are shortsighted" or "we are blind to the consequences of our actions" or "when it comes to poverty, our proposed solutions suffer from a poverty of ambition."

He offers an important critique of the public stigmatization of animal advocates as "profoundly delusional." While he perceives the ableism in using the term delusional in the conclusion to his post, he strives to defend his use of the term schizophrenia to stigmatize those who eat meat and exploit nonhuman animals by arguing that using terms such as cancer, shortsighted, and blind to describe a negative topic, event, or action is not ableist. On the contrary those who use such phrases, analogies, and comments <u>are</u> ableist; whenever someone is describing people in a negative or insulting manner by using terms that have been historically or are currently meant to describe people with physical or mental disabilities, that person is being ableist.

Francione (2009) strove to draw the parallel between cancer and schizophrenia, where one is a disease, while the other is a personal characteristic that makes up who that person is. In this ableist society both of them are disabilities. Therefore this term demeans those who have schizophrenia and reinforces that people should not be schizophrenic (as if there is a choice). Francione is certainly not the only ableist in the animal advocacy movement. There are many who use phrases such as "We must cripple capitalism," "Society is blind to the exploitation of animals," and "Vivisectors are idiots." Even many at the Conference for Critical Animal Studies at Brock University in St. Catherines, Canada, used Francione's term <u>moral schizophrenia</u>, which I addressed publicly. People who used the term at the conference took accountability and recognized their ableism.

A quick Google search can prove this, as people call each other "retard," "idiot," "crazy," "insane," "mentally ill," "freak," "mentally disturbed," "mentally unstable," "lame," "crippled," and so much more, emphasizing the four <u>D</u>s of dissent, which construct the individual as a <u>deviant</u>, <u>delinquent</u>, <u>demon</u>, or <u>disabled</u>. Dr. Stephanie Jenkins (personal communication, January 18, 2011) says there is a long history of relationships between and among the medical, criminal justice, legal, and psychiatric fields, in that they have a record of supporting each other's work. She adds that the largest minority group in the world is those with disabilities. They straddle all classes, nations, ages, genders, and races. For the most part they are nonviolent people, yet they are almost all portrayed as violent dangers to society.

I spoke with Jenkins a few weeks after the shooting in Arizona on January 8, 2011. She mentioned that the shooter, twenty-two-year-old Jared Lee Loughner, was identified as a person with a possible mental disability, although a full investigation of his background had not been conducted. She went on to say that this depiction was a common practice employed by media, society, and the government to convey that these types of violent actions are not acts of terrorism and therefore have no validity, rationality, or reason behind them. It is a common practice throughout society to label constructed social, political, interpersonal, or communal enemies as "disabled" (Corrigan 2006; Davis 1997, 2002; Nocella 2008; Snyder and Mitchell 2006).

Dr. Michael Loadenthal (personal communication, February 16, 2011) gave another example, of the shooter James Jay Lee, who had written a manifesto decrying what he perceived as the Discovery Channel's promotion of environmental destruction. CBS had labeled him an "environmental militant" (Effron and Goldman 2010). ABC's article "Environmental Militant Killed by Police at Discovery Channel Headquarters" (Effron and Goldman 2010) quotes witnesses who describe the activities in the event using ableist language, such as "insane," "crazy," and "nuts." Loadenthal states:

Whether Lee's critiques are valid or not, whether or not the Discovery Channel is contributing to global overpopulation or not was made kind of irrelevant. Immediately upon his attack, where he walked into the Discovery Channel building in Silver Spring, Maryland with two non-lethal starter pistols, held four hostages and was eventually killed by police, HIS POLITICAL ARGUMENT WAS MADE IRRELEVANT. How someone can be so angry about issues of overpopulation, and whether issues of overpopulation are a threat, and whether or not the Discovery

Channel is to be blamed, were not examined. The analysis immediately was why is this man "crazy" and "insane," why has this man gone this far, what led this man to this "extreme" end.

Dr. Jennifer Grubbs (personal communication, January 30, 2011) mentions the horrible shooting at Virginia Tech as yet another example of an individual who was stigmatized as having a mental disability but with little attention paid to the content of his video manifesto. It seems that, too often, these shooters in the United States are dismissed when identified as persons with mental illnesses and not as terrorists. This only reinforces the stigma that people with mental disabilities are violent and a physical threat to society, not to mention the social threat of being "abnormal."

For example, Dr. Colin Salter (personal communication, January 30, 2011) notes that many homeless people are people with disabilities who are regularly arrested, jailed, and deemed "abnormal" due to their socioeconomic situation. Swan (2002, 293) writes, "In the earlier scheme [the classic definition], disability described the degree to which one was restricted in performing an activity; handicap described the degree to which one could no longer fulfill a social or economic role." The term handicap reinforces the idea that people who have disabilities are poor and, furthermore, are dependent on others or are beggars. Dr. Liat Ben-Moshe's scholarship and activism focuses on the connection between the prison industrial complex and imprisoning people with disabilities. I asked her to tell me about the incarceration of people with disabilities; she responded, "Besides being labeled for life, you could be in a psych ward for life. You know, until the doctor pretty much says that you can go. So there is no end date for your imprisonment, unlike a criminal" (personal communication, January 20, 2011). Dr. Stephanie Jenkins (personal communication, February 16, 2011) suggests that people with disabilities are "labeled as being inferior, not happy, and being associated with certain kinds of pain, that is always assumed to be a negative." Stigmatization is a powerful tool used to imprison, silence, murder, perform tests on, and, of course, repress others (Corrigan 2006).

Deconstructing Disability

What is disability, and why does it have a negative connotation?[3] Disability is a negative term because it connotes being broken, not working properly, or being simply wrong. Disabled, crippled, lame, and retarded all mean similar things. They are all used commonly in U.S. society (Taylor 1996) to conjure negative images that are most often used to insult and label others. For example, these are common phrases: "You are being lame"; "You are so retarded"; "What, are you mad?"; "Don't be insane!"; and "What are you, crippled or something?" Thus "feebleminded," "retarded," "special needs," and "learning difficulties" are all examples of what Corbett (1995) calls "bad mouthing" (cited in Armstrong et al. 2000, 3). Goffman (1963, 1) writes, "The Greeks, who were apparently strong on visual aids, originated the term stigma to refer to bodily signs designed to expose something unusual and bad about the moral status of the signifier." All of these terms indicate stigmatization.

The classic label dumb is historically applied to both human and nonhuman animals. For example, in St. Thomas Aquinas's (2007, 2666) thirteenth-century tome Summa Theologica, one of the most influential works in Western culture, he writes, "Dumb animals and plants are devoid of the life of reason whereby to set themselves in motion; they are moved, as it were by another, by a kind of natural impulse, a sign of which is that they are naturally enslaved and accommodated to the uses of others." Here dumb is actually not the insult we see it as today; it indicates the nonhuman animal's inability to speak and also his or her lack of intelligence or sense of self. But <u>dumb</u> was most certainly a term used to dismiss those creatures labeled as such. Western rationalist philosophers after Aquinas would use the same terminology. More than just the import of the word itself, however, is the notion that because a being cannot speak the dominant language (i.e., human English) and process the world intellectually through the dominant framework (as white, human, able-bodied, heterosexual males), those individuals should become slaves, be used by others as food, clothing, or subjects for scientific experiments. This stigma against nonhuman animals is evident, but what is not as immediately apparent is the way the term similarly stigmatizes those with disabilities.

A rich example of stigma against people with disabilities is found in the movie <u>300</u> (Snyder 2006), in which the great warriors, the Spartans, battle the Persians, who are depicted as "uncivilized." A Greek who is strong and loyal but physically disabled approaches Leonidas and asks to join the Spartans. However, King Leonidas sees this man as a liability rather than a powerful and strong soldier with wit. The soldier with disabilities pleads his case to be part of the Spartans, but the king, after asking the soldier to perform a few defensive and offensive moves, says that he is not at the high level of a successful warrior. This devastates the soldier so much that he becomes a traitor for what the movie portrays as the uncivilized, "wild" Persians.

The meaning of the story is that the Spartans, as a "perfect" society, could never have a person with disabilities among them. But for the uncivilized, "wild" Persians, the movie portrays disability as acceptable. As all marginalized groups are the same, this implies that <u>non-Spartan</u> equals <u>nonperfect</u> or <u>not normal</u>. Based on the historical battle, the story has many imperialist lessons, one of them being that "civilized men" are more powerful than all of nature. This line of thinking carried over to the era of colonial empire rule, where the concept of disability was seen as a normalized level of physical and mental ability, while disability has at times been the justification to kill, test, segregate, abort, and abandon those with disabilities.

Disability, people with disabilities (using person-first language), or dis-ability (separating the prefix dis- from the root word ability, which I and many others do), are terms endorsed and used by dis-ability rights activists, theorists, advocates, and allies. As I noted earlier, there are negative connotations to the term disability, but the disability rights movement has reclaimed the term out of an understanding of the definition of disability and to whom it refers (Fleischer and Zames 2001). It is also the only term used to describe the differently abled, which holds significant legal and medical value, for it "appears to signify something material and concrete, a physical or psychological condition considered to have predominantly medical significance" (Linton 1998, 10). This does not suggest the term should and must be resisted. Most disability activists would not argue for doing so. However, while many in the movement embrace the term, others (including those who teach disability pedagogy) are now striving to promote new terms that connote positive values of difference, such as ability pedagogy. The classic predicament with all names for particular identities is that not everyone will understand the term or even be aware that it exists, thus forcing the focus group to put a great deal of energy into promoting the name and its correct and respected definition (Snyder et al. 2002).

Much of the theoretical work on disability studies is centered on terminology, because of the diverse array of imagery related to people with disabilities. There are currently two major points being made by the disability rights movement to correct negative perceptions of the differently abled. The first of these is that they are not disabled, meaning they are not deformed, lame, or broken, nor do they have something wrong with them that needs to be fixed. They are ideal the way they are. This point has two concerns. The first is that society's exclusion of difference and the reinforcement of the social construction of normalcy are a problem (Fulcher 1999) that allows capital to exclude people with disabilities from economic life. The second concern is that until all are accepted in society, there is truly an identifiable group that needs assistance and is challenged in our current exclusionary society (Snyder and Mitchell 2006).

The second main point is the theoretical understanding of all disability activists, which is that all people are different and have unique needs. This point is critical to understanding how society identifies people's roles. We must recognize that <u>normal</u>, <u>average</u>, and <u>able</u> are socially constructed terms that can and must change. Disability rights activists are also critical of the capitalist system insofar as it tries to reduce our humanity and citizenship functions to the roles of producer and consumer, both of which support capitalism. Consumption supports the engines of production because people have to work in order to buy, and ideologically capitalism captures their desires and economic support (Gramsci 1989; Marcuse 1969).

Similarly disability activists critique the norm of a "productive" employee, student, daughter, son, or parent. There is no measurement for an individual except within the context of that individual. Nothing is objective and able to be measured in a detached state. Let us analyze some of the standard definitions of the names given to those identified as disabled. <u>The American Heritage Dictionary of the English Language</u> (2009) defines <u>illness</u> as "poor health resulting from disease of body or mind; sickness," and <u>disease</u> as "a pathological condition of a part, organ, or system of an organism resulting from various causes, such as infection, genetic defect, or environmental stress, and characterized by an identifiable group of signs or symptoms." Disease is defined as "a condition or tendency, as of society, regarded as abnormal and harmful." Disability has traditionally been associated with illness and disease. Yet this socially constructed meaning cannot be understood without examining the notion of normalcy. Normal is defined as "relating to or characterized by average intelligence or development," and normalcy (derived from normal) means therefore "free[dom] from mental illness; sane. Conforming with, adhering to, or constituting a norm, standard, pattern, level, or type; typical." Fulcher (1999, 25) writes, "Disability is primarily a political construct rather than a medical phenomenon."

With this backdrop it comes as no surprise that disability is understood as "the condition of being disabled; incapacity"; that it is stigmatized as "a disadvantage or deficiency, especially a physical or mental impairment that interferes with or prevents normal achievement in a particular area" and is defined as "something that hinders or incapacitates." As the definitions build on each other we see the repeated theme of "something wrong with," incapable, harmful, or sick (The American Heritage Dictionary of the English Language 2009). In contemporary society these are the terms that are used interchangeably with disability. But by measuring everyone according to this imaginary notion of a "normal person," society is inclusive only of certain types of people, nonhuman animals, elements, and plants. Those that are excluded and identified as the abnormal include the wild, the savage, those with disabilities, the purely animalistic, and the violent. Put those five characteristics together and you construct what filmmakers and storytellers identify as monsters. Monsters are uncivilized savages; wild, not domestic; with disabilities, not able-bodied; violent, not peaceful; and animalistic, not humanistic.

The social constructions of terms such as normalcy, ableism, and civilization have been put in the service of domination for political power, economic gain, and social control. Those in power used them to establish a superior (dominator) versus inferior (dominated) binary, which has repeatedly played out in theories, beliefs, cultures, and identities. People are typically judged against the standard of a "normal" human; those who choose not to, or simply cannot strive toward the norm because of their identity, politics, or social and economic factors, are labeled "abnormal." Within this context ableism is a social construct, which suggests that society should manipulate those individuals whose capabilities fall outside the "norm" in an attempt to reach the same physical and mental abilities as those considered "normal," instead of being accepting and inclusive toward all.

While it has been used as a key term for unifying and bringing attention to the topic (e.g., disability studies), disability is still a term that has been challenged and manipulated by groups attempting to "take back" the terms and own them, similar to other marginalized groups owning terms previously considered derogatory. These newer fields of inquiry include disability studies, crip studies, and mad studies. Still disability studies in education can be regarded as the "new" special education field, which only reinforces a socially constructed binary. All are disabled in some way because of exclusionary social identities that limit one's life activities. These exclusionary practices are not due to various medical conditions or factors such as being a woman, tall, short, a person of color, young, elderly, LGBTQIA, non-Christian, not formally educated, a noncitizen of a country, someone with physical and mental differences, or any other nondominant identity. Unless and until we recognize this, disability will continue to be one of the most demeaning labels and identifications human or nonhuman animals, elements, plants, water, and air can be given, even more so than being called "wild" or "an animal," because disability is a label solely constructed by those in power to stigmatize and marginalize others as abnormal.

NOTES

1. I would like to thank Kim Socha for helping to edit this chapter and for her important input.
2. This section was adapted from my personal website biography, www .anthonynocella.org, and Nocella 2008.
3. This section was adapted from Nocella 2008.

REFERENCES

The American Heritage Dictionary of the English Language. 2009. 4th ed. Boston: Houghton Mifflin. http://www.thefreedictionary.com.

Amster, Randall, Abraham DeLeon, Luis Fernandez, Anthony J. Nocella II, and Deric Shannon, eds. 2009. Contemporary Anarchist Studies: An Introductory Anthology of Anarchy in the Academy. New York: Routledge.

Aquinas, Thomas. 2007. Summa Theologica. Vol. 3. New York: Cosimo.

Armstrong, Felicity, Derrick Armstrong, and Len Barton. 2000. Inclusive Education: Policy, Contexts and Comparative Perspectives. London: David Fulton.

Bauman, Zygmunt. 2001. Modernity and the Holocaust. Ithaca NY: Cornell University Press.

Ben-Moshe, Liat. 2011. Genealogies of Resistance to Incarceration: Abolition Politics within the Deinstitutionalization and Anti-Prison Activism in the U.S. Syracuse NY: Syracuse University.

Ben-Moshe, Liat, Dave Hill, Anthony J. Nocella II, and Bill Templer. 2009. "Dis-abling Capitalism and an Anarchism of 'Radical Equality' in Resistance to Ideologies of Normalcy." In Contemporary Anarchist Studies: An Introductory Anthology of Anarchy in the Academy, edited by Randall Amster, Abraham DeLeon, Luis Fernandez, Anthony J. Nocella II, and Deric Shannon, 113–22. New York: Routledge.

Best, Steven, and Anthony J. Nocella II. 2006. Igniting a Revolution: Voices in Defense of the Earth. Oakland CA: AK Press.

Binet, Alfred, and Theodore Simon. 1973. The Development of Intelligence in Children (the Binet-Simon Scale). New York: Arno Press.

Bodley, John H. 2005. Cultural Anthropology: Tribes, States, and the Global System. New York: McGraw-Hill.

Bogdan, Robert. 1988. Freak Show: Presenting Human Oddities for Amusement and Profit. Chicago: University of Chicago Press.

Bullard, Robert D., ed. 1993. Confronting Environmental Racism: Voices from the Grassroots. Boston: South End Press.

Center for Universal Design. 2010. "About." http://www.ncsu.edu/project/de-sign-projects/udilcenter-for-universal-design/.

Corbett, Jenny. 1995. Bad-Mouthing: The Language of Special Needs. New York: Routledge.

Corrigan, Patrick W. 2006. On the Stigma of Mental Illness: Practical Strategies for Research and Social Change. Washington DC: American Psychological Association.

Davis, Lennard. 1997. The Disability Studies Reader. New York: Routledge.

———. 2002. Bending over Backwards: Disability, Dismodernism and Other Difficult Positions. New York: New York University Press.

Derrickson, Scott, director. 2008. The Day the Earth Stood Still. Los Angeles: Twentieth Century Fox Film Corporation.

Dowbiggin, Ian Robert. 2003. Keeping America Sane: Psychiatry and Eugenics in the United States and Canada, 1880–1940. Ithaca NY: Cornell University Press.

Dunayer, Joan. 2004. Speciesism. New York: Lantern Books.

Effron, Lauren, and Russell Goldman. 2010. "Environmental Militant Killed by Police at Discovery Channel Headquarters." ABC News, September 1. http://abcnews.go.com/US/gunman-enters-discovery-channel-headquarters-employees-evacuated/story?id=11535128.

Fassbinder, Samuel, Anthony J. Nocella II, and R. Kahn. In press. Greening the Academy. Rotterdam, The Netherlands: Sense.

Fleischer, Doris Z., and Frieda Zames. 2001. The Disability Rights Movement: From Charity to Confrontation. Philadelphia: Temple University Press.

Francione, Gary L. 2000. Introduction to Animal Rights: Your Child or the Dog? Philadelphia: Temple University Press.

———. 2009. "A Note on Moral Schizophrenia." Animal Rights: The Abolitionist Approach, August 12. http://www.abolitionistapproach .com/a-note-on-moral-schizophrenia/#.V72WT5grKhc.

Fulcher, Gillian. 1999. Disabling Policies? A Comparative Approach to Education Policy and Disability. New ed. Sheffield, UK: Philip Armstrong.

Gaard, Greta. 1993. Ecofeminism: Women, Animals, Nature. Philadelphia: Temple University Press.

Goffman, Erving. 1963. Stigma: Notes on the Management of Spoiled Identity. New York: Simon & Schuster.

Gramsci, Antonio. 1989. Selections from the Prison Notebooks of Antonio Gramsci. New York: International.

Harding, Sandra, ed. 2003. The Feminist Standpoint Theory Reader: Intellectual and Political Controversies. New York: Routledge.

Linton, Simi. 1998. Claiming Disability: Knowledge and Identity. New York: New York University Press.

Marcuse, Herbert. 1969. An Essay on Liberation. Boston: Beacon Press.

Nocella, Anthony J., II. 2008. "Emergence of Disability Pedagogy." Journal for Critical Education Policy Studies 6, no. 2: 77–94.

Nocella, Anthony J., II, Judy K. C. Bentley, and Janet Duncan. 2012. Earth, Animal, and Disability Liberation: The Rise of the Eco-ability Movement. New York: Peter Lang.

Pfohl, Stephen. 2009. Images of Deviance and Social Control A Sociological History. 2d ed. Long Grove IL: Waveland Press.

Rosenau, Pauline M. 1992. Post-modernism and the Social Sciences: Insights, Inroads, and Intrusions. Princeton NJ: Princeton University Press.

Schou, Nick. 2006. Kill the Messenger: How the CIA's Crack-Cocaine Controversy Destroyed Journalist Gary Webb. New York: Nation Books.

Scott, Peter Dale, and Jonathan Marshall. 1998. Cocaine Politics: Drugs, Armies, and the CIA in Central America. Updated ed. Berkeley: University of California Press.

Smith, Robin M., and Jack P. Manno. 2008. "Disability Studies and the Social Construction of Environments." Social Advocacy and Systems Change 1, no. 1. http://webhost1.cortland.edu/sasc/wp-content /uploads/sites/12/2012/12/earth_smith_manno.pdf

Snyder, Sharon L., Brenda Jo Brueggemann, and Rosemarie Garland-Thomson. 2002. Disability Studies: Enabling the Humanities. New York: Modern Language Association of America.

Snyder, Sharon L., and David T. Mitchell. 2006. Cultural Locations of Disability. Chicago: University of Chicago Press.

Snyder, Zack, director. 2006. 300. Hollywood: Warner Bros. Pictures.

Swan, Jim. 2002. "Disabilities, Bodies, Voices." In Disability Studies: Enabling the Humanities, edited by S. L. Snyder, B. J. Brueggemann, and Rosemarie Garland-Thomson, 283–95. New York: Modern Language Association of America.

Taylor, Steve. 1996. "Disability Studies and Mental Retardation." Disability Studies Quarterly 16, no. 3: 4–13.

Tokar, Brian. 1997. Earth for Sale: Reclaiming Ecology in the Age of Corporate Greenwash. Boston: South End Press.

Torres, Bob, and Jenna Torres. 2010. Vegan Freak: Being Vegan in a Non-Vegan World: Version 2.0. Revised ed. Oakland CA: Tofu Hound Press.

van der Pijl, Kees. 2007. Nomads, Empires, States: Modes of Foreign Relations and Political Economy. Vol. 1. London: Pluto Press.

Webb, Gary. 1999. Dark Alliance: The CIA, the Contras, and the Crack Cocaine Explosion. New York: Seven Stories Press.

5

The Ecosomatic Paradigm in Literature
Merging Disability Studies and Ecocriticism

Matthew J. C. Cella

> Maps render foreign territory, however dark and wide,
> fathomable. I mean to make a map. My infinitely harder
> task, then, is to conceptualize not merely a habitable
> body but a habitable world: a world that wants me in it.
>
> —Nancy Mairs, <u>Waist-High in the World</u>

The cartographic metaphor that Mairs (1996) employs in the epigraph calls attention to the double-edged challenge that she faces as the result of her multiple sclerosis: as the number and severity of bodily impairments connected to her disease increase, Mairs must continually renegotiate both her sense of self and her place in the world. That is, not only does she have to reconcile herself to her changing body, but she also has to learn how to navigate a world that privileges the able-bodied and that is therefore a less habitable (and even disabling) world for those with physical and cognitive impairments. Through maps made of words—like each of the essays collected in <u>Waist-High in the World</u>, for example—Mairs is able to conceptualize a new way of being in the world, one that imagines her wheelchair-bound body at the middle of an ongoing collaboration between her changing body and the various places (built and wild) that she inhabits. In this way Mairs's cartographic metaphor highlights the deep entanglement of bodies and places. This deep entanglement—

the dialectic of embodiment and emplacement—is the central subject of this essay as this dialectic forms the basis for what I call the ecosomatic paradigm. The ecosomatic paradigm assumes contiguity between the mind-body and its social and natural environments; thus, under this scheme, the work of negotiating a "habitable body" and "habitable world" go hand in hand.

My primary contention is that the scrutiny of literary representations of the ecosomatic paradigm, particularly those focused on people with disabilities, provides a key method with which to deconstruct norms of embodiment while simultaneously promoting ethical treatment of the natural world. It is through the unearthing and analysis of the ecosomatic paradigm in literature that literary ecologists—who are already attuned to the importance of place—can best contribute to the ongoing work of disability studies and vice versa. Indeed the ecosomatic approach relies heavily on the cross-fertilization of ecocriticism and disability studies, and I believe these two fields of inquiry have much to offer each other.[1] In fleshing out the parameters of the ecosomatic paradigm in literature, I draw on two related concepts, both of which emphasize the inseparability of bodies and places: first, the sociocultural model of disability, which is the centerpiece of critical disability studies, and, second, the metaphor of "universal flesh," particularly as employed in Edward Casey's (1993) phenomenological study of the place-world and his defense of ecocentrism. In the first section of the essay I use the social model of disability to challenge the ableist premise of Casey's phenomenology of place, while simultaneously emphasizing the mutual ecosomatic concerns of the two theoretical approaches. I then read Cormac McCarthy's (2006) The Road as an allegory of the social model, one that demonstrates how a deeper consideration of environmental contexts can further trouble the able-bodied/disabled dyad. In the second section I return to Casey's work on the body and consider the "universal flesh," which he borrows from Merleau-Ponty (1969), as a powerful ecosomatic metaphor that has equally strong implications for renegotiating norms of embodiment as it does for promoting ethical and ecocentric encounters with the natural world. The dynamic interplay between embodiment and emplacement—and its implications for the natural world and its inhabitants—is central to Linda Hogan's (1997) novel <u>Solar Storms</u>, which I analyze in detail to further exemplify how an interrogation of the ecosomatic paradigm in literature can advance the goals of ecocritics and disability scholars alike.

Disability, Emplacement, and the Social Model

A mutual emphasis on place is a useful foundation upon which to establish a dialogue between disability studies and literary ecology. As Casey (1993) documents throughout his phenomenological analysis of place, the body is a pivotal component of the place-making process, to the point that embodiment and emplacement are almost synonymous. In the preface to <u>Getting Back into Place</u>, a philosophical and ecocritical examination of the place-world, Casey argues, "Place ushers us into what <u>already is</u>: namely, the environing subsoil of our embodiment, the bedrock of our being-in-the-world" (xvii). As he documents over the five parts of his book, this status of being-in-the-world is informed by our intellectual traditions concerning place, our ways of moving within space, our modes of dwelling in and around built places, our encounters with wilderness, and our experiences journeying between different places. Central to all of these aspects of place-experience is the body. Orientation and emplacement require a dialectical engagement between our lived bodies and our environment. Casey explains, "If I am to get oriented in a landscape or sea-scape (especially one that is unknown or subject to a sudden or unpredictable variation), I must bring my body into conformity with the configurations of the land or the sea. . . . The conjoining of the surface of my body with the surface of the earth or sea—their common integumentation—generates the interspace in which I become oriented" (28). The alternative is displacement and desolation, a kind of "place pathology" (38).

A key part of the emplacement equation, Casey contends, is the body-in-motion. Our understanding of the multidimensionality of place—here and there, up and down, near and far, and so on—occurs through a series of ongoing movements, precipitated by the body, in and between places. Casey writes, "My body continually takes me into place. It is at once agent and vehicle, articulator and witness of being-in-place. Although we rarely attend to its exact role, once we do we cannot help but notice its importance. Without the good graces and excellent services of our bodies, not only would we be lost in place—acutely disoriented and confused—we would have no coherent sense of place itself" (48). It is important here to call attention to the fact that Casey's phenomenology of place more or less presumes a compulsory able-bodiedness; this is to say that as thorough as his examination of the body's experience of place is, he does not account for the disabled body. The theoretical body that he imagines in his calculations is one much like his own. In fact many of the illustrations he uses to flesh out his narrative of the place-world come from his own able-bodied experiences, which he takes as the default. In his chapter on directionality, for example, he alludes to the importance of sight as the primary sense in the place-making and orientation process, noting how "the primacy of vision contributes powerfully to the dominance of the forward direction" (84). This raises questions about how emplacement works for those who are born blind and how relationships to place change for those who become blind later in their lives. Furthermore Casey builds his case for ecocentrism in the penultimate chapter of his book by positing the acts of "walking" and "ambling," particularly as described by Henry David Thoreau and John Muir, as powerful metaphors for the dialectic between body and environment and proscribes them as ideal processes through which we get back into place. What happens when bodily impairments alter or severely limit motion? Are such bodies doomed to suffer eternally from place pathology, forever disoriented and displaced?

By posing such hyperbolic questions, I do not mean to discount Casey's analysis of the place-world; while stemming from an able-bodied perspective, his mapping of the relationship between embodiment and emplacement provides a steady foundation for an inclusive ecosomatic paradigm. What I hope to draw attention to in raising these questions is the perhaps too obvious fact that not all mind-bodies are the same. The larger question, then, is: How might we modify the narrative of place to account for a wider variety of bodies and even for the multiple variations a single body might go through as it changes due to aging, illness, or accidents? For example, Casey highlights how transitions between places are often accompanied by feelings of desolation and displacement, as the embodied subject mourns the place she is leaving behind. Considering the deep entanglement of bodies and environments, it logically follows that changes to the subject's body may also bring on this feeling of displacement, even if the embodied subject remains in a place familiar to her. Again, as Mairs's comment in the epigraph suggests, changes to the body lead to subsequent changes in one's perception of and experience with being in the world. The title of Mairs's (1996) book, Waist-High in the World, is a nod toward this very notion, as Mairs remaps the world from the point of view of her impaired, wheelchair-bound body.

What adding a disability perspective to place-studies draws attention to most powerfully, however, is not the disabled subject's emotional and intellectual process of re/emplacement but the disabling elements of the built environment. In this sense issues of place are a central aspect of recent scholarship on disability, particularly those strands that rely upon the social model, with its emphasis on the spatial and place-based contexts that define disability. With origins in "Fundamental Principles of Disability," published in 1976 by the Union of the Physically Impaired against Segregation (UPIAS), the social model has continued to take shape over the past three decades and has developed many branches, often complementary but sometimes contradictory. As a whole, however, the various strands of social model theory share the fundamental principles as first outlined by the UPIAS. In her overview of the evolution of the social model, Claire Tregaskis (2002, 457) summarizes these principles, noting their emphasis on the need to "[challenge] disabled people's own internalized oppression by enabling them to make sense of their experience in a way which explains that it is not, after all, 'their own fault' that they face discrimination and social exclusion. Instead, responsibility for that exclusion is placed at the door of a normalizing society that has rigidly developed and maintained structures to . . . reward those who most closely conform to socially prescribed models of appearance and behavior." In essence the social model provides a vehicle for the important work of redefining disability and taking it out of the purview of medical discourse. As Simi Linton (1998, 11) argues in her landmark book, <u>Claiming Disability: Knowledge and Identity</u>, "the medicalization of disability casts human variation as deviance from the norm, as pathological condition, as deficit, and, significantly, as an individual burden and personal tragedy." Disability studies, on the other hand, recasts disability as something <u>created</u> by discriminatory social, political, and economic practices and environments. So rather than focus on treating "the condition and the person with the condition," disability activists instead spotlight "'treating' the social processes and policies that constrict disabled people's lives" (11).

One of the derivatives of this shift from a medical definition of disability to a social definition is that the social model places great emphasis on the <u>contexts</u> that create disability; that is, it moves the focus away from viewing the impaired mind-body as an isolated phenomenon and instead highlights the mind-body's relationship to the places it occupies. Admittedly this shared concern in disability studies and ecocriticism for spatial (or, more broadly, environmental) contexts provides somewhat tenuous ground for a coalition between the two fields. The problem has to do with the divide between the decidedly sociopolitical schema of disability studies and the alleged asocial tendencies of ecological criticism. The environmental contexts that disability studies scholars are most concerned with are, after all, predominantly social ones: the built environments and sociopolitical transformations of space into places that create disability. The earliest versions of social model theory developed by scholars like Michael Oliver and Vic Finkelstein examined how "the experience of disability depends on the sort of society we live in" and pointed out, for example, the disabling effects of capitalism in Great Britain (Tregaskis 2002, 460). The focus, in other words, tends to be on how social systems and policies create disability by placing barriers on individuals with physical and mental impairments. Understandably there is little need to consider the nonhuman community, or at least dimensions of the natural world that are unsocialized. To put it simply, looking at Yellowstone National Park through a disability studies lens means not focusing on the flora and fauna that define the place but instead examining whether the National Park Service's management of the park's facilities limits or promotes access for those with physical or mental impairments. So while the consideration of place is a necessary aspect of both theoretical approaches, this factor alone is not enough to bridge the gap between disabilities studies and ecological criticism. But it is, I contend, a starting point: if a shared emphasis on place is not a bridge, it is at least an important connecting thread.

As a metaphor, a way of organizing human perceptions about the natural world, the ecosomatic paradigm has the potential to reorient our way of thinking about the relationship between the body and the social and natural environments it inhabits. It presents an ideal model for eradicating disability in the manner imagined and theorized by scholars like Tregaskis, who pursue a social constructionist approach to disability. As Solveig Mangus Reindal (2010, 127) notes, Tregaskis represents an extreme idealistic position wherein she argues that disability could be outright eliminated if society was reorganized in such a manner that it accounted for the needs of every one of its members. In this vein Peter Freund (2001, 689), for example, has suggested ways in which "transport-public space" might be structured to accommodate the majority of human mind-body types that maneuver through space in different ways, whether walking or in wheelchairs. He asks us to "move from asking what <u>bodies</u> can function in a particular context . . . to asking what types of structures can accommodate the widest range of bodies" (691). To this end Freund advances the "architectural paradigm" of "universal design"—a "minority voice in the chorus of architects"—to illustrate the practical ways in which, "over time, deconstructing and reconstructing the social organization of space would benefit many bodies, not merely those that are impaired. . . . We must <u>universalize</u> non-disabling spatial organization" (704).[2] Whether it is the architecture of individual buildings or the broader architecture of urban and regional planning, the idea is that social and political organization needs to structure and restructure space to universalize access.

Many within and outside of disability studies have questioned, and rightly so, the viability of this idealistic approach. Indeed much of the criticism concerning the social model in general stems from what Reindal (2010, 127) refers to as the "over-socializing of the phenomenon of disability." While most disability studies scholars agree that social barriers are a major impediment to the lives of people with disability, many express concern that the social model does not fully or properly account for the experience of impairment and the limitations that such impairments impose on disabled people's lives no matter what the social environment.[3] As J. R. Richards argues, a paraplegic may very well maneuver with ease around a town structured on the principles of universal design, but still "there would be problems about trying to keep with a party climbing in the Himalayas" (qtd. in Reindal 2010, 127). One cannot theorize away limitations imposed by bodily impairments.

I am not an architect, nor a sociologist or regional planner, for that matter, so I am not equipped to address the practical applications or implications of a "universal design" approach to disability. And I agree with critics of the social model who call for greater attention to the experience of impairment and who emphasize what Tobin Siebers (2001, 747) calls "the new realism of the body." I am particularly interested, though, in exploring the dialectic between the body (and the experience of the subject) and the structure of the social and natural environments in which it is situated; the social model, particularly in Freund's (2001, 691) sociomaterial analysis of it, ultimately "recognizes the inseparability of the body from its social structural, material integument." I am interested, then, in how the social model underscores the experiential and theoretical contiguity of the body and its surrounding environment. I think there is room to develop the social and ecological applications that such an idea as contiguity makes possible. Furthermore I think there is much to be gained by taking an ecological approach to the social model to see how the land community operates as an organizing structure and to examine what kind of potential such an approach has for redefining disability.

McCarthy's (2006) Pulitzer Prize–winning novel, The Road, is particularly instructive here because it documents how modes of embodiment and emplacement must be renegotiated by the novel's protagonists in the face of environmental devastation. In this manner McCarthy's novel may be read as an allegory for the social model, one that employs the ecosomatic paradigm to both deconstruct conventional norms of embodiment and to offer a cautionary tale about impending environmental degradation. The action of the novel can be summed up as follows: In the aftermath of an unspecified apocalyptic event, the world has become an ashen and cold place where most living things have died. Those who are still alive can be broken down into two basic categories: those who cannibalize ("the bad guys," as McCarthy's protagonists label them) and those who do not (those who "carry the fire"). The narrative follows an unnamed father and son as they travel through this barren landscape—what was once the southern Appalachians—hoping to find better and warmer conditions near the coast. The journey to the coast is a hazardous one, simultaneously tragic and beautiful as the father and son confront the best and worst of humanity.

The postapocalyptic setting is an intriguing one from a social model perspective because it represents an environment stripped of all but the most rudimentary social structures. This stripped-down environment and the various figures that move across it help to demonstrate the power of place within the social model in a couple of significant ways. First, the human body's relation to space and place in this postapocalyptic landscape is altered completely, as the relationship between signs and the signified that existed in the preapocalyptic world—ostensibly our world—has been unalterably deconstructed. The narrator reveals this fact by describing the status of this new world, its defining nondefinitiveness: "Everything uncoupled from its shoring. Unsupported in the ashen air" (11). This semiotic erosion is a tragic circumstance of the postapocalyptic world, particularly from the point of view of the father, whose ties to the forms that defined the old world are a constant source of sorrow and loss. It is also a difficult, near-impossible place to inhabit. But it is a difficult, near-impossible place to inhabit for all bodies, from the young to the old and from the healthy to the infirm. Furthermore because the landscape is devoid of meaningful physical or social structures, it presents an intriguing reverse example of the "universal design" metaphor, that ideal mode of spatial organization that seeks to accommodate as many mind-body types as possible. Because the ashen wilderness makes its demands equally on all comers, the category of disability is, like most other things in The Road's world, stripped of its meaning.

Second, from a social model perspective, the unmade (or remade) world in The Road destabilizes the notion of a normative mind-body and thereby explodes the distinction between able-bodiedness and dis-ability. Particularly instructive is Rosemarie Garland-Thomson's (1997, 9) coinage of the term normate, which "designates the social figure through which people can represent themselves as definitive human beings." The normate is a "constructed identity" that grants authority and power based on a series of overlapping hierarchies involving gender, race, sexuality, and mind-body types; thus the normative heterosexual, able-bodied, Caucasian male provides the model through which alternative configurations are perceived as deviations. Such a construction is responsible for a series of economic and political oppressions that limit the agency of those who cannot claim normate status. Within the fictional world of The Road the figure of the normate in the preapocalyptic world—the healthy and unimpaired body—is reinscribed by McCarthy in the new world as a sign of moral corruption. The blood cults, whose members manifest healthy bodies by the old normative standard, must be viewed as anything but normal. Their vigor and average body weight signal their cannibalism and designate them as the "bad guys." Conversely the emaciated and weakened bodies of the "good guys" represent the new standard, redefining emaciation, at least on a symbolic level, as a sign of strength and moral fortitude. Such a reversal, of course, is hard to conceive when measured by the standards familiar to us in the here and now. But this reversal powerfully reveals the central claim of the social model: the social-environmental context has the power to disable the impaired body. If you change the context, you can liberate the body by eliminating disability as a defining marker of difference. In the postapocalyptic world that McCarthy imagines in The Road, the dramatic changes wrought by environmental ruination even work to cast deviant forms of embodiment—bodies wracked to the point of near death—as beautiful.

This environmentally influenced redefinition of the norms of embodiment is subtly reinforced by McCarthy's emphasis on the troubling effects of the father's normative color perception. One of the recurring sources of sorrow and nostalgia for the father is connected to the fact that the world as he knew it has literally lost its color. First, most things, living and built, have burned to ash; second, the ubiquity of ash in the atmosphere blocks the sunlight and casts a grayish hue over the whole landscape. The novel is replete with descriptions of the grayscale reality of the postapocalyptic world: the opening two sentences alone contain four references to the <u>dark</u> and <u>gray</u> cast to the landscape, only to be followed in the third sentence with a simile that compares seeing in the new world to "some cold glaucoma dimming away the world" (3). Just as this postapocalyptic world establishes emaciation and sickness as the new norm, it also establishes impaired vision (and what we might call color deficiency) as the new standard of seeing—one not shaped by biological determinants (there are no Ishihara tests to measure such things after an apocalypse, after all), but one determined instead by the environment. For the boy, who was raised under these conditions, the subtraction of color does not necessarily detract from his aesthetic experience of the world; although disappointed that the ocean is gray and not blue (as his father told him it used to be), the boy still establishes a connection to the sea and is eager to go for a swim. For the father, however, memories of the Technicolor world continually enter his consciousness and agitate his state of being comfortable in the new world. Early in the novel, for example, he stares in awe at the orange flames of a forest fire, and the limited omniscient narrator explains, "The color of it moved something in him long forgotten. Make a list. Recite a litany. Remember" (31). His nostalgia for the once colorful world is moving, and his need to commit this old world to memory is heroic; however, this same nostalgia upends his ability to fully adapt to the conditions of the new world. As he nears death toward the end of the novel, the father's dreams are increasingly driven by a longing to return to the world-as-it-was: "In the nights sometimes he'd wake in the black and freezing waste out of softly colored worlds of human love, the songs of birds, the sun" (272). While the colors of the postapocalyptic environment are muted, the birds likely gone forever, and the sun blotted out by the clouds of ash, these realities do not affect the son in the same way as they do the father because, again, such conditions are all the son has ever known. That the son's evolution as an embodied subject is shaped by these conditions is a key factor in his survival.

The son's survival, beyond merely deconstructing the figure of the normate, establishes an ecosomatic paradigm of identity that privileges interdependence and cooperation. What ultimately passes as ideal behavior in the new world resides in establishing connections among the "good guys" and forging a community defined by a shared need to survive and adapt to the challenges proffered by the postapocalyptic physical environment. It is on this point that the father and son differ in their approach to the new world order. The son's compassion toward the fellow travelers they meet on the road—including a lost boy and an old man who has been struck by lightning—reveals a deep understanding of the body-environment relationship. Born and raised in this postapocalyptic world, the boy implicitly understands how the ashen environment equalizes all mind-bodies that inhabit it. The father, on the other hand, largely in an effort to protect his son and himself, devises a social structure that places their family at the center (a kind of myopic normative standard) and then defines all others as falling into two equally problematic categories: burdensome or cannibalistic. The son understands that there is a difference between those who hunt humans and those who do not, but he otherwise operates from a paradigm of equality, seeing the need to form coalitions with the other survivors. He is more trusting and open than his father, in part because he is younger but also because he approaches his situation and environment without the baggage of old protocols and without mourning the old forms. The boy's instinct toward cooperation and community—forged in the wild and barren environment that is and has always been his home place—ultimately saves him, as he is absorbed into a new family he meets along the coast after his father dies.

Reading McCarthy's novel through a bifocal lens that merges disability studies and literary ecology ultimately raises some interesting questions worth pursuing. To what degree does the physical environment model the principles of universal design, and what might ecology contribute to the advancement of social model theory? What is to be gained by defining the variety of mind-body configurations not by their individual characteristics alone but also by their relationships with and dependencies upon other bodies, human and nonhuman? What might also be gained when these relationships and dependencies are recognized as central components of both embodiment and emplacement?

These are the kinds of questions an ecosomatic approach to literature seeks to answer, and it does so, as I have already suggested, by foregrounding the dialectical relationship between the individual subject and its ecological context. What the social model and Freund's (2001) use of universal design draws attention to is the very notion at the core of the ecosomatic paradigm: places function as contact zones between the human mind-body and its environment so that the embodied subject is part of, and not separate from, the places it inhabits and moves through. One of the implications of this deep association is that the goal of liberating the mind-body (a primary objective of disability studies) is concomitant with the goal of ecological stewardship (a primary objective of ecological criticism). As I document in the following section, Casey's (1993) expansion of the "universal flesh" concept establishes a firm foundation upon which to build a coalition between disability studies and ecological criticism.

The "Universal Flesh": Bodies in the Place-World

It is in the "Going Wild in the Land" chapter that Casey (1993) most fully articulates the significance of the body-environment dialectic, which is a vital component of his overall defense of an ecocentric ethic. In this chapter he considers and ultimately rejects two extreme ways of approaching the nature/culture dyad: one that views wilderness as "culture-free" (233) and the other that sees wilderness as utterly "culture bound" (235). What he ultimately concludes is that the two, nature and culture, are impossible to separate: "Rather than thinking of Nature and Culture as antipodes between which we must make a forced choice, we ought to regard them as coexisting in various forms of commixture within a middle realm, a genuine 'multifarious between,' in which the partners are in a relation of 'consanguinity'" (242).

The most concrete sign of this "middle realm" is the embodied subject who is both natural—as in a part of nature—and culturally conditioned. He builds off of Merleau-Ponty's (1969) idea of the "universal flesh," seeing such a notion as the culmination of what he argues throughout the book. Casey (1993, 255) writes, "In this encompassing circumstance, there is a co-emplacement of the natural and the cultural such that each can be said to flesh out the other or to give the other consistency and substance. Or more exactly, each is a phase or region of a more encompassing flesh. If 'the world is universal flesh,' such flesh is neither matter alone nor mind alone but something running through both, a common 'element,' as it were." To conceive of the world as such is to see that our bodies and the natural world, as Casey argues, "are not just conterminous but continuous with each other" (255). To imagine this universal flesh and the layers of bodies and places that make up the encompassing world is akin to imagining a universal design that accommodates the full spectrum of mind-body types. While a frigid breeze or the physical strain of crossing a rugged, rocky terrain—or even the pain and discomfort associated with physical impairment—might consistently jar us into an awareness of our body as distinct and separate from our surroundings, our contiguity with the wild and built places cannot be denied since even these experiences of disconnection are themselves situated in place. The ecosomatic paradigm foregrounds the inseparability of ecological context and somatic experience; as a metaphor it calls into consciousness and makes tangible the ways in which our bodies and the places we inhabit are "continuous with each other." This contiguity, as I will outline in my discussion of Hogan's (1997) novel, has obvious ethical consequences related to how we interact with other bodies and the places that encompass them.

The ecosomatic paradigm builds on the assumption that the association between people and places, as Francesco Loriggio (1994, 6) contends, is part of an ongoing process predicated on the "dialectic of what there is and what people believe or imagine there is." What we "believe or imagine" is shaped and articulated, in large part, by literary art and certainly by the stories we tell, hear, and repeat. Literature and storytelling are powerful forces in shaping our individual and collective environmental imaginations. Casey (1993, 254) would refer to the work that literature does as "thickening," the label he uses to describe the process wherein "something <u>emerges</u> from the . . . dense coalescence of cultural practices and natural givens." An ecocritic might call this process "developing a sense of place"—envisioning the deep entanglement between the natural and cultural parameters of place. As the geographer J. Nicholas Entrikin (1991, 5) explains, narrative is one of the most effective tools for explaining and investigating the complex nature of our relationships with places: "To understand place requires that we have access to both an objective and a subjective reality. From [a] decentered vantage point . . . place becomes either location or a set of generic relations and thereby loses much of its significance for human action. From the centered view-point of the subject, place has meaning only in relation to an individual's or a group's goals and concerns.

Place is best viewed from points in between." Because narrative provides a form that allows for the synthesis of the decentered (natural, objective) and centered (social, subjective) dimensions of place, it offers perhaps the clearest view of this in-betweenness. In narrative, storytellers can pull together the disparate elements of place into a representative whole. Literary narrative provides a means to organize and mediate this complicated process of emplacement. Although Entrikin's overall aim is to emphasize the usefulness of a narrative-like approach to the geographical study of place, his conclusions also make clear the value of place-oriented literary ecology precisely because literary narrative can provide insight into both the human endeavor of place-making (and unmaking and remaking) and how this endeavor is influenced by the overlapping social, historical, and ecological contexts in which it is undertaken.

As David Mitchell and Sharon Snyder (2000) have persuasively shown, literary narrative also gives us fodder for understanding the place of disability within our culture. Through much of their work, particularly Narrative Prosthesis: Disability and the Dependencies of Discourse, they point to "the prevalence of disability representation [in narrative art] and the myriad meanings ascribed to it" (4). They refer to this prevalence as "narrative prosthesis," which "mediates between the realm of the literary and the realm of the body" and therefore provides a "way of situating a discussion about disability within a literary domain while keeping watch on its social context" (7, 9). While "stereotypical portrayals and reductive metaphors" abound in literature, Mitchell and Snyder contend that with the right methodology and interpretive schema there is much to be learned about disability and norms of embodiment from our stories (163). A crucial aspect of the methodology involves paying attention to the social and historical contexts of narratives that employ disability as a metaphor or trope or that feature characters with disabilities. They write, "Since the seemingly abstract and textual world affects the psychology of individuals (and, thus, the cultural imaginary), the interpretation of these figures and their reception proves paramount to the contribution of the humanities to disability studies. One cannot assess the merits or demerits of a literary portrait, for example, without understanding the historical context within which it was constructed and imbibed" (42). In historicizing literary representations of disability, the literary critic performs work that has the potential to liberate and expand our understanding of embodiment.

The ecosomatic approach to literature I am proposing here is an extension of the narrative prosthesis idea, one that scrutinizes the ecological as well as social-historical contexts of literary representations of embodiment. That is, the ecosomatic approach recognizes the variety of somatic experience and seeks to nullify the able-bodied/disabled dyad by emphasizing the metaphorical power of considering the impaired body in relation to its environmental situatedness. Ultimately literary narratives that incorporate an ecosomatic imperative highlight the role the mind-body plays in the process of emplacement and thereby have the capacity to reorient our sense of and behavior toward both the human body and the natural world. We see this capacity in McCarthy's novel about a possible future world that explodes norms of embodiment; as I demonstrate in the section that follows, we also see this capacity in Hogan's environmental justice narrative, Solar Storms, which traces her narrator's ecosomatic awakening and reveals the kind of cultural work literary ecology can accomplish when paired with insight from disability studies.

Dams and Disability in Linda Hogan's Solar Storms

Hogan's (1997) third novel, Solar Storms, like most of her work, is widely recognized as a powerful narrative of environmental justice, one that emphasizes, as Silvia Schultermandl (2005, 67) puts it, "the interconnectedness between the domination of the Native American tribal culture and the exploitation of the nonhuman biosphere."[4] Even a cursory examination of the novel's plot reveals the centrality of the environmental justice thread. The novel is narrated by Angel Jensen, a young woman of mixed Cree and Inuit descent who has deep scars on the bottom half of her face—physical wounds that reify the anger, fear, and emotional emptiness that characterize the course of her early life. As an infant Angel was wounded by her own mother, an act of violence that forces the state to intervene and take Angel away from her family and her homeland in the Boundary Waters between Minnesota and Canada. Funneled through the foster care system, Angel leads a vagabond existence for much of her childhood and adolescence, and begins to find herself only when she returns to the Boundary Waters seeking answers about her scars and about the woman who gave them to her. When she does return to her family and her ancestral homeland, Angel finds that the Boundary Waters landscape, like her own body, is also broken and scarred, ravaged by an ambitious hydroelectric development project that has altered the face of the region. The process of recovering from and making sense of this double disfigurement—of the human body and the nonhuman landscape—becomes the focus of Angel's Bildungsroman narrative, as she partakes in a journey from damage to healing. As Catherine Rainwater (1999, 94) points out, the novel contains twenty chapters that are neatly divided along an axis of suffering and redemption: "The first ten relate Angel's flight from the world and her angry preoccupation with her scarred face and blighted inner self . . . while the last ten portray the girl's healthy return to community after soul-healing experiences on the land, among family." Critics like Schultermandl (2005), Laura Virginia Castor (2006), and Jim Tarter (2000) have focused on Angel's status as an Indian woman and the role race and gender play in Hogan's environmental politics. While many have also commented on the symbolic significance of Angel's disfigurement, I think a fuller consideration of her status as a woman with a disability is warranted.[5] Indeed Angel's physical wounds and the profound role they play in the outcome of her life makes Hogan's novel particularly valuable as a vehicle through which to illustrate how the concerns of literary ecology and disability studies overlap.

To this end I want to foreground the parallels between Angel's changing sense of her own body, her emergent awareness of her body's connection to the land community, and her concurrent, steady awakening to political consciousness as a Native woman. That is, her liberation stems from a shift in perspective that allows her to understand the correspondence between embodiment and emplacement. Through a consideration of how Angel's disfigurement is inextricably linked to the novel's overall environmental concerns, I want to emphasize the ways Hogan employs discursive strategies that correlate with what I have been calling the ecosomatic paradigm. Ultimately, like McCarthy's The Road, Hogan's novel subverts normative classifications of able-bodiedness by reconstituting the concept of wholeness as a dynamic, relational process wherein the human mind-body interacts on a psychosomatic level with the land communities it inhabits. For Hogan this ecosomatic paradigm is based on a Native-centered spirituality, which views the human body as part of a broader ecological matrix.

This ecosomatic paradigm emerges from two trajectories of damage and healing that commence upon Angel's return to Adam's Rib and her subsequent voyage north with her relatives to protest the building of dams on the land of her people, the Fat Eaters. The first trajectory follows Angel's growing acceptance of her body, particularly the deep scars on her face that mark her as physically different, while the second trajectory traces the evolution of her bioregional consciousness and her concomitant growth as an environmental activist. As we shall see, the ideological forces that threaten the integrity and health of the Boundary Waters bioregion are ultimately the same forces that mark Angel, with her wounds, as an Other. Ultimately it is in her physical, political, and emotional struggle to counter the tide of "progress" set in motion by the dam builders that Angel comes to feel more comfortable in her skin and in the world.

The source of Angel's facial disfigurement is unknown to her; she knows only that she received her wounds from her mother and that it was because of her mother's violence that she was sent away from Adam's Rib. The important thing is that the scars become, in many ways, the defining feature of Angel's life. She explains, "My ugliness, as I called it, had ruled my life. My need for love had been so great I would offer myself to any boy or man who would take me. . . . There was no love in it, but I believed any kind of touch was a kind of love. . . . It would heal me, I thought. It would mend my heart. It would show my face back to me, unscarred" (54). Her "ugliness" ultimately affects her on two levels. The first has to do with social stigmatization; as a sign of her difference from the "normal" body, her scarred face is a source of shame, which she unsuccessfully attempts to correct by hiding her scars with her hair and makeup or by seeking validation of and approval for her body by engaging in meaningless sexual relationships. The second effect of the scars is more directly emotional: rooted as they are in her personal origins and in the mysteries surrounding her abusive mother, the scars represent Angel's sense of detachment, which exacerbates this drive toward any kind of human contact. As Hogan's novel unfurls, what Angel learns about the complex origins of her mother's violence imbues her wound with a deeper historical significance, as she comes to understand that her mother's behavior is a manifestation of a larger cycle of personal, cultural, and ecological exploitation and violence perpetrated by the Euro-American settlers who colonized the Boundary Waters region. In this sense the personal becomes political, as the story of Angel's wounds fosters Hogan's engagement with issues of environmental justice and Native sovereignty.

The function of Angel's impairment within the broader semiotic system that Hogan creates to address her social concerns qualifies it as an example of narrative prosthesis. As Mitchell and Snyder (2000, 48) explain, writers often use disability as a trope to address a variety of social concerns, though "they rarely take up disability as an experience of social or political dimensions." This is to say that within mainstream literature the disabled body has been appropriated to address just about every social issue imaginable except the social construction of disability itself. Given the prevalence of disability in our stories, however, even stereotypical representations of disability, if unpacked with the right methodology, can offer insight into the social experience of disability. That Hogan draws a distinct correlation between Angel's scar and the ravages of settler colonialism suggests that on the surface Angel's disability is merely a trope, a vehicle to transmit the author's environmental justice message. However, I would argue that it is precisely through this linkage between Angel's body and the colonized landscape that Hogan enacts a double critique, wherein she plots a path away from colonialism and toward environmental justice while simultaneously positing a theoretical and spiritual framework that explodes the normal/abnormal dichotomy upon which disability is typically constructed. In looking at Angel's transformation through an ecosomatic lens, it becomes apparent that Hogan's novel offers what Mitchell and Snyder refer to as a "disability counternarrative" (164).

The correlation between Angel and the Boundary Waters landscape is emphasized throughout Solar Storms, perhaps most potently in descriptions that highlight their shared disfigurement. For example, in the second half of the book, when Angel arrives in the northern lands of her ancestors, she observes, "It was a raw and scarred place, a land that had learned to survive, even to thrive on harshness. At first it seemed barren to me, the trees so thin and spindly, the soil impoverished, but soon I felt a sympathy with this ragtag world of seemingly desolate outlying places and villages. . . . Like me, it was native land and had survived" (224). What the land has survived—and what it continues to survive—are the cataclysmic effects of the hydroelectric power project, loosely related to the actual James Bay Project in Quebec, where the construction of dams and power stations has altered the landscape and destroyed much of the native habitat.[6] On one level, of course, Angel sympathizes with this ragtag and scarred landscape because she is viewed by others as herself ragtag and scarred; on another level her emerging appreciation for the transcendent beauty of the land—its endurance in the face of alteration and destruction—indicates a process of reconditioning that involves constructing new ways of viewing her own body.

Her evolving intimacy with the land and her recognition of it as a "living creature," a view she adopts from her great-great-grandmother, Dora-Rouge, stands in stark contrast to the dam builders' perspective on the land. As Angel comes to realize, the debate over the dam project ultimately manifests a much deeper collision of ideologies, loosely divided along Native and non-Native lines. In recalling the defenses of the hydroelectric proposal levied by the government and corporation officials, she explains that "their language didn't hold a thought for the life of water, or a regard for the land that sustained people from the beginning of time. They didn't remember the sacred treaties between humans and animals. . . . For the builders, it was easy and clear-cut. They saw it only on the flat, two-dimensional world of paper" (279). In their evaluation the builders read the land in terms of its economic viability or by how well it fits the paradigm of industrial capitalism. As an outlying place with a complex network of rivers and lakes, the Boundary Waters region does not possess this economic value of its own accord, as it repels the forces of agricultural and commercial development; for a developed nation like Canada, however, the region is ripe for hydroelectric development.

This is where the language employed in disability studies comes into play to further establish the contiguity between Angel's body and the land. Garland-Thomson's (1997) notion of the normate is again instructive here: if we apply this theoretical approach to the land community, we can see how the strategies used to define and represent the disabled body as a deviant Other have been employed (and continue to be employed) to direct the development of natural resources and the exploitation and destruction of whole ecosystems. For example, for much of the nineteenth century surveyors and settlers characterized the arid American West as essentially disabled, defined by what it supposedly lacked: water and trees. The failure of the western grasslands to measure up to normative standards embodied by the woodlands east of the Mississippi initiated a centuries-long battle to "reclaim" this abnormal terrain; it was a process managed by the Bureau of Land Reclamation, which was created specifically to diagnose and treat the problem of the arid terrain. To "reclaim" in this instance means to actually alter the land from its natural state so that after irrigation it looks and produces like an economically viable, agricultural landscape. As it is with the arid West, so it is with the remote Boundary Waters region. In both cases the dam, as a tool of reclamation, can be read as a prosthetic device, a contraption meant to correct a presumably abnormal and disabled landscape so that it conforms to normative standards of economic utility.

Angel's early attempts to hide her scars and the hydroelectric company's attempt to correct the Boundary Waters both fit within a medical-model scheme that reads difference as deficiency. As the novel progresses, Angel adapts to the cultural rhythms of her blood relatives and witnesses and experiences a way of being in the world that follows instead the contours of natural cycles. As a result of these experiences she moves away from the divisive and hierarchical paradigm of the dominant culture and toward an ecosomatic ideal. This transformation is cemented as Angel commits herself to defending the "ragtag and scarred" land of her ancestors, an activism that culminates in public statements she makes against the dam project, which are broadcast over the radio. Hers is therefore a manifold conversion experience, a spiritual, political, ecological, and cultural coming of age that is manifest in the new name she is given by the Fat Eaters, Maniki, which means "the girl who turned human" (295). This of course is precisely the point: what Angel learns, or relearns, is what it means to be human, and she does so not by changing herself but by refashioning the mirror in which she views herself and her body. She comes to understand the physical environment, and her embodiment within it, as part and parcel of what Casey classes as the "universal flesh." She comes to see emplacement and embodiment as intertwined. Castor (2006, 160) identifies the central role that place plays in developing empathy within and for Hogan's narrative: "Place . . . gives shape and proportion to the narrator's feelings in a way that provides her with enough critical distance from her pain to allow her to create imaginative spaces for a more defined yet flexible sense of identity to emerge." By coming to "live in the body where the land spoke," as Angel puts it, she breaks down the barrier between herself, her community, and the world. She bears witness to the conterminous nature of the social and the natural, the individual and the ecological, as implied by the metaphor of the universal flesh. She achieves an ecosomatic unity that dissolves the split between nature and culture and that understands the inexorable link between the two. In reconstructing her idea of humanity and resisting normative standards, her wounds lose their power to define her as deviant and instead become a visual marker of her new humanity. Birgit Hans (2003, 98) too notes that, formerly a "mark of isolation, Angela's [sic] scarred face, has become one of belonging." She reevaluates her body from an ecological, and not simply social, context and therefore erases not her physical scars but the worn-out meanings that others would attach to her scars.

This personal victory over her body corresponds to the victory Angel and the protestors achieve in their fight against the hydroelectric company, bringing a halt to the building of further dams. Angel explains, "It was too late for the Child River, for the caribou, the fish, even for our own children, but we had to believe, true or not, that our belated victory was the end of something. Yes, the pieces were infinite and worn as broken pots . . . but we'd thrown an anchor into the future and followed the rope to the end of it, to where we would dream new dreams, new medicines, and one day, once again, remember the sacredness of every living thing" (344). These new dreams and new medicines are grounded in an ecosomatic definition of wholeness—one that accounts for fluidity and change. Ultimately, to deconstruct the figure of the normate, whether applied to the human body or the natural landscape, is a pursuit that has benefits from both a disability studies and an ecocritical perspective. The ecosomatic paradigm exhibited in Angel's transformation promotes the ideal of, indeed the life-sustaining need for diversity—of bodies, minds, and landscapes. It is significant, of course, that her transformation occurs as the result of an accumulation of stories that realign her relationships toward the human and nonhuman communities of which she is a part. It is also significant that her activism takes the form of public storytelling in her interview broadcast over the radio. Hogan's novel ultimately affirms the power that stories have to give shape to the world and to condition our behavior toward it. This faith in stories is essential to the ecocritical enterprise in general and to literary ecology in particular. Whether it is the story Angel hears about the source of her scars, or Hogan's story about Angel's coming of age, or even the story I am telling here about what Hogan's novel might teach us about our connection to place and the role of the body in connecting to place, stories structure the world for us and can dictate how, or even whether, we care for it. The process of emplacement, Casey (1993) tells us, is one that requires guidance from something or someone else. Much of this guidance comes from the contours of the land community itself, "the lay of the land," but Casey reminds us that "human beings rely on intermediary presences," be it a map, a local guide, or a work of imaginative fiction (250).

Narrative and metaphor give us ways to conceptualize and make tangible the richness of the wild and built places we inhabit. They "thicken" our experience of places, as Casey puts it, adding layers of meaning to our encounters with the natural world. Even when the stories are about places we've never been, even if they are about fictional places that never were, they still have the power to shape our sense of place and to make us care about places that are real and that we do inhabit. This is a crucial ingredient and a critical idea to grasp. At the end of her essay calling for the incorporation of the disability perspective into the environmental movement, Alison Kafer (2005, 145) proclaims, "We cannot forge a movement based on the assumption that only those of us who can scale the mountain can care about the mountain." Compassion for the mountain—or the prairie, ocean, forest, or urban green space—comes from many sources and from many different types of stories. The beauty in contiguity is this: our love of place, wherever it may come from, is transferrable not only from one place to another but also from page to place and back again.

NOTES

1. Exploration of a meaningful collaboration between the disability and environmental movement is already under way. Alison Kafer (2005), for example, has already suggested some practical "points of contact" between the disability and environmental concerns. At the end of "Hiking Boot and Wheelchairs," in which she criticizes ecofeminism's "unspoken but assumed requirement" of able-bodiedness, Kafer outlines three "possible grounds of coalition" that could bring the goals of ecofeminism and disability studies into alignment (133). The first has to do with the issue of protecting biodiversity and how this environmentalist concern might be extended to include the "formidable battle against genetic/eugenic attempts to eradicate many disabilities" (142). The second is focused on the possibility of the greening of the adaptive technology industry and health care facilities. The third basis for coalition would be to "address the complicated relationships among poverty, race, illness and pollution," including an emphasis on "how the effects of soil and water contamination and toxic waste tend to be felt most severely by poor communities, which are disproportionately composed of [people of] color" (144). Because the toxification of these communities creates illness and impairment, it is an issue of concern for both disability activists and environmental justice activists. This integration of the disability perspective into the environmental justice movement is also the subject of a recent special issue of the journal Local Environment, edited by Rob Imrie and Huw Thomas (2008). In the introduction to the issue the editors assert, "Any social change pursued successfully in relation to either disability or sustainability will have

implications for the other" (481). The essays in the collection bear out this contention, exploring how concerns about disability and sustainability coalesce in multiple facets of social life, including transport, architecture, urban and suburban planning, and learning centers.

2. For more information on universal design and its relationship to disability, see the websites of the Institute for Human Centered Design (http://www.adaptenv.org/) and the Center for Universal Design (https://www.ncsu.edu/ncsu/design/cud/).

3. See, for example, Hughes and Paterson 1997; Siebers 2001. Reindal (2010) also offers a succinct overview of and response to external and internal critiques of social model theory. Because of its failure to incorporate the centrality of the body and how it shapes the experience of disability, disability scholars who want to emphasize both the social construction of disability and the role of the body often refer to a "cultural model" of disability.

4. For other ecocritical readings of Solar Storms, see especially Castor 2006; Donaldson 2003; Hans 2003; Rainwater 1999; Tarter 2000.

5. Angel's status as a disabled woman is admittedly debatable, particularly as her facial scars do not necessarily limit her functioning. As Linton (1998, 12) notes, however, "the question of who 'qualifies' as disabled is as answerable or as confounding as questions about identity status. One simple response might be that you are disabled if you say you are." As I outline below, for much of her early life Angel was defined by her scars, and while she never comes out and says so, this disfigurement produced disabling mental and social conditions. What matters most for my purpose here is Angel's status as a literary representation of disability, as someone whose body is marked, through her disfigurement, as a deviation from the normate.

6. Tarter (2000) offers the most detailed examination of the ways the events in Hogan's novel correlate and make use of the historical James Bay Project. The damming of rivers on Native lands is a major concern within the environmental justice movement, as it raises issues concerning Native sovereignty and land rights as well as competing paradigms of land use drawn along cultural lines: Euro-American agriculture and industrial development versus Native fishing and hunting practices. For some historical context on this

issue, see Colombi 2005; Oberly 1995; Lawson 2010. Oberly's history of the Lac Courte Oreilles battle against a dam project in Winter, Wisconsin, has some relevance to Hogan's novel as it documents an experience that possesses some geographic parallels to Hogan's fictional account of Native resistance to damming.

REFERENCES

Casey, Edward. 1993. Getting Back into Place: Toward a New Understanding of the Place World. Bloomington: University of Indiana Press.

Castor, Laura Virginia. 2006. "Claiming Place in Wor(l)ds: Linda Hogan's Solar Storms." MELUS 31, no. 2: 157–80.

Colombi, Benedict J. 2005. "Dammed in Region Six: The Nez Perce Tribe, Agricultural Development, and the Inequality of Scale." American Indian Quarterly 29, nos. 3–4: 560–89.

Donaldson, Laura. 2003. "Covenanting Nature: Aquacide and the Transformation of Knowledge." Ecotheology 8: 110–18.

Entrikin, J. Nicholas. 1991. The Betweenness of Place: Towards a Geography of Modernity. Baltimore: Johns Hopkins University Press.

Freund, Peter. 2001. "Bodies, Disability and Spaces: The Social Model and Disabling Spatial Organisations." Disability & Society 16, no. 5: 689–706.

Garland-Thomson, Rosemarie. 1997. Extraordinary Bodies: Figuring Physical Disability in American Culture and Literature. New York: Columbia University Press.

Hans, Birgit. 2003. "Water and Ice: Restoring Balance to the World in Linda Hogan's Solar Storms." North Dakota Quarterly 70, no. 3: 93–104.

Hogan, Linda. 1997. Solar Storms. New York: Scribner's.

Hughes, Bill, and Kevin Paterson. 1997. "The Social Model of Disability and the Disappearing Body: Towards a Sociology of Impairment." Disability & Society 12, no. 3: 325–40.

Imrie, Rob, and Huw Thomas. 2008. "Guest Editorial: The Interrelationship between Environment and Disability." Local Environment 13, no. 6: 477–83.

Kafer, Alison. 2005. "Hiking Boots and Wheelchairs: Ecofeminism, the Body, and Physical Disability." In Feminist Interventions in Ethics and Politics: Feminist Ethics and Social Theory, edited by Barbara S. Andrew, Jean Clare Keller, and Lisa H. Schwartzmann, 131–50. Lanham MD: Rowman.

Lawson, Michael. 2010. Dammed Indians Revisited: The Continuing History of the Pick-Sloan Project and the Missouri River Sioux. Pierre SD: SDHS.

Linton, Simi. 1998. Claiming Disability: Knowledge and Identity. New York: New York University Press.

Loriggio, Francesco. 1994. "Regionalism and Theory." In Regionalism Reconsidered: New Approaches to the Field, edited by David Jordan, 3–28. New York: Garland.

Mairs, Nancy. 1996. Waist-High in the World: A Life among the Disabled. Boston: Beacon.

McCarthy, Cormac. 2006. The Road. New York: Knopf.

Merleau-Ponty, Maurice. 1969. The Visible and the Invisible. Chicago: Northwestern University Press.

Mitchell, David T., and Sharon L. Snyder. 2000. Narrative Prosthesis: Disability and the Dependencies of Discourse. Ann Arbor: University of Michigan Press.

Oberly, James W. 1995. "Tribal Sovereignty and Natural Resources: The Lac Courte Oreilles Experience." In Buried Roots and Indestructible Seeds: The Survival of Indian Life in Story, History, and Spirit, edited by Mark A. Lindquist and Martin N. Zanger, 127–53. Madison: University of Wisconsin Press.

Rainwater, Catherine. 1999. "Intertextual Twins and Their Relations: Linda Hogan's Mean Spirit and Solar Storms." Modern Fiction Studies 45, no. 1: 93–113.

Reindal, Solveig Mangus. 2010. "Redefining Disability: A Rejoinder to a Critique." Etikki i praksis: Nordic Journal of Applied Ethics 4, no. 1: 125–35.

Schultermandl, Silvia. 2005. "Fighting for the Mother/Land: An Ecofeminist Reading of Linda Hogan's Solar Storms." Sail 17, no. 3: 67–84.

Siebers, Tobin. 2001. "Disability in Theory: From Social Constructionism to the New Realism of the Body." American Literary History 13, no. 4: 737–54.

Tarter, Jim. 2000. "'Dreams of Earth': Place, Multiethnicity, and Environmental Justice in Linda Hogan's Solar Storms." In Reading under the

Sign of Nature: New Essays in Ecocriticism, edited by John Tallmadge, 128–47. Salt Lake City: University of Utah Press.

Tregaskis, Claire. 2002. "Social Model Theory: The Story So Far." *Disability & Society* 17, no. 4: 457–70.

Union of the Physically Impaired against Segregation. 1976. "Fundamental Principles of Disability." London: Union of the Physically Impaired against Segregation/Disability Alliance.

6

Bodies of Nature

The Environmental Politics of Disability

Alison Kafer

> The creatures that populate the narrative space called "nature" are key characters in scientific tales about the past, present, and future. Various tellings of these tales are possible, but they are always shaped by historical, disciplinary, and larger cultural contexts.
>
> —Jennifer Terry, "'Unnatural Acts' in Nature"

Although concern with the environment has long been an animating force in disability studies and activism, "environment" in this context typically refers to the built environment of buildings, sidewalks, and transportation technologies. Indeed the social model of disability is premised on concern for the built environment, stressing that people are disabled not by their body but by their inaccessible environment. (The wheelchair user confronting a flight of steps is probably the most common illustration of this argument.) Yet the very pervasiveness of the social model has prevented disability studies from engaging with the wider environment of wilderness, parks, and nonhuman nature because the social model seems to falter in such settings. Stairs can be replaced or supplemented with ramps and elevators, but what about a steep rock face or a sandy beach? Like stairs, both pose problems for most wheelchair users, but, argues Tom Shakespeare, "it is hard to blame the natural environment on social arrangements." He asserts that the natural environment—rock cliffs, steep mountains, and sandy beaches—offers proof that "people with impairments will always be disadvantaged by their bodies"; the social model cannot adequately address the barriers presented by those kinds of spaces.[1] I too recognize the limitations of the social model and the need to engage with the materiality of bodies, but I am not so sure that the "natural environment" is as distinct from the "built environment" as Shakespeare suggests. On the contrary, the natural environment is also "built": literally so in the case of trails and dams, metaphorically so in the sense of cultural constructions and deployments of "nature," "natural," and "the environment."

Disability studies could benefit from the work of environmental scholars and activists who describe how "social arrangements" have been mapped onto "natural environments." Many campgrounds in the United States, for example, have been designed to resemble suburban neighborhoods, with single campsites for each family, clearly demarcated private and public spaces, and layouts built for cars. Each individual campsite faces the road or common area so that rangers (and other campers) can easily monitor others' behavior. Such spacing likely discourages, or at least pushes into the cover of darkness, outwardly queer acts and practices.[2] Environmental historians such as William Cronon explain that indigenous people were removed from parklands and evidence of their communities was destroyed so that the new parks could be read as pristine, untouched wilderness.[3] Nature writers such as Carolyn Finney and Evelyn White explain that African Americans are much less likely than whites to find parks and open spaces welcoming, accessible, or safe; histories of white supremacist violence and lynchings in rural areas make the wilderness less appealing. Park brochures, wilderness magazines, and advertisements for outdoor gear have, in turn, tended to cater overwhelmingly to white audiences.[4] As these examples attest, the natural environment is also a built environment, shaped by and experienced through assumptions and expectations about gender, sexuality, class, race, and nation. As Mei Mei Evans argues, "One way of understanding the culturally dominant conception of what constitutes 'nature' in the United States is to ask ourselves who gets to go there. Access to wilderness and a reconstituted conception of Nature are clearly environmental justice issues demanding redress."[5]

How might we begin to read disability into these formations? How have compulsory able-bodiedness/able-mindedness shaped not only the environments of our lives, both buildings and parks, but our very understandings of the environment itself? One way to address these questions is by examining the deployment of disability in popular discourses of nature and environmentalism; another would be to uncover the assumption of able-bodiedness and able-mindedness in writings about nature. I follow both paths in this essay, unpacking the work of disability and able-bodiedness/able-mindedness in cultural constructions of nature, wilderness, and the environment. As with the visions of a "better" future found in discussions of reproduction, childhood, community, and cyborgs, visions of nature are often idealized and depoliticized fantasies, and disability plays an integral, if often unmarked, role in marking the limit of these fantasies. Whether we focus on nature writing or trail construction (the subjects of the first two sections), disabled people are figured as out of place.

Given the often exclusionary dimensions of "nature" and "wilderness," it is important to explore how those considered out of place find ways of engaging and interacting with nature. As Evans argues, the "culturally dominant conception of what constitutes 'nature'" becomes more clear when we encounter the narratives of those who are not expected or allowed "to go there."[6] In the final section, then, I explore the possibility of a cripped environmentalism, one that looks to disabled bodies and minds as a resource in thinking about our future natures differently. I argue that the experience of illness and disability presents alternative ways of understanding ourselves in relation to the environment, understandings which can generate new possibilities for intellectual connections and activist coalitions.

Natural Exclusions

We tend to think of the definitions of terms such as <u>nature</u>, <u>wilderness</u>, and <u>environment</u> as self-evident, assuming their meanings to be universal, stable, and monolithic. However, as Cronon argues, "'nature' is not nearly so natural as it seems."[7] On the contrary, our encounters with wilderness are historically and culturally grounded; our ideas about what constitutes nature or the natural and unnatural are completely bound up in our own specific histories and cultural assumptions. What is needed, then, is an interrogation of these very assumptions.[8] Instead of taking for granted the qualities we attribute to wilderness experiences, such as spiritual renewal or physical challenge, we can ask, as Linda Vance does, "Whose values are these? What do they assume about experience, and whose experience is the norm? What other social relations depend on or produce these values? What is their historical context?"[9] We can extend the scope of these questions to include an examination of ableism and compulsory able-bodiedness/able-mindedness: Whose experiences of nature are taken as the norm within environmental discourses? What do these discourses assume about nature, the bodymind, and the relationship between humans and nature? And how do notions of disability and able-bodiedness/able-mindedness play a key role in constructing values such as "spiritual renewal" and "physical challenge" in the first place?

In this section I examine three sites of able-bodiedness/able-mindedness: a canonical environmental memoir, a controversial ad in a mainstream hiking magazine, and an autobiographical essay in ecofeminist philosophy. These are three vastly different texts, with different agendas and from different time periods. I bring them together in order to sketch out the role disability plays in constructions of the natural environment. In the first two selections the figure of disability is explicitly invoked in order to be immediately disavowed, making clear that disability has no place in the wilderness. Both hail the able body, or the nondisabled body, as the proper denizen of the outdoors; they deploy the figure of disability to further cultural representations of nature as a rugged proving ground, making disability the dystopic sign of human failure, or potential failure, in nature. The final example, the ecofeminist essay, shares the presumption of able-bodiedness that runs through the first two representations, this time presenting the nondisabled body as the grounds through which we arrive at ecofeminist insight. Reading each of these examples through a critical disability lens reveals the ways we assume the environmental body to be a very particular kind of body.

One of the most explicit articulations of a compulsorily able-bodied/able-minded environmentalism is found in Edward Abbey's cult classic, Desert Solitaire: A Season in the Wilderness, first published in 1968.[10] In this highly acclaimed memoir Abbey offers a polemic against "industrial tourism" in national parks, a phenomenon that is destroying wilderness areas across the country and robbing all of us of our ability to access nature. Abbey repeatedly draws on disability metaphors to make his case, most notably when he refers to cars as "motorized" or "mechanized wheelchairs."[11] He thus presents cars as having a literally crippling effect on our ability to experience nature. The motorized wheelchair becomes the epitome of technological alienation, of technology's ability to alienate us from our own wild nature and the wilderness around us. Sarah Jaquette Ray calls this pattern the "disability-equals-alienation-from-nature trope," arguing that Abbey's text relies on disability as "the best symbol of the machine's corruption of . . . harmony between body and nature."[12]

This representation becomes even more clear later in the book, when Abbey exhorts everyone to get out of their cars/wheelchairs and walk: "Yes sir, yes madam, I entreat you, get out of those motorized wheelchairs, get off your foam rubber backsides, stand up straight like men! like women! like human beings! and walk-walk-WALK upon our sweet and blessed land!" Although Abbey elsewhere allows for travel by bicycle and horse, he frequently hails walking as the only way to access "the original, the real" nature.[13] His assertion that we must get out and walk, that truly understanding a space means moving through it on foot, presents a very particular kind of embodied experience as a prerequisite to environmental engagement. Walking through the desert becomes a kind of authorizing gesture; to know the desert requires walking through the desert, and to do so unmediated by technology. In such a construction there is no way for the mobility-impaired body to engage in environmental practice; all modalities other than walking upright become insufficient, even suspect. Walking is both what makes us human and what makes us at one with nature.[14]

Abbey's framing has been influential. As Ray notes, the environmental movement is deeply attached to the notion of "the solitary retreat into nature as the primary source of an environmental ethic."[15] It is common to find ecocritics making connections and deriving insight from hiking trips and other adventures in the wilderness. By implying that one must have a deep immersion experience of nature in order to understand nature, ecocritics create a situation in which some kinds of experiences can be interpreted as more valid than others, as granting a more accurate, intense, and authentic understanding of nature. They ignore the complicated histories of who is granted permission to enter nature, where nature is said to reside, how one must move in order to get there, and how one will interact with nature once one arrives in it.[16] (As we will see, these assumptions then play a huge role in struggles over increasing disability access in parks and public lands.)

This kind of exclusionary framing of nature is on full display in a provocative advertisement for Nike's Air Dri-Goat shoe. The advertisement ran in eleven different outdoor magazines in the fall of 2000, reaching a combined circulation of approximately 2.1 million readers. It featured a picture of the shoe against a hot-pink background, with this accompanying text:

> Fortunately, the Air Dri-Goat features a patented goat-like outer sole for increased traction, so you can taunt mortal injury without actually experiencing it. Right about now you're probably asking yourself, "How can a trail running shoe with an outer sole designed like a goat's hoof help me avoid compressing my spinal cord into a Slinky' on the side of some unsuspecting conifer, thereby rendering me a drooling, misshapen non-extreme-trail-running husk of my former self, forced to roam the earth in a motorized wheelchair with my name, embossed on one of those cute little license plates you get at carnivals or state fairs, fastened to the back?"
>
> To that we answer, hey, have you ever seen a mountain goat (even an extreme mountain goat) careen out of control into the side of a tree?
>
> Didn't think so.

In the first two days after publication Nike received over six hundred complaints about the ad, and the company withdrew it from further circulation. Three public apologies followed, each one containing more cause for offense.[17] The perceived need for multiple apologies testifies to the blatant offensiveness of the ad. It is not surprising that the ad came under attack: it paints an incredibly negative portrait of people in wheelchairs, trivializes and mocks the experiences of those who have survived spinal cord injuries, and dehumanizes disabled people. Most important for my exploration of crip futures, however, are its assumptions about disability and nature, or, more to the point, its assumptions about the place of a disabled person in nature.

First, in running this advertisement Nike has assumed that the readers of <u>Backpacker</u> and similar magazines are neither disabled nor allies of the disabled, casting outdoor enthusiasts and disabled people as two mutually exclusive groups.[18]

Second, the advertisement assumes that disability prohibits encounters with nature, dooming one to roam "carnivals or state fairs" rather than mountain ranges. It is perhaps no accident that Nike's advertisement conjures an image of disabled people at the fair or carnival, buying accoutrements for their wheelchairs. From the 1840s through the 1940s in the United States, disabled people were frequently exhibited in public at traveling sideshows and carnivals, cast as "freaks," "freaks of nature," and, in a blending of ableist, racist, and colonialist narratives, "missing links."[19] Freak shows were one of the few places where one could see disabled people in public, and the Nike advertisement extends this depiction of the carnival as the proper terrain of the disabled body. Conversely it makes clear that once one becomes disabled, mountain ranges and wilderness areas are out of reach.

Third, it reminds nondisabled hikers that they must be ever vigilant in protecting themselves from disability, denying any trace of disability in or on their body. These last two assumptions are interrelated, in that nondisabled hikers must deny disability precisely because it (allegedly) prohibits encounters with nature. In other words, the advertisement is explicitly invoking a disabled body in order to reassure readers of their own able-bodiedness. As Rosemarie Garland-Thomson argues, the figure of disability "assures the rest of the citizenry of who they are not while arousing their suspicions about who they could become."[20]

Thus two distinct bodies appear in this text. The first is the nondisabled body ostensibly shared by both Nike associates (the advertisement's "we") and Nike consumers ("you"). The text tells its readers little about this nondisabled body; it takes shape only when juxtaposed with the second body in the text. Unlike the first body, which is unmarked, the second, disabled body is described with utmost specificity: readers learn of its appearance ("drooling, misshapen," and "forced" into a wheelchair), its inabilities ("non-extreme-trail-running"), its quality of life (a "husk of my former self"), and its home ("carnivals or state fairs"). The disabled body appears in the text only as the specter of impending tragedy; one can allegedly ward it away by assertively and aggressively staking one's claim to nature, by "taunting mortal injury" and celebrating one's alleged hyperability. As Ray suggests, it is the "threat of disability" that makes "the wilderness ideal body meaningful"; part of the thrill of adventure is risking—yet ultimately avoiding—disablement.[21] Thus disability exists out of time, as something not-yet and, with the right equipment, not-ever. In order to belong to the text's "us," one must deny any physical limitations or inabilities, casting oneself as separate from and superior to the disabled figure. "We" are not drooling or misshapen disabled people, the text proclaims; we are hikers, and never the twain shall meet. Nike explicitly repudiates the disabled body, casting it as the antithesis of the hiker's body, which is the body "we" all have and want to preserve.

The hiker's body as imagined by both Nike and Abbey is necessary because it is only through it that we are able to truly experience nature (or to experience true nature). Nature, wilderness, mountain ranges: all are described as separate from "us," but we can bridge or transcend that separation by rugged, masculine individualism; disability serves both to illustrate that separation between human and nature and to exacerbate it. Although my third site, an ecofeminist essay, does not rely on this kind of explicit ableism, it continues the narrative of separation from nature. Its reliance on this trope is harder to recognize, as it comes in the context of a much more critical approach to nature and wilderness than that found in Abbey or Nike.

In her essay "Ecofeminism and the Politics of Reality," Vance traces her political and theoretical development as an ecofeminist. Vance weaves accounts of her own hiking experiences into the essay, revealing how her experiences in and through nature have played an important role in her journey toward ecofeminism. For most of the essay Vance writes in the first person, describing her personal experiences with nature (e.g., "I hike through the Green Mountains"), but there is one passage in which she shifts to the third person, writing about "an ecofeminist": "On a bad day, then, say when she's hiking through a spruce bog trying to convince herself that being a food source for mosquitoes and black flies is an ecologically sound role, an ecofeminist can despair, and start to feel like she is the least loved cousin of just about everyone, and sister to no one. Except, of course—and here she pauses, a boot heavy with black muck arrested in mid-step, and she looks around—except, of course, nature. Sister. Sister Nature."[22] In this passage Vance's phrasing itself suggests that "hiking" and "being an ecofeminist" are related activities:

by shifting from a description of her own particular experiences to the adventures of an unnamed ecofeminist, she positions the figure as a stand-in for all ecofeminists. Moreover she suggests that it is through this kind of rugged activity that "an ecofeminist" comes to understand herself in relation to nonhuman nature. Vance's ecofeminist comes to a key realization as she hikes through the muck; indeed the act of stepping through the bog is what spurs her insight. Hiking, according to this passage, is vital to an ecofeminist's development of her relationship with and understanding of nature; without such hikes "an ecofeminist" will remain in some way separate from nature. Once again able-bodiedness is necessary in order to bridge or transcend the essential separation between human and nature.

Ecofeminism for Vance is a complex theoretical and conceptual framework deeply invested in activist practices; she would likely oppose Abbey's assumption that cities are unnatural and impure while wilderness is not.[23] However, the passage under consideration here reflects an assumption not far from Abbey's, that one must immerse oneself in nature in order to understand it and one's relationship to it. In describing an ecofeminist's hike through the mucky bog, Vance suggests that people need to have personal, physical experiences of the wilderness in order to understand, appreciate, and care for nature. But what kind of experiences render one qualified to understand and care about nature? Are all experiences of nature equally productive of such insights? And how do we define "experiences of nature" in the first place?

These questions lead me back to Shakespeare's assumption that the natural environment is completely separate from social arrangements. Each of the selections I have examined here—Abbey, Nike, Vance—operates under a similar assumption, at least when it comes to the body of the hiker. These accounts take for granted the existence of trails that accommodate one's body, presenting access to nature not only as necessary to personal growth or renewal but also as apolitical. Abbey is the extreme here, making clear that the hiker's access to parks and wilderness is natural, but everyone else's (those in "motorized wheelchairs," for example) is political, debatable, and ideally stoppable. To tell a tale of a lack of appropriate access—no trails wide enough for a wheelchair or level enough for crutches—would be to insert the all-too-human into the wilderness, thereby violating the persistent dualisms between the human and the natural and the natural and the political.

Thus what is needed in ecofeminism, ecocriticism, and environmentalism in general are the narratives of people whose bodies and minds cause them to interact with nature in nonnormative ways. How might a deaf ecofeminist understand her position within the natural world differently than a hearing one? What can narratives about negotiating trails on crutches reveal about the ways all trails, not just "accessible" ones, are constructed and maintained? How do concepts of nature, wilderness, and ecofeminism shift when elaborated by an ecofeminist who experiences nonhuman nature primarily through sound, smell, and touch rather than sight, or by an ecofeminist who draws more on sounds and sensations than on words? In what ways would ecofeminist activism be transformed by someone whose chronic fatigue and pain prevent her from traveling more than a few blocks from her house but do not hinder her environmental organizing, lobbying, and fundraising efforts? How might the use of a service dog affect an ecofeminist's understanding of his relationship with nonhuman nature?

One of my hopes in writing this essay is that nondisabled ecofeminists will supplement these questions with queries of their own: How might reflecting on her able-bodied status affect a nondisabled ecofeminist's understanding of the ecofeminist project? In what ways would he alter his concepts of nature and politics after thinking through his position in an ableist culture? Making space for these kinds of questions expands the domain of ecofeminism and environmental movements, challenging the representation of nondisabled experience as the only possible way to interact with nonhuman nature. Such challenges will necessarily entail expanding our understandings of nature as well, which will, in turn, affect the environments around us. Our conceptions of nature and the natural, in other words, play a direct role in how we shape parks and other public lands.

Accessible Trails and Other (Un)Natural Disasters

Ableist assumptions about the body certainly influence the concrete realities of access, thereby affecting disabled and non-disabled people alike. Steep, narrow, and root-filled trails are barriers not just for people with mobility or vision impairments but also for some seniors and families with young children. Similarly nature education has developed around the needs of the nondisabled, as attested by the dearth of interpretive materials available in formats such as Braille, large print, or audiotape.[24] The lack of maps, guidebooks, park brochures, and explanatory markers in large print affects not only those who identify as disabled, however, but all people with low vision. Thinking through these issues can help deconstruct the ableist assumptions embedded in contemporary and historical ideas about nature. Ecofeminists can then begin the process of tracing the impact those assumptions have had on the design of trails and park materials, designs that have determined who is able to use such resources. Rob Imrie and Huw Thomas argue, "These contexts may be thought of as perpetuating forms of environmental injustice, in which inappropriate and thoughtless design means that disabled people cannot use significant parts of the environment."[25]

Mobility is one of the key issues of trail access, and proposals to create wheelchair accessibility are often met with suspicion, as if such access were inherently more damaging to the environment than access points for nondisabled people. Plans to build an accessible canoe launch on Maine's Allagash Wilderness Waterway, for example, encountered opposition from environmental groups who claimed such a launch would damage the waterway.[26] Although some critics were clear that they opposed any new access points on the waterway, regardless of their design, others seemed more concerned about the level of accessibility offered by this proposal; there was a sense that an accessible launch would be more damaging to the environment than an inaccessible one. But most canoe launches are created by clearing away brush, altering the gravel or sand level near the water, and constructing parking areas and toilets, raising doubts as to whether accessible launches are really more detrimental than inaccessible ones. An accessible site may differ from an inaccessible site only slightly, having wider doors on the bathroom and a wider and more level path to the water, changes that are not necessarily more disruptive or damaging.

When I was visiting a wildlife refuge in Rhode Island in the spring of 2007, one of the staff recounted a recent outcry from the local community about making trails within the refuge wheelchair accessible. According to their complaints, both the materials used in such a trail (in this case crushed asphalt) and the users of such trails (presumably people with wheelchairs or other mobility aids) would be too noisy; birds that nested in the area would be scared away by the trail's imagined new users. However, given how frequently hikers use cell phones, talk loudly with their companions, or yell to a child, it is hard to believe that noise is the real fear here. While birders may dislike those interruptions as well, they were not advocating for barriers to keep them out; children were permitted in the park without having to undergo some kind of silencing or muting practice. (Moreover I would imagine a crushed stone trail or, especially, a paved trail would be much quieter than one made of thick gravel or covered in dry, brittle leaves and branches.)

To take another example: in 2000, when a group of disabled and nondisabled hikers made a trek to the newly accessible hut at Galehead in the White Mountains, they were met with derision on the trail by a nondisabled hiker who accused them of taking up too much room and harming the terrain. In a letter to the editor of the New York Times, Dan Bruce condemned those involved with the hike, charging them with "selfishness": "Wheelchairs do incredible damage to trails in these fragile areas. Did anyone in the group do an environmental assessment before attempting the exploit or consider that the damage done to the trail by their wheeled equipment may take years for nature to repair?"[27] What interests me about Bruce's letter and the comments from the hiker on the trail is the presumption that wheelchair users inevitably damage trails more than other hikers do.

It was not just the disabled hikers' presence on the trail that garnered criticism, however, but the very idea that a backcountry cabin would be retrofitted with a wheelchair ramp and accessible bathroom. Challenging the need for the ramp, one reporter asked "why people in wheelchairs could drag themselves up the trail and not drag themselves up the steps to the hut."[28] If the hikers were able to complete such an arduous hike, in other words, surely they were capable of crawling up the steps to the cabin. This challenge to the appropriateness of the Galehead ramp exemplifies how nondisabled access is made invisible while disabled access is made hypervisible. Steps are themselves an accommodation, just one made for a different kind of body; as Jill Gravink notes, rather than focus on ramps as being out of place, the reporter could just as easily have focused on stairs, demanding of nondisabled hikers, "Why bother putting steps on the hut at all? Why not drag yourself in through a window?"[29]

Those who protest the development of accessible trails and services consistently use the language of protection in making their claims; in their view increasing disability access and protecting the environment are irreconcilable. But the fact that it is often only <u>disability</u> access that comes under such interrogation suggests an act of ableist forgetting. As the steps/ramp question shows, the development of trails and buildings that suit very particular bodies goes unmarked as access; it is only when atypical bodies are taken into account that the question of access becomes a problem. The rhetoric of ecoprotection then seems to be more about discomfort with the artifacts of access: ramps, barrier-free pathways, and the bodies that use them. Trails, which are mapped, cut, and maintained by human beings with tools and machinery, are seen as <u>natural</u>, but wheelchair-accessible trails are seen as <u>unnatural</u>. The very phrasing of these sentences reveals the differences in valence: trails, by definition (or, more to the point, <u>naturally</u>), are not wheelchair accessible; they need no modifier. Reading for disability opens up these assumptions, making visible the ways in which the constructedness of <u>all</u> trails is covered over by focusing on the constructedness of <u>some</u> trails.

Some disability organizations, such as the California-based Whole Access, have countered these assumptions, stressing that, while all trails affect the land, well-designed trails can both minimize that impact and maximize accessibility for all people, including those with mobility disabilities.[30] For example, installing boardwalks over fragile land, as has been done in the Florida Everglades, Cape Lookout National Seashore, and Yellowstone

National Park, promotes access for people with mobility impairments and people with small children while also protecting delicate terrain from direct traffic. People are less likely to step off the boardwalk and walk through prohibited or protected areas than they are on a trail. In collaboration with California State Parks, Whole Access documented how trails that follow the natural contours of the land (as opposed to steeper trails that cut vertically through a slope) tend to reduce erosion, require less maintenance, and increase accessibility because of their more gentle slopes and inclines.[31]

Access to the wilderness, as many disability activists and advocates argue, is not an all-or-nothing endeavor. Some accessible trails and entry points are better than none, and trails that cannot be brought into full compliance with accessibility guidelines can often be easily modified to permit some disability access. Don Beers, a district supervisor with California State Parks, explains, "The big thing was changing my mindset that [accessibility] had to be all or nothing. . . . The thought now is, let's look at every trail to make it as accessible as possible."[32] Beers's instruction to make every trail "as accessible as possible" can be interpreted narrowly; like the call for "reasonable" accommodation under the Americans with Disabilities Act, it can potentially be used as a way to rule out some changes as too extreme (as "unreasonable"). But read radically, making every trail "as accessible as possible" means that every trail needs to take every kind of body and way of movement into account. That doesn't mean that every single trail will actually accommodate every single body; there will be terrain too rocky or too steep for some bodies and modalities. But this is true for all bodies, disabled and nondisabled. What shifts in this view is that trails are no longer designed for only one single body and that decisions about trails are recognized as decisions, ones that can be changed, extended, modified.

Moreover making every trail as accessible as possible disrupts the long-standing pattern of making visitors' centers and very short nature trails accessible while ignoring disability access everywhere else. Such a model of access, argues Ann Sieck, a wheelchair hiker who has long been involved in attempts to improve wheelchair access in Bay Area parks, sends "the alienating—if unintended—message that for disabled people the outdoors is available only at 'special' facilities. It is hard to describe how painful it is to be excluded through simple indifference, or through the ignorance of planners who see no need to maximize the usability of trails that are not designated 'whole access.'"[33]

Yet, as Laura Hershey recounts, even when wheelchair hikers discover trails for themselves, their experiences are often not incorporated into official park literature. Hiking in Yosemite with her lover and their attendant, Hershey came upon a sign with "a red circle and bar canceling out the universal wheelchair access symbol." After much discussion Hershey and her companions chose to continue, and after a difficult and bumpy ride they arrived at a magnificent view of a waterfall. Hershey included a description of the hike in "Along Asphalt Trails," an essay for National Parks, the magazine of the National Parks Conservation Association. Prior to publication, however, an editor cut that section of the essay because it might encourage readers to ignore posted signs.[34] Yet, as Hershey's story demonstrates, such signs are based on ableist assumptions about what "accessible" trails look like. I have hiked on the trail Hershey describes, and it was more rugged than I could handle in my manual chair; I made it to the waterfall only with generous help and my willingness to crawl on the ground. It is inaccessible to many folks with mobility impairments (and perhaps also to adults traveling with small children, or elderly hikers, or those uninterested in such a strenuous hike), but not all. What seems important in Hershey's story is its insistence that disabled hikers have the same opportunities as nondisabled hikers to make their own decisions about access, including unsuccessful (or even risky) decisions.

Thus the problem of assuming access to be an all-or-nothing endeavor extends beyond the construction and maintenance of trails to the training given park rangers and wildlife docents. As long as they are talking to nondisabled hikers park rangers are full of detailed information about hiking trails in the area. I have often observed rangers asking hikers what kind of terrain they want, how long they want to hike, and what level of difficulty best suits their needs. As a wheelchair user, however, I am seldom asked these kinds of questions, as if my desired level of difficulty were self-evident. As Sieck notes, "park rangers are also unable to answer questions about a trail's usability—it's either designated as accessible or not, end of discussion."[35] This lack of information is mirrored in park maps and other material that make no mention of accessible facilities or, more often, assume accessible facilities to mean only one kind of experience.

Scrambling, Climbing, Touching, Holding:
How to Crip the Trail Map

Loss is a topic disabled people are typically reluctant to discuss, and for good reason. Disability is all too often read exclusively in such terms, with bitterness, pity, and tragedy being the dominant registers through which contemporary U.S. culture understands the experiences of disabled people. Why encourage such attitudes by speaking publicly about our inabilities, frustrations, and limitations? Yet loss is undeniably one of the motivations behind this essay, behind my concern with trails and beaches and access. Prior to my injuries I was a runner, and running was an activity I loved largely for its solitude. Running gave me the adrenaline high of physical exertion, but more importantly it served as a meditative practice, as a way to be outside alone in nature. I ran along the beach in eastern North Carolina, through the woods in upstate New York, next to farmland in northern California; I used these experiences to clear my head, to make sense of my thoughts, to maintain my mental and physical health. When Vance writes about discovering herself in nature, feeling at one with the ecosystem, or developing relationships with nonhuman nature by wading through a bog, I know exactly what she is talking about; I feel it in my bones. Although I agree with environmental critics in their deconstruction of the nature experience and their insistence that there is no bright line between nature and culture, I cannot deny that I feel different outside, away from traffic and exhaust pipes and crowds of people. That I have been conditioned to feel this way does not change the fact that I feel more at peace in my body when perched on the side of a cliff, or gazing over a meadow, or surrounded by sequoias.

Loss factors into all of this because such experiences are made much more difficult with the body I have now, the body that relies primarily on a wheelchair for mobility. It is hard to find an isolated yet accessible trail that will grant me the solitude I seek; it is hard to get out to the water's edge or up to the cliff's peak. Part of this difficulty is due to the histories of trail development and access discussed earlier, the assumption that only certain kinds of bodies need to be accommodated in parks and on trails, but it is also due to the terrain itself. There simply are hills too steep, creeks too rocky, soil too sandy for a wheelchair; or, rather, ensuring access to some locations would mean so drastically altering those locations that the aesthetic and environmental damage to the area would be profound. (The same is true, of course, for nondisabled access to some areas.)

Thus this kind of project entails reckoning with loss, limitation, inability, and failure. Indeed I long to hear stories that not only admit limitation, frustration, even failure but that recognize such failure as grounds for theory itself. What might Vance's ecofeminist have learned about her connection to nonhuman nature if she had fallen in that mucky bog? How might her framing of nature shift if she had turned around that day, finding the bog too slippery for her loping gait? Moving outward from ecofeminism, we can occasionally find disability in popular nature writing, but almost always as something to be overcome, and overcome spectacularly. The story of Erik Weihenmayer's blind ascent of Mount Everest, for example, relies on disability to hold our interest, but the narrative's very structure assumes that our interest is dependent on disability eventually being vanquished.

Weihenmayer's memoir, <u>Touch the Top of the World</u>, suggests that successfully hiking Everest was a way for him to "transcend" his blindness. His story would lose its thread if it ended not with the successful ascent but with Weihenmayer discovering that the peak was simply too high, or the climb too dangerous, or the risks too great. He does mention two instances when he and his climbing partner turned back, failing to reach the summit of Humphrey's Peak in Arizona and, later, of Long's Peak in Colorado. But these two stories appear in the first few pages of the book and only in passing; their function in the narrative is to make Weihenmayer's later successes all the more remarkable.[36]

Weihenmayer's climb—not to mention his career as a motivational speaker—exemplifies the narrative of the "supercrip," the stereotypical disabled person who garners media attention for accomplishing some feat considered too difficult for disabled people. (Depending on the kind of impairment under discussion, supercrip acts can include anything from rock climbing to driving a car.) Weihenmayer is familiar with the supercrip narrative and at times seems wary and tired of it, but his book cannot easily be read through any other lens. Its narrative structure repeats the overcoming tale over and over again, both within and between chapters, and everything about the marketing of the book, from its cover images to its promotional blurbs, reiterates this interpretation of Weihenmayer. Supercrip stories rely heavily on the individual/medical model of disability, portraying disability as something to be overcome through hard work and perseverance. And a disabled person accomplishing an amazing adventure in the wilderness is one of the most pervasive supercrip narratives; such stories are popular because of their twinned conquests: both disability and wilderness are overcome by individual feats of strength and will. As Petra Kuppers notes, "The same language of overcoming used traditionally in relation to nature conquests also informs much writing about disability: conquest and vanquishing, lording over or being lorded over, climbing the mountain or perishing on its slopes."[37] It is the very combination of these barriers that makes the stories work.

To return to my earlier questions: What stories get effaced by this focus on the supercrip's achievements? Can we imagine a crip interaction with nature, a crip engagement with wilderness, that doesn't rely on either ignoring the limitations of the body or triumphing over them? In asking these questions I am motivated by a desire to write myself back into nature even as I unpack the binary of nature and self, nature and human. Discussions about the practicalities of access, such as Whole Access's advocacy for universally designed trails, is certainly a necessary part of this work; the sooner we recognize that all trails are built interventions on the landscape, and as such can be reimagined or reconceived, the sooner we can make room for a fuller range of bodies, including but not limited to disabled people. Equally important, however, is a willingness to expand our understanding of human bodies in nonhuman nature, to multiply the possibilities for understanding nature in and through our bodies. If, as

Catriona Sandilands argues, queer ecology means "seeing beauty in the wounds of the world and taking responsibility to care for the world as it is," then perhaps a feminist, queer, crip ecology might mean approaching nature through the lenses of loss and ambivalence.[38]

There are disabled people and disability studies scholars doing exactly this kind of reimagining. In Exile and Pride: Disability, Queerness, and Liberation, poet Eli Clare provides a moving reflection on the diverse ways human bodies interact with non-human nature. He begins with a tale of hiking New Hampshire's Mount Adams:

> The trail divides and divides again, steeper and rockier now, moving not around but over piles of craggy granite, mossy and a bit slick from the night's rain. I start having to watch where I put my feet. Balance has always been somewhat of a problem for me, my right foot less steady than my left. On uncertain ground, each step becomes a studied move, especially when my weight is balanced on my right foot. I take the trail slowly, bringing both feet together, solid on one stone, before leaning into my next step. . . . There is no rhythm to my stop-and-go clamber.

Clare scrambles up and down the mountain, climbing on all fours when he cannot trust his feet. As do other ecocritics and ecofeminists, Clare uses his experiences as a ground for theory, in his case moving from this particular hike to a longer meditation on the politics of bodies, access, and ableism. In other respects, however, Clare's narrative of the mountain stands in stark contrast to the prevailing narrative of moving through nature without any difficulties. In his ascent of Mount Adams he must eventually reckon with the limitations of his own body.

As the afternoon wears on, Clare and his friend realize they will probably need to turn around before reaching the summit, given Clare's slow pace and the remaining hours of daylight. Such a decision doesn't come easily, however, and Clare shares his frustrations with his reader:

> I want to continue up to treeline, the pines shorter and shorter, grown twisted and withered, giving way to scrub brush, then to lichen-covered granite, up to the sun-drenched cap where the mountains all tumble out toward the hazy blue horizon. I want to so badly, but fear rumbles next to love next to real lived physical limitations, and so we decide to turn around. I cry, maybe for the first time, over something I want to do, had many reasons to believe I could, but really can't. I cry hard, then get up and follow Adrianne back down the mountain. It's hard and slow, and I use my hands and butt often and wish I could use gravity as Adrianne does to bounce from one flat spot to another, down this jumbled pile of rocks.

He goes on to discuss his ambivalence with this decision, an ambivalence stemming from his own internalized ableism. He cannot help but feel that he should have gone on, he should have overcome his limitations:

> I climbed Mount Adams for an hour and a half scared, not sure I'd ever be able to climb down, knowing that on the next rock my balance could give out, and yet I climbed. Climbed surely because I wanted the summit, because of the love rumbling in my bones. But climbed also because I wanted to say, "Yes, I have CP [cerebral palsy], but see. See, watch me. I can climb mountains too." I wanted to prove myself once again. I wanted to overcome my CP . . . . The mountain just won't let go.

Clare uses this experience to reflect on the ways disabled people hold ourselves up to norms that we can never achieve, norms that were based on bodies, minds, or experiences unlike our own. We want to believe that if we accomplish the right goals, if we overcome enough obstacles, we can defend ourselves against disability oppression.[39] The mountain, both literal and metaphorical, becomes a proving ground rather than a site of connection or relation, and it is this characterization that Clare challenges throughout the book.

The mountain as proving ground is a terrain of fierce independence: "In the wilderness myth, the body is pure, 'solo,' left to its own devices, and unmediated by any kind of aid."[40] Cripping this terrain, then, entails a more collaborative approach to nature. Kuppers depicts human-nonhuman nature interactions not in terms of solo ascents or individual feats of achievement but in terms of community action and ritual. Describing a gathering of disabled writers, artists, and community members, she writes, "We create our own rhythms and rock ourselves into the world of nature, lose ourselves in a moment of sharing: hummed songs in the round, shared breath, leanings, rocks against wood, leaves falling gentle against skin, bodies braced against others gently lowering toes into waves, touch of bark against finger, cheek, from warm hand to cold snow and back again."[41] In this resolutely embodied description, the human and nonhuman are brought into direct contact, connecting the fallen leaf to the tree or the breath to the wind. What entices me about this description is that it acknowledges loss or inability—she goes on to describe the borders of parking lots and the edges of pathways as the featured terrain, not cliff tops and crevices—and suggests alternative ways of interacting with the world around us. Rather than conquering or overcoming nature Kuppers and her comrades caress it, gaze upon it, breathe with it. Such forms of interaction are made more possible by recognizing nature as (and in) everything around us. The edges of the park, the spaces along its borders, are a part of nature too.

Moreover Kuppers's "we" is an acknowledgment of the ways in which our encounters with nature include and encompass relations with other people. Humans are interdependent, and our relationships with each other play a role in our understanding of the nonhuman world. Samuel Lurie, who is nondisabled, hints of this interdependence in an essay about his relationship with Clare:

> On one of our first hikes in Vermont, on a steep, slippery trail, the kind where Eli moves especially slowly—he was shrugging off my outstretched hand, not wanting any help. But I was only offering it in part to provide balance. "We're lovers out on a hike," I reasoned, "you're supposed to want to hold my hand." He laughed, relaxing, the tension breaking. . . .
>
> We hike more easily now, Eli referring to my hand serving as that "third point of contact"—stabilizing and comforting.[42]

How might this story of interdependence, of moving through nonhuman nature in relationship, expand the realm of ecofeminism? How might it bolster the claims of ecocritics who reject popular distinctions between humans and nature by presenting other humans as part of our encounters with nature? What happens to theory when it is no longer based primarily on tales of individuals' encounters with nature but on experiences of interdependence and community? Hiking with a small child, assisting an elderly relative through the woods, or sitting with a neighbor in a city park—all activities we might be doing already—can transform our ideas about nature and about ourselves. Recognizing our interdependence makes room for a range of experiences of human and nonhuman nature, disrupting the ableist ideology that everyone interacts with nature in the same way.

In her video In My Language, A. M. (Amanda) Baggs offers a visual and aural description of her interactions with the world around her, a description that radically expands econormative conceptions of both nature and interaction. To be clear, the video is not "about" nature and the environment; rather it is an autobiographical account of living with autism. Yet in this self-portrait Baggs interacts fully with her surroundings, challenging implicit assumptions that nature exists only "out there" as opposed to in the everyday spaces around us. In the first half of the video the only sounds we hear are Baggs's wordless songs and noises; the second half features a script Baggs wrote that is voiced by her computer. Throughout we watch Baggs touch, smell, listen to, look at, and tap objects around her. In one scene she gently moves her fingers through the water coming out of a faucet. These images are accompanied by text scrolling across the bottom of the screen, and Baggs's computer voices the words she has typed: "It [my language] is about being in a constant conversation with every aspect of my environment. Reacting physically to all parts of my surroundings. . . . The water doesn't symbolize anything. I am just interacting with the water as the water interacts with me."[43] The images confirm Baggs's syntax: the water spills across her fingers, shifting its flow in response to her movements. In foregrounding this mutual interaction between fingers and water, between self and stream, she pushes us to expand our conceptions of both language and nature; indeed the two are intimately related. Language is about interaction with our environment, a mutual interaction that does not, cannot, occur only in spoken words or written text.

Yet, as Baggs reminds us, spoken words and written text are almost always the only forms of communication recognized and valued as language. Similarly only certain kinds of interactions with the environment are recognized as such; swimming in the ocean and wading in mountain streams are more likely to be understood as meaningful ways to interact with water, while running one's fingers in the water under a faucet is not. But why not? The answer lies partly in long-standing assumptions that nature and the environment exist only "out there," outside of our houses and neighborhoods; the answer lies too in long-standing—and even less visible—assumptions that only certain ways of understanding and acting on one's relation to the environment (including other humans) are acceptable. These assumptions have significant material effects. Seeing nature as only out there or faucet water as categorically different from ocean water makes environmental justice work all the more difficult. And as Baggs argues in her video, seeing her diverse interactions with her environment as strange or abnormal makes it all too easy to ignore the institutionalization and abuse of people on the autism spectrum or people with intellectual disabilities.

Artist Riva Lehrer offers more visual images of crip approaches to nature, representations that argue for human-nonhuman relationships based on the very limitations or variations of the body that are typically ignored in environmental literature. In In the Yellow Woods (figure 6.1), a woman kneels on the ground, peeling the bark from a branch with her knife. She looks down, concentrating on her work, completely focused on the task before her. On the ground around her are scattered bones, bones she has carved herself from tree branches and trunks. A perfect pelvis, a rib cage, random bits of leg and spine—all lie next to her on the ground. She is literally carving a body from the trees. The painting, and the woman, seem inhabited by loss; the intensity of her concentration suggests the necessity of these new bones, untouched by pain or surgery or breakage. And yet the scattered placement of the bones suggests that this work is not about creating wholeness, not about finding the cure in this forest; she has not arranged the bones in the shape of a body, and she is not inserting them into her skin. Rather the bones seem to sink into the fallen leaves, to become part of the autumn landscape.

Bones become roots, linking this woman—her body, her self—to the landscape, literally grounding her in space and time. And time itself is in play here, as these bones vary in their coloration, marking time across their surfaces. The pelvis gleams white, new, untouched by rain and storm, while some of the longer bones—rib, clavicle, femur—bear the marks of time, calling to mind fossils of previous generations, suggesting that these bones are not for her only. By the same token, the dress pattern tacked to the tree in the background suggests a future project, a sign of additional work to come, a guideline for other bodies. Although she is depicted alone in this forest, signs of other bodies, other figures, echo around the woman.

It is the process captured in the painting that captures me, that draws me in to the figure's meditative practice. How does this painting simultaneously offer a new map of the body and a new map of nature? How might it open up new avenues of understanding ourselves in relationship to nonhuman nature? How does it blur the very line between the human and the nonhuman? Reading this painting from a cripped ecofeminist perspective, I see a woman making a connection between caring for the body and caring for the earth, suggesting an expanded view of health that looks beyond the boundaries of the body. This is not a supercrip story of triumphing over disability, and it's not an ableist story of bodies without limitation. It's a story of recognizing ourselves in the world around us, recognizing common structures of bone, flesh, oxygen, and air.

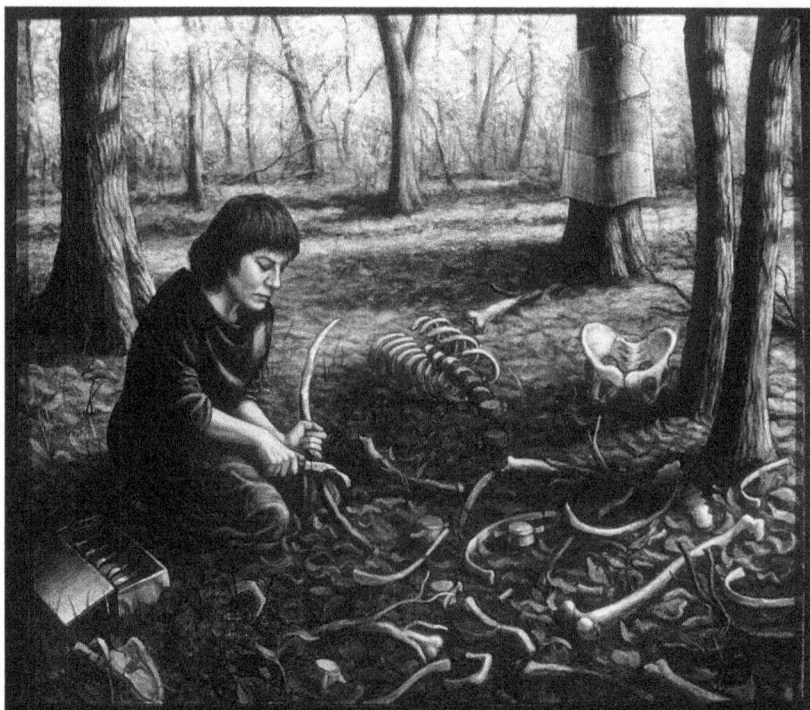

Fig. 6.1. Riva Lehrer, <u>In the Yellow Woods</u>, 1993, acrylic on panel.

These connections manifest again in Lehrer's portrait of Eli Clare, part of her <u>Circle Stories</u> series of paintings chronicling the lives of disability artists, activists, and intellectuals. In this 2003 painting (figure 6.2) Clare crouches on the ground, one knee touching the sandy soil, the other bracing his body. In the background is a river lined by trees, trees that are reflected in the surface of the water. The detail with which the flora is represented is telling, making clear that the plants are as important as the person. In fact person and plant are not easily distinguished, as evidenced by the young sapling emerging out of Clare's chest. The tree is rooted firmly in the ground before Clare, and it curves to snake through his shirt. It's not clear if Clare has buttoned

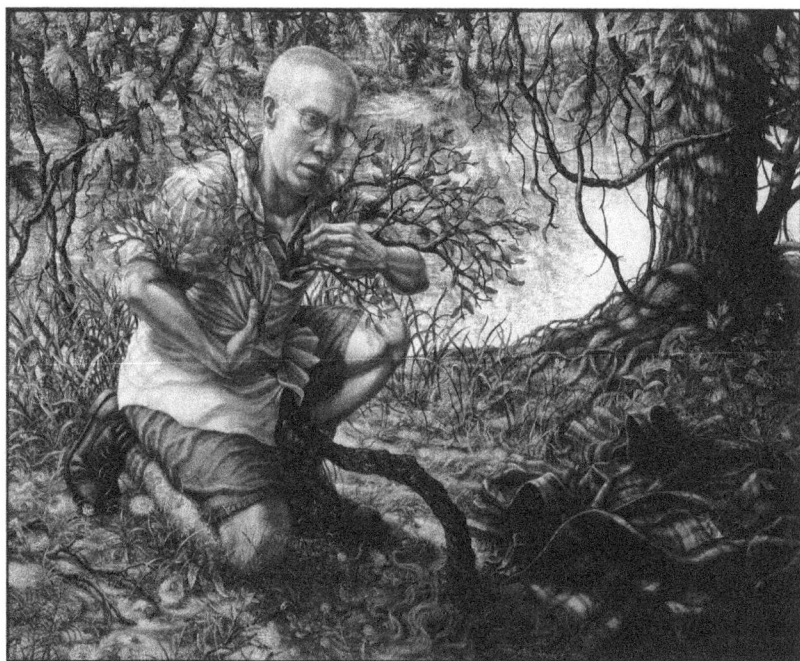

Fig. 6.2. Riva Lehrer, Circle Stories #10: Eli Clare, 2003, acrylic on panel.

his shirt around the tree, clutching it to his chest, or if the tree made its own way onto Clare's skin, the two figures moving upward together. The painting is breathtaking in its conjuring of an entire ecosystem, one that recognizes humans as inextricably part of nature. Its power also lies in its mythology, in its blending together of environmental, disability, and gender politics.

As Lehrer makes clear in her artist's statement, her Circle Stories paintings are intensely collaborative. She meets repeatedly with her subjects, studying and discussing their work and brainstorming potential imagery. Lehrer's work with Clare coincided with his transition from butch female to genderqueer to transman (the collaboration lasted approximately two and a half years), and it seems no accident that this young tree explodes from the site of Clare's changed chest. The image implicitly challenges easy depictions of technology as bad, as encroaching on the alleged purity of nature. This tree is healthy, vibrant; advanced biomedicine hasn't stunted its growth. On the ground before Clare are long locks of red hair, even a piece of a braid, suggesting that he has shed traces of femininity just as the trees around him will drop their leaves. The site of nature serves as a site of transformation in this painting, the clutched tree rooting Clare in his history but also exploding outward in new directions.

These tales of the gendered body intertwine with tales of the crip body. Clare writes poignant prose and poetry about living in a body marked by tremors and an uneven gait, signs of his cerebral palsy. Knowing these histories of Clare's body, I can't help but notice that it is his right hand that clutches the tree to his chest, his right hand that pulls the shirt closed around his sapling. In an essay titled "Stolen Bodies, Reclaimed Bodies," Clare writes, "Sometimes I wanted to cut off my right arm so it wouldn't shake. My shame was that plain, that bleak."[44] This image serves as an antidote to that memory, a reclaiming of that right arm. The steady sureness of the sapling—rooted, curving into Clare's body without breaking or splintering—becomes linked to the sure shaking of his body, so that the tremors become rooted in both the body and the place. Like the bone woman in the forest, Clare isn't connecting with nature in order to be cured of his allegedly broken body; rather he is solidly locating that body in space and time. He's not getting rid of the tremor but locating it, grounding it; it's as much a part of his body as the tree. As in In the Yellow Wood, Lehrer again presents a model of embodied environmentalism, of a concern with how we can get on together, earth, bone, and body.

I bring these paintings into my exploration of disability and environmentalism because they conjure images of nature-human relationships that not only allow for the presence of bodies with limited, odd, or queer movements and orientations, but they literally carve out a space for them, recognizing them as a vital part of the landscape. The content of Clare's and Lehrer's work as activists encourages my paying attention to these images, facilitates my placing them within the discourse of ecological feminism and environmentalism. Both of them are longtime advocates for environmental causes: Exile and Pride is a complex meditation on relationships among race, class, poverty, labor politics, gender, and environmental destruction and conservation in the Pacific Northwest, and Lehrer is a longtime supporter of animal rights movements.[45] Moreover they both make explicit connections between these environmental projects and their location in disability communities. Clare writes poignantly about the disabling effects of logging on bodies and ecosystems and of coming to understand his crip body on the rural roads and creek sides of rural Oregon. His book, which bears the subtitle Disability, Queerness, and Liberation, is dedicated "to the rocks and trees, hills and beaches," suggesting a direct link between his understanding of queer disability and the landscapes around him. Similarly Lehrer's paintings often combine landscapes with portraits, and nonhuman animals are a common presence. In two of her most recent series, Family and Totems and Familiars, she showcases relationships between human and nonhuman animals; in the latter she depicts Nomy Lamm and other crip artists alongside their animal familiars, which serve as alter egos or sources of strength. The cultural productions of artists such as Clare and Lehrer enact alternative versions of nature and of humans' position within it. They are imagining and embodying new understandings of environmentalism that take disability experiences seriously, as sites of knowledge production about nature. Their future visions, because grounded in present crip communities, recognize disability experiences and human limitations as essential, not marginal or tangential, to questions about nature and environmental movements.

NOTES

1. Shakespeare, <u>Disability Rights and Wrongs</u>, 45, 46.
2. Mortimer-Sandilands and Erickson, introduction to Queer Ecologies, 19. The authors discuss Joe Hermer's work on campgrounds in their thorough examination of queer ecologies.
3. Cronon, introduction to <u>Uncommon Ground</u>; Cronon, "The Trouble with Wilderness." See also Chaia Heller, "For the Love of Nature: Ecology and the Cult of the Romantic," in <u>Ecofeminism: Women, Animals, Nature</u>, edited by Greta Gaard (Philadelphia: Temple University Press, 1993), 219–42; Lauret Savoy, "The Future of Environmental Essay: A Discourse," <u>Terrain</u>, Summer–Fall 2008, online.
4. White, "Black Women and the Wilderness." On Carolyn Finney's work, see Barry Bergman, "Black, White, and Shades of Green," <u>Berkeleyan</u>, November 28, 2007, http://berkeley.edu/news/berkeleyan/2007/11/28_finney.shtml. Surveys of park-goers support these claims, revealing that visitors to wilderness parks such as Yosemite and Yellowstone tend overwhelmingly to be white. A survey conducted at Yosemite in 2009 found white people constituted 77 percent of park visitors; 11 percent were Latino, 11 percent were Asian, and only 1 percent were black. Mireya Navarro, "National Parks Reach Out to Blacks Who Aren't Visiting," <u>New York Times</u>, November 2, 2010, http://www.nytimes.com/2010/11/o3/science/earth/o3parks.html?scp=2&sq=race+national+parks&st=nyt. See also Jason Byrne and Jennifer Wolch, "Nature, Race, and Parks: Past Research and Future Directions for Geographic Research," <u>Progress in Human Geography</u> 33, no. 6 (2009): 743–65; John Grossmann, "Expanding the Palette," <u>National Parks</u> 84, no. 3 (2010): 1.
5. Evans, "'Nature' and Environmental Justice," 191–92.
6. Evans, "'Nature' and Environmental Justice," 191, 192.
7. Cronon, introduction to <u>Uncommon Ground</u>, 25.
8. I am excited by the rethinking of materiality taking place in feminist theory and environmental studies; I agree we need, in Stacy Alaimo's

framing, "investigations that account for the ways in which nature, the environment, and the material world itself signify, act upon, or otherwise affect human bodies, knowledges, and practices" (<u>Bodily Natures</u>, 7–8). Although here I focus more on discursive constructions of nature, I see my project as a necessary complement to that work, as we have yet to reckon closely with relationships between disability, ability, and nature.

9. Vance, "Ecofeminism and Wilderness," 71.
10. According to blurbs on the book's cover, the <u>New Yorker</u> called the book "an American masterpiece," while the <u>New York Times Book Review</u> praised it for its "power and beauty." This is not to say that Abbey is without critics; on the contrary Abbey has long been challenged for his views on women and immigration. He himself describes <u>Desert Solitaire</u> as "coarse, rude, bad-tempered, violently prejudiced, unconstructive," and likely to draw criticism from "serious critics, serious librarians, serious associate professors" (<u>Desert Solitaire</u>, xii). I thank Cathy Kudlick for pushing me to engage with this text.
11. Abbey, <u>Desert Solitaire</u>, 49, 51, 233.
12. Ray, "Risking Bodies in the Wild," 271, 272.
13. Abbey, <u>Desert Solitaire</u>, 233, 49.
14. The genre of nature writing relies heavily on the epistemological assumption that walking brings knowledge. As both Hart ("'Enough Defined'") and Ray ("Risking Bodies in the Wild") note in their discussion of nature writing, walking is the privileged method of attaining a sense of unity and wholeness with nature.
15. Ray, "Risking Bodies in the Wild," 260. Abbey was himself influenced by Thoreau and other writers who came before him.
16. For a discussion of such exclusions, see Giovanna Di Chiro, "Nature as Community: The Convergence of Environment and Social Justice," in <u>Uncommon Ground: Toward Reinventing Nature</u>, edited by William Cronon (New York: Norton, 1995), 298–319; Evans, "'Nature' and Environmental Justice"; Gaard, "Ecofeminism and Wilderness"; Vance, "Ecofeminism and the Politics of Reality"; Richard T. Twine, "Ma(r)king Essence: Ecofeminism and Embodiment," <u>Ethics and the Environment</u> 6, no. 2 (2001): 31–57.
17. Nike issued its first apology on October 24, 2000, expressing regret for the offensive nature of the ad and stressing its own connec-

tion to the disability community, a connection embodied by the fact that a former Nike executive was "confined to a wheelchair." The company tried again a day later, stating that disabilities "are no laughing matter" and that disabled people "demonstrate more courage in a day than most of us will in a lifetime." Striking some activists as condescending for its assumption that any attempt to live with disability is worthy of praise, that apology was followed shortly thereafter with a more straightforward one. Taken together the group of apologies maps out the overlapping models of disability available to Nike: disability as tragedy, disabled people as inspiration to others, disability as the site of pity. The apologies were all posted on Nike's website, although disability activists argued that Nike should print its apologies in the same publications in which the ad originally appeared; only then could the company begin to rectify the damage of the original ad. The ad and the apologies have since been removed from the company's website.

My understanding of the Nike controversy comes from the following: Bruce Steele, "Faculty Member Encourages Boycott over Ad," University Times (University of Pittsburgh), November 22, 2000; "Crip Community Outraged at Nike Ad," Ragged Edge Online Extra, 2000, http://www.ragged-edge-mag.com/extra/nikead.htm; "Nike Issues Formal Apology, Ragged Edge Online Extra, 2000, http://www .ragged-edge-mag.com/extra/nikead.htm. On the use of disability and disabled people in advertising, see Rosemarie Garland-Thomson, "Seeing the Disabled: Visual Rhetorics of Disability in Popular Photography," in The New Disability History: American Perspectives, edited by Paul K. Longmore and Lauri Umansky (New York: New York University Press, 2001), 335–74.

18. Nike has long had a reputation for running edgy advertisements, and they very well may have suspected that the ad would generate some controversy (and thereby garner some free publicity). But even that strategy would rely on the assumption that they could offend or anger disability communities without alienating their consumers or affecting their bottom line.

19. Although the freak show did not disappear in the 1940s, it was no longer as acceptable or as widespread as it had been in the previous decades. For accounts of this history, see, for example,

Leslie Fiedler, Freaks: Myths and Images of the Secret Self (New York: Simon and Schuster, 1978); Robert Bogdan, Freak Show: Presenting Human Oddities for Amusement and Profit (Chicago: University of Chicago Press, 1988); Rosemarie Garland-Thomson, ed., Freakery: Cultural Spectacles of the Extraordinary Body (New York: New York University Press, 1996); Garland-Thomson, Extraordinary Bodies; Leonard Cassuto, The Inhuman Race: The Racial Grotesque in American Literature and Culture (New York: Columbia University Press, 1997); Rachel Adams, Sideshow U.S.A.: Freaks and the American Cultural Imagination (Chicago: University of Chicago Press, 2001).

20. Garland-Thomson, Extraordinary Bodies, 41.
21. Ray, "Risking Bodies in the Wild," 263.
22. Vance, "Ecofeminism and the Politics of Reality," 133.
23. See, for example, Vance, "Ecofeminism and Wilderness."
24. According to a survey of people with learning disabilities and cognitive impairments, a lack of materials in alternative formats is one of the more alienating dimensions of public parks (Mathers, "Hidden Voices"). The survey covered only urban parks, but it seems likely that the same would be true of wilderness parks.
25. Imrie and Thomas, "Interrelationships between Environment and Disability," 477.
26. For a discussion of the access battles at Maine's Allagash Waterway, see A. J. Higgins, "Canoe Launch Divides Environmentalists, Disabled," Boston Globe, June 4, 2000; Joe Huber, "Accessibility vs. Wilderness Preservation: Maine's Allagash Wilderness Waterway," Palaestra: Forum of Sport, Physical Education, and Recreation for Those with Disabilities 16, no. 4 (2000), online (Huber's article has since been removed from the Palaestra site). For a more general discussion of accessibility, wilderness, and the law, see Jennie Bricker, "Wheelchair Accessibility in Wilderness Areas: The Nexus between the ADA and the Wilderness Act," Environmental Law 25, no. 4 (1995): 1243–70.
27. Bruce was responding to a front-page article in the Times about the modifications to the hut at Galehead and the integrated hiking team. Carey Goldberg, "For These Trailblazers, Wheelchairs Matter," New York Times, August 17, 2000; Dan Bruce, letter to the editor, New

York Times, August 21, 2000, http://www.nytimes.com/2000/08/21
/opinion/l-destructive-hiking-748404.html.

28. Quoted in "Trailblazing in a Wheelchair," 52.

29. Quoted in Goldberg, "For These Trailblazers." Gravink was the director of the Northeast Passage program at the University of New Hampshire, the organization sponsoring the hike.

30. Whole Access was founded in 1983 by Phyllis Cangemi; although the group often served as a clearinghouse for individuals interested in accessible trails, its primary goal was to educate park managers and planners about accessibility. Cangemi, who served as the executive director of the organization, died in 2005, and Whole Access closed not long after.

31. Steep trails (which hinder the use of wheelchairs) tend to collect water and create erosion channels, eventually damaging the trail and surrounding terrain (Cangemi, "Trail Design," 4).

32. "Accessibility Guidelines for Trails."

33. Sieck, "On a Roll." See also Claire Tregaskis, "Applying the Social Model in Practice: Some Lessons from Countryside Recreation," Disability and Society 19, no. 6 (2004): 601–11.

34. Hershey includes the excised section of the essay on her website, as well as a brief description of her exchange with the editor. Hershey, "Along Asphalt Trails (The Rest of the Story)"; Hershey, "Along Asphalt Trails."

35. Sieck, "On a Roll."

36. Weihenmayer, Touch the Top of the World, 5–7.

37. Kuppers, "Outsides," 1.

38. Sandilands, "Unnatural Passions?"

39. Clare, Exile and Pride, 4, 5, 8–9.

40. Ray, "Risking Bodies in the Wild," 265.

41. Kuppers, "Outsides," 2.

42. Lurie, "Loving You Loving Me," 85.

43. Baggs, In My Language.

44. Clare, "Stolen Bodies, Reclaimed Bodies," 362.

45. The relationship between disability rights and animal rights movements, not to mention the overlaps and gaps between the categories of disability and animality, is a rich site for analysis. Philosopher

Peter Singer's use of cognitive disability to make arguments for animal rights has long been criticized by disability studies scholars and activists (and with good reason), and the representation of disabled people as animals has a deep and troubling history that is thoroughly entwined with scientific racism and eugenics. At the same time there are exciting possibilities for political and theoretical collaboration between disability studies and animal studies. Several sessions of the Society for Disability Studies conferences in recent years have addressed the potential for animal rights–disability rights alliances, and there are scholars, activists, and artists working to deconstruct and reimagine the relationship between animality and disability. See, for example, Licia Carlson, The Faces of Intellectual Disability (Bloomington: Indiana University Press, 2010); Mel Y. Chen, Animacies: Biopolitics, Racial Mattering, and Queer Affect (Durham NC: Duke University Press, 2012); Nora Ellen Groce and Jonathan Marks, "The Great Ape Project and Disability Rights: Ominous Undercurrents of Eugenics in Action," American Anthropologist 102, no. 4 (2001): 818–22; Sunaura Taylor, "Beasts of Burden: Disability Studies and Animal Rights," Qui Parle: Critical Humanities and Social Sciences 19, no. 2 (2011): 191–222; Cary Wolfe, "Learning from Temple Grandin, or, Animal Studies, Disability Studies, and Who Comes after the Subject," New Formations 64 (2008): 110–23. See also the artwork of the painter Sunaura Taylor, whose Animal exhibition at the Rowan Morrison Gallery in Oakland, California in October 2009 tracked the overlapping visual iconography of freak shows, medical textbooks, and butcher-shop diagrams. Images from the show are available on Taylor's website, http://www.sunaurataylor.org/portfolio/animal/.

BIBLIOGRAPHY

Abbey, Edward. Desert Solitaire: A Season in the Wilderness. New York: Touchstone, 1990.

"Accessibility Guidelines for Trails." Universal Design Newsletter, July 1999, 5.

Alaimo, Stacy. Bodily Natures: Science, Environment, and the Material Self. Bloomington: Indiana University Press, 2010.

Baggs, A. M. In My Language. YouTube, January 14, 2007, https://www .youtube.com/watch?v=JnylM1hI2jc.

Cangemi, Phyllis. "Trail Design: Balancing Accessibility and Nature." Universal Design Newsletter, July 1999, 4.

Clare, Eli. Exile and Pride: Disability, Queerness, and Liberation. Boston: South End Press, 1999.

———. "Stolen Bodies, Reclaimed Bodies: Disability and Queerness," Public Culture 13, no. 3 (2001): 359–65.

Cronon, William. Introduction to Uncommon Ground: Toward Reinventing Nature, edited by William Cronon, 23–56. New York: Norton, 1995.

——— "The Trouble with Wilderness; or, Getting Back to the Wrong Nature." In Uncommon Ground: Toward Reinventing Nature, edited by William Cronon, 69–90. New York: Norton, 1995.

Evans, Mei Mei. "'Nature' and Environmental Justice." In The Environmental Justice Reader: Politics, Poetics, and Pedagogy, edited by Joni Adamson, Mei Mei Evans, and Rachel Stein, 191–92. Tucson: University of Arizona Press, 2002.

Gaard, Greta. "Ecofeminism and Wilderness." Environmental Ethics 19, no. 1 (1997): 5–24.

Garland-Thomson, Rosemarie. Extraordinary Bodies: Figuring Physical Disability in American Culture and Literature. New York: Columbia University Press, 1997.

Hart, George. "'Enough Defined': Disability, Ecopoetics, and Larry Eigner." Contemporary Literature 51, no. 1 (2010): 152–79.

Hershey, Laura. "Along Asphalt Trails." National Parks 82, no. 4 (2008): 22–24.

———. "Along Asphalt Trails (The Rest of the Story)." Blog, September 18, 2008. http://www.laurahershey.com/?p=4.

Huber, Joe. "Trailblazing in a Wheelchair—An Oxymoron?" Palaestra: Forum of Sport, Physical Education, and Recreation for Those with Disabilities 17, no. 4 (2001): 52.

Imrie, Rob, and Huw Thomas. "The Interrelationships between Environment and Disability." Local Environment 13, no. 6 (2008): 477–83.

Kuppers, Petra. "Outsides: Disability Culture Nature Poetry." Journal of Literary Disability 1, no. 1 (2007): 22–33.

Lurie, Samuel. "Loving You Loving Me." In Queer Crips: Disabled Gay Men and Their Stories, edited by Bob Guter and John R. Killacky, 83–86. New York: Harrington Park Press, 2004.

Mathers, A. R. "Hidden Voices: The Participation of People with Learning Disabilities in the Experience of Public Open Space." Local Environment 13, no. 6 (2008): 515–29.

Mortimer-Sandilands, Catriona, and Bruce Erickson. Introduction to Queer Ecologies: Sex, Nature, Politics, Desire, 1–47. Bloomington: Indiana University Press, 2010.

Ray, Sarah Jaquette. "Risking Bodies in the Wild: The 'Corporeal Unconscious' of American Adventure Culture." Journal of Sport and Social Issues 33, no. 3 (2009): 257–84. .

Sandilands, Catriona. "Unnatural Passions? Toward a Queer Ecology." Invisible Culture, no. 9 (2005). http://www.rochester.edu/in_visible_culture/Issue_9/sandilands.html.

Shakespeare, Tom. Disability Rights and Wrongs. New York: Routledge, 2006.

Sieck, Ann. "On a Roll: A Wheelchair Hiker Gets Back on the Trail." Bay Nature, October 1, 2006. http://baynature.org/articles/on-a-roll.

Terry, Jennifer. "'Unnatural Acts' in Nature: The Scientific Fascination with Queer Animals." GLQ: A Journal of Lesbian and Gay Studies 6, no. 2 (2000): 151–93.

Vance, Linda. "Ecofeminism and the Politics of Reality." In Ecofeminism: Women, Animals, and Nature, edited by Greta Gaard, 118–45. Philadelphia: Temple University Press, 1993.

———. "Ecofeminism and Wilderness." NWSA Journal 9, no. 3 (1997): 60–76.

Weihenmayer, Erik. Touch the Top of the World: A Blind Man's Journey to Climb Farther than the Eye Can See. New York: Plume, 2002.

White, Evelyn C. "Black Women and the Wilderness." In The Stories That Shape Us: Contemporary Women Write about the West, edited by Teresa Jordan and James Hepworth, 376–83. New York: Norton, 1995.

7

Notes on Natural Worlds, Disabled Bodies, and a Politics of Cure

Eli Clare

Prairie

You and I walk in the summer rain through a thirty-acre pocket of tallgrass prairie that not so long ago was one big cornfield. We follow the path mowed as a firebreak. You carry a big flowered umbrella. Water droplets hang on the grasses. Spiderwebs glint. The bee balm hasn't blossomed yet. You point to numerous patches of birch and goldenrod; they belong here but not in this plenty. The thistle, on the other hand, simply shouldn't be here. The Canada wild rye waves, the big bluestem almost open. Sunflowers cluster, spots of yellow orange amid the gray green of a rainy day. The songbirds and butterflies have taken shelter. For the moment the prairie is quiet. Soon my jeans are sopping wet from the knees down. Not an ocean of grasses but a start, this little piece of prairie is utterly different from row upon row of corn.

With the help of the Department of Natural Resources you mowed and burned the corn, broadcast the seed—bluestem, wild rye, bee balm, cornflower, sunflower, aster—sack upon sack of just the right mix that might replicate the tallgrass prairie that was once here. Only remnants of the original ecosystem remain in the Midwest, isolated pockets of leadplants, milkweed, burr oaks, and switchgrass growing in cemeteries, along railroad beds, on remote bluffs, somehow miraculously surviving.

You burn; you plant; you root out thistle and prickly ash. You tend, save money for more seed, burn again. Over the past decade and a half of labor you've worked to undo the two centuries of damage wrought by plows, pesticides, monoculture farming, and fire suppression. The state of Wisconsin partners in this work precisely because the damage is so great. Without the massive web of prairie roots to anchor the earth; bison to turn, fertilize, and aerate the earth; and lightning-strike fire to burn and renew the earth, the land now known as Wisconsin is literally draining away. Rain catches the topsoil, washing it from field to creek to river to ocean. Prairie restoration reverses this process, both stabilizing and creating soil. So you work hard to restore this eight-thousand-year-old ecosystem, all the while remembering that the land isn't yours or the dairy farmer's down the road; it was stolen a mere century and a half ago from the Dakota people. The histories of dirt, grass, genocide, bison massacre float here.

We have taken this walk a dozen times over the past fifteen years, at noon with the sun blazing, at dusk with fireflies lacing the grasses, at dawn with finches and warblers greeting the day. My feet still feel the old corn furrows. As we walk I think about the words natural and unnatural, normal and abnormal. Does this fragment of land in transition from cornfield to tallgrass prairie define what natural is? If so, how do we name the overabundance of birch and goldenrod, the absence of bison? What was once normal here? What can we consider normal now? Normal and natural dance together, while unnatural and abnormal bully, threaten, patrol the boundaries. Of course it's an inscrutable dance. How does unnatural technology repair so-called abnormal bodies to their natural ways of being? Dismissing the distinctions between normal and abnormal, natural and unnatural, as meaningless would be lovely, except they wield extraordinary power.

Abnormal, Unnatural

It is not an exaggeration to say that the words <u>unnatural</u> and <u>abnormal</u> haunt me as a disabled person. Or maybe, more accurately, they pummel me. Complete strangers ask me, "What's your defect?" Their intent is mostly benign. To them my body simply doesn't work right, <u>defect</u> being another variation of <u>broken</u>, supposedly neutral. But think of the things called defective: the boom box that won't play a CD, the car that never started reliably, the calf born with three legs. They end up in the back of the closet, the trash heap, the scrap yard, the slaughterhouse. Defects are disposable and <u>abnormal</u>, bodies to eradicate.

Or complete strangers yell at me down the road, across the playground, "Hey, retard!" Their intent is often malicious. Sometimes they have thrown rocks, sand, and rubber erasers. Once on a camping trip with my family I joined a whole crowd of kids playing tag in and around the picnic shelter. A slow and clumsy nine-year-old, I quickly became "it." I chased and chased but caught no one. The game turned. Kids came close, ducked away, yelling "Defect, retard." Frustrated, I yelled back for a while. "Retard" became "monkey"; became a circle around me; became a torrent, "Monkey defect retard you're a monkey monkey monkey"; became huge gulping sobs of rage, frustration, humiliation, shame; became not knowing who I was. My body crumpled. It lasted two minutes or two hours until my father appeared and the circle scattered. Even as the word <u>monkey</u> connected me to the nonhuman <u>natural</u> world, I became supremely <u>unnatural</u>.

Or complete strangers pat me on the head. They whisper platitudes in my ear, clichés about courage and inspiration. They enthuse about how remarkable I am. They declare me special. Once a woman wearing dreamcatcher earrings, a big turquoise necklace, and a fringed leather tunic with a medicine wheel painted on the back confided that I was, like all people who tremor, a <u>natural</u> shaman. She grabbed me in a long hug and advised that if I were trained, I could become a great healer. Before this woman, sporting a mishmash of Indigenous symbols, jewelry, and clothing, released me from her grip, she directed me never to forget my specialness. Oh, how <u>special</u> disabled people are: we have <u>special</u> education, <u>special</u> needs, <u>special</u> restrooms, <u>special</u> parking spots. That word drips condescension. It's no better than being defective. As <u>special</u> people, we are still <u>abnormal</u> and disposable.

Or complete strangers offer me Christian prayers or crystals and vitamins, always with the same intent; to touch me, fix me, mend my cerebral palsy, if only I will comply. They cry over me, wrap their arms around my shoulders, kiss my cheek. Even now, after five decades of these kinds of interactions, I still don't know how to rebuff their pity, how to tell them the simple truth that I'm not broken. Even if there were a cure for brain cells that died at birth, I'd refuse. I have no idea who I'd be without my specific tremoring, slurring, tense body. Those strangers assume my body is <u>unnatural</u>, want to make me <u>normal</u>, take for granted the need and desire for cure. <u>Unnatural</u> and <u>abnormal</u> pummel me every day.

Restoration

As an ideology seeped into every corner of Western thought and culture, cure rides on the back of <u>normal</u> and <u>natural</u>. Insidious and pervasive, it impacts many, many bodies. In response we need a politics of cure: not a simple or reactive belief system, not an anti-cure stance in the face of the endless assumptions about bodily difference, but rather a broad-based politics mirroring the complexity of all our bodies and minds.

The American Heritage Dictionary defines cure as "restoration of health." In developing a politics of cure based on this definition it would be all too easy to get mired in an argument about health, trying to determine who's healthy and who's not, as if there's one objective standard. As an alternative I want to bypass the questions of who defines health and for what purposes. So many folks are working to redefine health, struggling toward a theory and practice that will contribute to the well-being of entire communities. But I won't be joining them with a redefinition of my own. Instead I want a politics of cure that speaks from inside the intense contradictions presented by the multiple meanings of health.

Today in the white Western world dominated by allopathic medicine, health ranges from individual and communal bodily comfort to profound social control. Between these two poles a multitude of practices exist. Health promotes both the well-being sustained by good food and the products sold by the multimillion-dollar diet industry. It endorses both effective pain management for folks who live with chronic pain and the policed refusal to prescribe narcotic-based pain relief to people perceived as drug seeking. It both saves lives and aggressively markets synthetic growth hormone to children whose only bodily "problem" is being short.

Rather than offer a resolution to this whole range of contradictory, overlapping, and confused meanings of health, I want to follow the word restoration. To restore an object or an ecosystem is to return it to an earlier, often better condition. We restore a house that's falling down, a prairie that's been decimated by generations of monoculture farming and fire suppression. In this return we try to undo the harm, wishing the harm had never happened. Talk to anyone who does restoration work—a carpenter who rebuilds 150-year-old neglected houses, a conservation biologist who turns cornfields back to prairie—and she'll say it's a complex undertaking. A fluid, responsive process, restoration requires digging into the past, stretching toward the future, working hard in the present. And the end results rarely, if ever, match the original state.

Restoring an ecosystem means rebuilding a dynamic system that has somehow been interrupted or broken, devastated by strip mining or clear-cut logging, taken over by invasive species, unbalanced by the loss of predators, crushed by pollution. The work is not about re-creating a static landscape somehow frozen in time but rather about encouraging and reshaping dynamic ecological interdependencies, ranging from clods of dirt to towering thunderheads, tiny microbes to herds of bison, into a self-sustaining system of constant flux. This reshaping mirrors the original or historical ecosystem as closely as possible, but inevitably some element is missing or different. The return may be close but is never complete.

The process of restoration is simpler with a static object, an antique chair, or old house. Still, if the carpenters aren't using ax-hewn timbers of assorted and quirky sizes, mixing the plaster with horse hair, building at least a few walls with chicken wire, and using newspaper, rags, or nothing at all for insulation, then the return will be incomplete, possibly sturdier and definitely more energy efficient but different from the original house. Even though restoration as a process is never complete, it always requires an original or historical state in which to root itself, a belief that this state is better than what currently exists, and a desire to return to the original.

Thinking about the framework of restoration, I circle back to the folks who offer disabled and chronically ill people prayers, crystals, and vitamins, believing deeply in the necessity of cure. A simple one-to-one correspondence between ecological restoration and bodily restoration reveals cure's mandate of returning damaged bodies to some former, and nondisabled, state of being. This mandate clearly locates the problem, or damage, of disability within individual disabled or chronically ill bodies.

To resist the ableism in this framing a disability politics has emerged in the past forty years. It asserts that disability is lodged not in paralysis but in the stairs without an accompanying ramp, not in blindness but in the lack of Braille. Disability itself does not live in depression or anxiety but rather exists in a whole host of stereotypes, not in dyslexia but in teaching methods unwilling to flex, not in lupus or multiple sclerosis but in the belief that certain bodily conditions are a fate worse than death. In short, disability politics establishes that the problem of disability is not about individual bodies but about social injustice.

But for some of us, even if we accept disability as harm to individual bodies, restoration still does not make sense, because an original non-disabled body does not exist. How would I, or the medical establishment, go about restoring my body? The vision of me without tremoring hands and slurred speech, with more balance and coordination, does not originate from my body's history. Rather it arises from an imagination of what my body should be like, some definition of <u>normal</u> and <u>natural</u>.

Not Simple

To reflect the multilayered relationships between disabled and chronically ill bodies and restoration, a politics of cure needs to be as messy and visceral as our bodies. To reach into this messiness, I turn to story.

You and I know each other through a loose national network of queer disability activists, made possible by the Internet. Online one evening I receive a message from you containing the cyber equivalent to a long, anguished moan of physical pain. You explain that you're having a bad pain day, and it helps just to acknowledge the need to howl. Before I log off I type a good-night to you, wish you a little less pain for the morning. The next day you thank me for not wishing you a pain-free day. You say, "The question isn't whether I'm in pain but rather how much." Later, as I get to know you in person, you tell me, "I read medical journals hoping for a breakthrough in pain treatment that might make a difference." You wait, trying to get doctors to believe your pain and, once you get the appropriate scripts, working to find the right balance of narcotics. The rhetoric of many disability activists declares, "There's nothing wrong with disabled bodies and minds, even as they differ from what's considered normal." I have used this line myself more than once, to which you respond, "Not assuming our bodies are wrong makes sense, but the chronic fatiguing hell pain I live with is not a healthy variation, not a natural bodily difference."

I pause, thinking hard about natural. In disability community we sometimes half-sarcastically call non-disabled people tempo-rarily able-bodied, or TABS, precisely because of the one instant that can disable any of us. Are these moments and locations of disability and chronic illness natural as our fragile, resilient human bodies interact with the world? Is it natural when a spine snaps after being flung from a car; when a brain processes informa-tion in fragmented ways after being exposed to lead, mercury, pesticides, uranium tailings; when a body or mind assumes its own shape with withered muscles or foreshortened limbs, brittle bones or ears that do not hear sound, after genes settle into their own particular patterns soon after conception? And when are those moments and locations of disability and chronic illness unnatural, as unnatural as war, toxic landfills, and poverty? Who, pray tell, determines natural and unnatural? I'm searching for a politics of cure that grapples both with the pain, brokenness, and limitation contained within disabled bodies and with the encompassing damage of ableism.

I return to story. You and I sit in a roomful of disabled people, slowly inching our way toward enough familiarity to start telling bone-deep truths. And when we arrive there, you say, "If I could wake up tomorrow and not have diabetes, I'd choose that day in a heartbeat." I can almost hear the stream of memory: the daily insulin; the tracking of blood sugar level; the shame; the endless doctors judging your weight, your food, your numbers; the seizures; the long-term unknowns. You don't hate your body or equate diabetes with misery. You're not waiting desperate, half-panicked. All the time and money spent on research rather than universal health care, a genuine social safety net, an end to poverty and hunger pisses you off. At the same time you're weary of all the analogies: the hope that one day AIDS will become as treatable and manageable as diabetes, the equating of trans-sexual hormone replacement therapy with insulin. You want to stamp your feet and say, "Pay attention to this specific experi-ence of Type I diabetes: my daily dependence on a synthesized hormone, my life balanced on this chemical, the maintenance that marks every meal." You'd take a cure tomorrow, and at the same time you relish sitting in this room.

In creating a politics of cure, we need to hold both the desire to restore a pancreas to its typical functioning and the value bodily difference, knowing all the while that we will never live in a world where disability does not exist. How do we embrace the brilliant imperfection of disability and what it has to offer the world while knowing that very few of us would actively choose it to begin with?[1]

I return again to disability community. You and I talk, as we so often do, over food, this time pasta, bread, and olive oil. It would be a cliché to start with a description of your face across from mine, a story of color and texture, which I both see and don't. Certainly I observe the vivid outline of your birthmark, its curve of color, but that colored shape does not become your entire being. I know from your stories that your face precedes you into the world, that one visible distinction becoming your whole body. You say, "I don't know why I stopped wearing that thick waxy makeup; why after a childhood of medical scraping, burning, tattooing, I didn't pursue laser surgery; don't know when I stopped cupping face in hand, shielding the color of my skin from other humans. I listen as you try to make sense, track your body's turn away from eradication toward a complicated almost-pride. You research beauty, scrutinize the industry of birthmark removal, page through medical textbooks, see faces like yours, swallow hard against shame. You've started meeting with other people with facial distinctions; talking about survival and desire, denial and matter-of-factness. Tonight you wear a bright shirt, earrings to match; insist on your whole body with all its color.

I ask again: What becomes <u>natural</u> and <u>normal</u>? Who decides that your purple textured skin is <u>unnatural</u>, my tremoring hands <u>abnormal</u>? How do those life-changing decisions get made? I don't want a politics of cure that declares anyone's specific bodily experience <u>normal</u> or <u>abnormal</u>, <u>natural</u> or <u>unnatural</u>.

I turn yet again to story in disability community. We end up in a long conversation about shame and love. Military pollution in the groundwater in your childhood neighborhood shaped your disabled body, toxins molding neurons and muscles as you floated in utero. Most of the time when you talk about the military dumping of trichloroethylene and its connection to you, folks look at your body with pity (Taylor and Taylor 2006). As you tell me this story I think of all the ways disabled bodies are used as cautionary tales: the arguments against drunk driving, drug use, air pollution, lead paint, asbestos, vaccines, and on and on.

So many public campaigns use the cultural fear and hatred of disability to make the case against environmental degradation. You want to know how to express your hatred of military dumping without feeding the assumption that your body is bad, wrong, unnatural. No easy answers exist. You and I talk intensely; both the emotions and the ideas are dense. We arrive at a slogan for you: "I hate the military and love my body."

As simplified and incomplete as it is, this slogan is also profound. How do we witness, name, and resist the injustices that reshape and damage all kinds of bodies—plant and animal, organic and inorganic, nonhuman and human? And alongside our resistance how do we make peace with the reshaped and damaged bodies themselves, cultivate love and respect for them? Inside this work, these stories, the concepts of unnatural and abnormal stop being useful.

Loss

The desire for restoration is bound to bodily loss and yearning—the sheer loss of bodies and bodily functions, whether it be human, bison, dirt, or an entire ecosystem. For many disabled and chronically ill people there is a time before our particular bodily impairments, differences, dysfunctions existed.

What we remember about our bodies is seductive. We yearn; we wish; we regret; we make deals. We desire to return to the days before immobilizing exhaustion or impending death; to the nights thirty years ago when we spun across the dance floor; to the years before depression descended, a thick, unrelenting fog; to the long afternoons curled up with a book before the stroke, before the ability to read vanished in a heartbeat. We feel grief, bitterness, regret. We remain tethered to the past. We compare our bodies to those of neighbors, friends, lovers, models in Glamour and Men's Health, and we come up lacking. We feel inadequate, ashamed, envious. We remain tethered to images outside ourselves, to Photoshopped versions of the human body. Tethered to the gym, the diet plan, the miracle cure. But can any of us move our bodies back in time, undo the lessons learned, the knowledge gained, the scars acquired? The desire for restoration, the return to a bodily past—whether shaped by actual history, imagination, or the vice grip of <u>normal</u> and <u>natural</u>—is complex.

Even those of us who live with disability or chronic illness as familiar and ordinary and have settled into our bodies with a measure of self-love, even those of us who have no non-disabled past, deal with yearning. Sometimes I wish I could throw my body into the powerful grace of a gymnast, rock climber, cliff diver, but that wish is distant, dissolving into echo almost as soon as I recognize it. Sometimes the frustration of not being able to do some task right in front of me roars up, and I have to turn away again from bitterness and simply ask for help. But the real yearning for me centers upon bodily change. As my wrists, elbows, and shoulders grow chronically painful, I miss kayaking, miss gliding on the rippling surface of a lake, miss the rhythm of a paddle dipping in and out of the water. Restoration can be a powerful way of dealing with loss. Cure—when desired, possible, and successful—offers the return some of us sometimes yearn for.

Of course the connections among loss, yearning, and restoration are not only about human bodies. Many of us mourn the swamp once a childhood playground, now a parking lot. We fear the wide-reaching impacts of global warming as hurricanes grow more frequent, glaciers melt, and deserts expand. We yearn for the days when bison roamed the Great Plains in the millions and Chinook salmon swam upstream so numerous that rivers churned frothy white. We yearn for a return, and so we broadcast just the right mix of tallgrass prairie seeds, raise and release wolves, bison, whooping cranes. We tear up drainage tiles and reroute water back into what used to be wetlands. We pick up trash, blow up dams, root out loosestrife, tansy ragwort, gorse, Scotch broom, bamboo, and a multitude of other invasive species. Sometimes we can return a place to some semblance of its former self before the white colonialist, capitalist, industrial damage was done. And in doing so we sometimes return ourselves as human animals to the natural world, moving from domination to collaboration. When it works, restoration can be a powerful antidote to grief, fear, despair.

Restoration's possibilities grow even more inviting as loss extends beyond individual bodies and places to entire communities and ecosystems. I remember bison herds hunted to near extinction, carcasses left to rot. White hunters sold bison tongue and skin. Later homesteaders collected the bones. Then ranchers with cattle and farmers with plows tore up the grasslands; beef animals, wheat, corn, and soybeans replaced prairie. In a photo from 1870 a man stands atop an immense pile of bison skulls waiting to be ground up for fertilizer (Bison Skull Pile). The immensity of this mountain of bone is irrevocable. I remember whole forests of towering Douglas fir, western red cedar, Sitka spruce, and redwoods leveled. Loggers left slash piles, clear-cuts, and washouts in their wake. In a photo from the late 1800s, fourteen men stand, sit, and lounge in the deep cross-cut of a single redwood tree in the process of being felled (Ericson 1890). The breadth of this stump provides a window into the forests demolished. I remember mountaintops removed wholesale in Kentucky. Miners cleared, blasted, dug, and blasted some more in the southern Appalachian Mountains, extracting layer upon layer of coal, creating huge, open gashes. In a photo from 2003 the mountaintop has been leveled into a pit that stretches out toward the horizon, the scale large enough that I can't quite make sense of what I see (Stockman).

As evidence of ecosystems destroyed, all three of these photos measure magnitudes of loss, a sheer loss of bodies—animal, grass, tree, earth, mountain. This devastation includes, of course, human bodies. The mass slaying of bison interweaves with the genocide of Indigenous peoples who depended on those big shaggy animals and open prairie for material and cultural sustenance. So many loggers broke their backs, lost their limbs, damaged their hearing as they cut down the titan trees. The bulldozers displaced working-class and poor folks from their multigeneration homes, turning both people and mountaintops into rubble to push over the edge.

But how do we deal with bodily and ecological loss when restoration in its various manifestations is not the answer? Sometimes viable restoration is not possible. Sometimes restoration is a bandage trying to mend a gaping wound. Sometimes restoration is an ungrounded hope motivated by the shadows of natural and normal. Sometimes restoration is pure social control. I want us to tend the unrestorable places and ecosystems that are ugly, stripped down, full of toxins, rather than considering them unnatural and abandoning them. I want us to respect and embrace the bodies disabled through environmental destruction, age, war, genocide, abysmal working conditions, hunger, poverty, and twists of fate, rather than deeming them abnormal bodies to isolate, fear, hate, and dispose of. How can bodily and ecological loss become an integral conundrum of both the human and non-human world, accepted in a variety of ways, cure and restoration only a single response among many? When the woman whose body has been shaped by military pollution declares, "I hate the military and love my body," she is saying something brand new and deeply complex.

Monocultures and Biodiversities

In pursuing the analogy between restoration of health and restoration of ecosystems, curious questions begin to emerge. Are disabled bodies akin to cornfields? After all, both kinds of restoration, the one grounded in medical science and the other in environmental science, arise from the certainty that cornfields and disabled bodies are damaged and need to change. Restoration declares that cornfields need to return to a natural, self-sustaining, interdependent ecological balance and disabled or chronically ill bodies to a normal, independent functioning.

I remember walking a cornfield in early autumn. The leaves, stalks, husks rattle and sway overhead. Rows envelop me, the whole world a forest of corn beginning to turn brown. I step into the furrows between rows, onto the mounds upon which the stalks grow. Sound, sweat, and an orderly density of the same plant over and over fill the space. Nothing chirps or rasps, squawks or buzzes; the cicadas and grasshoppers have gone dormant for the season. I hear no warblers, finches, sparrows; I see no traces of grouse, pheasant, fox. The earth is laced with petroleum-based fertilizers and the air laden with pesticide residue. In spite of the damage they embody, cornfields are also beautiful on the surface, lushly green and quivering in the humid Midwest summer before they dry up in the fall, becoming brown and brittle. The stalks stand tall and sturdy, tassels silky and the color of honey, kernels of corn plump and hidden. Little tastes better than ears of sweet corn fresh from the field, husked, boiled, and buttered. But this beauty is deceptive; the monoculture of a cornfield has brought nothing but soil depletion and erosion; a glut of nonnutritious, corn-based processed foods; and wholesale destruction of prairie ecosystems. Restoration is not just a pleasant environmental pastime but a desperate need.

Let me return to my prompting question: Are disabled human bodies akin to cornfields? The ideology of cure answers with a resounding yes. Speaking through the medical establishment and dozens of cultural assumptions and stereotypes, cure declares that the need for the restoration of health is just as urgent as the restoration of tallgrass prairies. From this point of view, disabled bodies are as damaging to culture as cornfields are to nature.

Distrustful of this answer, including the easy separation of nature and culture, I turn my question inside out and ask: Are restored prairies like disabled bodies? Certainly the tallgrass prairie that my friends tend is a diverse ecosystem that is whole, but not as whole as it once was or could be, quirky and off-kilter, almost self-sustaining and entirely interdependent, imperfect and brilliant all at the same time. These descriptors apply equally well to disability communities.

I remember departing from a large disability gathering. It is late spring in the San Francisco airport, an environment as bland as a cornfield. I walk a long corridor toward the plane that will take me home. I have been in the foggy Bay Area for a long weekend with three hundred LGBT disabled people, queer crips, as many of us like to call ourselves. I meander through the airport, people streaming around and by me. I know something is missing, but I don't know what. I let my exhaustion and images from the weekend roll over me until all of a sudden I realize everyone passing me looks the same in spite of the myriad cultural differences held within these walls. A white businessman with a rainbow sticker on his briefcase strides past an African American woman and her grandson; a Latino man speaking quiet Spanish into his cell phone stands next to a white teen speaking twangy English with her friends; an Asian American woman pushes her cleaning cart, stopping to empty the trash can. In spite of all these differences everyone has two arms and two legs. They are walking rather than rolling; speaking with their lips, not their hands, speaking in even, smooth syllables, no stutters or slurs. They have no canes, no crutches, no braces; their faces do not twitch or their hands flop; they hold their back straight, and their smile is not lopsided. In some profound way they all look the same.

It would be all too convenient and neat to suggest that without disability, humans re-create ourselves as a monoculture—a cornfield, wheat field, tree farm—lacking some fundamental biodiversity. Environmentalists have named biodiversity a central motivation for ecosystem restoration and a foundation for continued life on the planet. But to declare the absence of disability as synonymous with a monoculture disregards the multiplicity of cultures among humans. It glosses over the ways culture and nature have been set against each other in the white Western world, as if the human ferment we call culture and the wild, interdependent messiness we call biodiversity are distinct and opposing entities. It does not acknowledge how culture dictates which bodily characteristics are considered disability and which are considered natural variation.

At the same time the absence of disability, even the desire for its absence, diminishes human experience and the inextricable interweaving of bio- and cultural diversity. Certainly the desire to eradicate disability runs deep. Even the most progressive of activists and staunchest of environmentalists have for the past 150 years envisioned an end to disability as a worthy goal. But the white Western drive to eradicate unnatural and abnormal bodies and cultures has never targeted disability alone. Patriarchy, white supremacy, and capitalism have twined together in ever-changing combinations to make eradication through genocide, incarceration, institutionalization, sterilization, and wholesale assimilation a reality in many marginalized communities. It is this long-standing, broad-based desire for and practice of eradication that threaten to create human monocultures.

I return to my prompting question turned inside out: Are restored prairies like disabled bodies? Ecological restoration is one powerful way to repair the damage wrought by monocultures and to resist the forces of eradication. A radical valuing of disabled and chronically ill bodies—inseparable from black and brown bodies; queer bodies; poor and working-class bodies; transgender, transsexual, and gender-nonconforming bodies; immigrant bodies; women's bodies; young and old bodies; fat bodies—is another part of the same repair and resistance. In this way a commitment to bio- and cultural diversity coupled with a multi-issue disability politics answers my question with a resounding yes. Simply put, the bodies of both disabled and chronically ill people and restored prairies resist the impulse toward and the reality of monocultures.

Illogic

Both kinds of restoration—one of ecosystems and the other of health—appear to value and prioritize the natural over the unnatural, yet they arrive at opposing conclusions about disabled bodies. The contradiction and lack of logic could simply mark the point at which the analogy between cure and ecological restoration falls apart. Or they could point to the profound difference between a complex valuing of disability as cultural and ecological diversity and a persistent devaluing of disability entirely as damage. Or they could underline the multiple, slippery meanings of natural and unnatural, normal and abnormal—a fundamental illogic rooted in the white Western framework that separates human animals from nonhuman nature.

This framework has rarely valued and prioritized the <u>natural</u> world, meaning largely intact, flourishing ecosystems, some of which include humans and others of which do not. Out of these values has emerged an out-of-control greed for and consumption of coal and trees, fish and crude oil, water and land. This framework despises and destroys the <u>natural</u> when it is not human. It declares cornfields more productive than prairies, tree farms and second-growth forest more sustaining to wildlife than old-growth forest, open coal pits more necessary than intact mountaintops and watersheds. Within this system of values the <u>civilized</u> is named and celebrated in opposition to the <u>savage</u>, the former rising above nature and the latter remaining mired in it.

The illogic grows as these values turn toward the human world, as the pairing of <u>savage</u> and <u>natural</u> collides with what is deemed <u>unnatural</u> and <u>abnormal</u>. Throughout the centuries rich white men have determined people of color, poor people, LGBT people, women, indigenous people, immigrants, and disabled people to be <u>savages</u>, nonhuman animals, close to nature. But in the same breath this long litany of peoples has also been held up as Other, <u>unnatural</u>, and <u>abnormal</u>. The illogic names certain humans both <u>natural</u> and <u>unnatural</u>, using each designation by turn as justification to enslave, starve, study, exhibit, and eradicate entire communities and cultures.

I return to the word <u>monkey</u>. As a taunt, a freak show name, a scientific and anthropological designation for human animals, this word drips with the illogic of <u>natural</u> and <u>unnatural</u>. So many disabled people or people of color (or both) have lived publicly and privately, in the spotlight and not, with <u>monkey</u> and paid dearly. Let me pause and step into a river of names: Ota Benga, William Henry Johnson, Krao Farini, Barney Davis, Hiram Davis, Simon Metz, Elvira Snow, Jenny Lee Snow, Maximo, Bartola, Sarah Baartman, and on and on. In 1906 Ota Benga, a Batwa man from central Africa, was forced to live in the Bronx Zoo monkey house. The sign on the cage he shared with an orangutan read:

> The African Pigmy, "Ota Benga." Age, 23 years. Height, 4 feet 11 inches. Weight,103 pounds. Brought from the Kasai River, Congo Free State, South Central Africa, by Dr. Samuel P. Verner. Exhibited each afternoon during September. (Bradford and Blume 1992, 181)

This sign makes Benga's situation stunningly clear: he was imprisoned in a zoo exactly because he was considered a curiosity, a specimen, a primate. His display was neither the first nor the last, but simply one in a long, long litany. P. T. Barnum exhibited William Henry Johnson as the "What-Is-It" and the "Missing Link." Freak show posters named Krao Farini "Ape Girl." Barney and Hiram Davis worked for decades as savages, the "Wild Men from Borneo." Freak show managers sold "Maximo" and "Bartola" as the "last of the ancient Aztecs," and anthropologists studied, measured, and photographed them naked as "throwbacks" to an earlier time in human evolution. White men caged, displayed, and studied Sarah Baartman as the "Hottentot Venus." These folks—all of them intellectually disabled or people of color (or both)—became monkeys or near monkeys in the white Western framework of scientific racism.

The brutality of monkey arises in part precisely because it removes particular bodies from humanity and places them among animals in the natural world. Scientific racism of the 1800s made this removal overt. Scientists declared that "the negro race . . . manifestly approaches the monkey tribe" (qtd. in Lindfors 1983, 9). They decided that "microcephalics [intellectually disabled people with an impairment medically known as microcephaly] must necessarily represent an earlier developmental state of the human being" (qtd. in Rothfels 1997, 158). They twined racism, colonialism, and ableism together until it was impossible to tell where one ended and the other began. And this thinking has not disappeared; it has just become more subtle most of the time, more subtle until a bully hurls the word monkey across the schoolyard, calling upon centuries of scientific racism, whether he knows it or not.

Monkey categorizes the bodies of white disabled people and people of color, both disabled and not, as savage and natural. Within this categorization these bodies become subject to the profound disconnect, disregard, and destruction with which the white Western world treats nonhuman animals and nature. The disabled painter, writer, and animal rights activist Sunaura Taylor (2011, 194–95) puts it this way: "I find myself wondering why animals exist as such negative points of reference for us. . . . In David Lynch's 1980 classic Elephant Man, John Merrick yells out to his gawkers and attackers, "I am not an animal!" . . . No one wants to be treated like an animal. But how do we treat animals? . . . At the root of the insult in animal comparisons is a discrimination against nonhuman animals themselves." At the same time these savage bodies, these monkey bodies, these natural bodies are also Other and abnormal, to be studied and gawked at exactly because of their abnormality. And in their Otherness and abnormality these bodies also become unnatural. Monkey seamlessly engages with the illogic of natural paired with abnormal and abnormal paired with unnatural. But the illogic does not stop here.

Natural slides again, pairing up with what is considered civilized. Certain other bodies—white, non-disabled, heterosexual, male, cisgender, rich bodies—have been established as good and valuable, as the standard of both natural and normal. Corporate advertising sells natural beauty, natural strength, natural sexiness, natural skin, natural hair every day, as if natural were a product to sell. The medical establishment provides technology to ensure normal height, normal weight, normal pregnancy and birth, normal walking, normal breathing, as if normal were a goal to achieve. The pressure to conform individually and systemically to these standards of natural and normal is immense. Whether it is curing disabled bodies or straightening kinky hair or lightening brown skin or making gay, lesbian, and bi people heterosexual, the priorities are clear. In this illogic normal bodies are natural and natural bodies are normal.

In all its arbitrary and illogical meanings natural names both what is dominated and who does the dominating. Natural establishes some bodies as radically abnormal and others as hypernormal. The illogic holds what is natural and dominated as abnormal and unnatural. And it insists that those who dominate are both normal and natural. Do not try to make sense of the illogic; it is nonsensical. These four concepts—natural, normal, unnatural, and abnormal—in all their various pairings form a matrix of intense contradictions, wielding immense power in spite of, or perhaps because of, the illogic.

Prairie

I return in early fall to the thirty acres of restored tallgrass prairie in Wisconsin. I walk, thinking not of concepts but of bodies. The grasses swish against my legs. A few swallowtail butterflies still hover. Coyote scat appears next to the path. The white-throated sparrows sing. The grasses rustle, and I imagine a white-footed mouse scurrying and a red fox pouncing. Above vultures circle on the thermals. A red-tailed hawk cries not so far away. I am one body, a tremoring, slurring human body, among many different kinds of bodies. Could it all be this complexly woven yet simple? The answer comes back an inevitable yes and no.

Right now, in this moment, the prairie both contains and is made up of myriad bodies. But just over the rise another cornfield turns brown and brittle. Just over the rise are a barbed-wire fence, a two-lane dirt road, and an absence of bison. Just over the rise is the human illogic of <u>natural</u> and <u>unnatural</u>, <u>normal</u> and <u>abnormal</u>. Just over the rise we grapple with loss and desire, with damaged bodies and deep social and ecological injustices. Just over the rise are the bullies with their rocks and fists, the words <u>monkey</u> and <u>retard</u>. Just over the rise we need to choose between monocultures, on one hand, and bio- and cultural diversities, on the other, between eradication and uncontainable flourishing. In so many ways the prairie cannot be a retreat but the ground upon which we ask all these questions.

NOTE

1. The idea of brilliant imperfection as a way of knowing, understanding, and living disability or chronic illness is one of hundreds of things I have learned in disability communities. In particular I want to thank Sebastian Margaret for this phrase.

REFERENCES

<u>Bison Skull Pile</u> (1870). Detroit Public Library. <u>Wikimedia Commons</u>. Online.

Bradford, Phillips Verner, and Harvey Blume. 1992. <u>Ota Benga: The Pygmy in the Zoo</u>. New York: St. Martin's Press.

Ericson, Augustus William. 1890. <u>Among the Redwoods</u>. Humboldt State University Library, Arcata. Cathedral Grove. Online.

Lindfors, Bernth. 1983. "Circus Africans." <u>Journal of American Culture</u> 6, no. 2: 9–14.

Rothfels, Nigel. 1997. "Aztecs, Aborigines, and Ape-People: Science and Freaks in Germany, 1840–1900." In <u>Freakery: Cultural Spectacles of the Extraordinary Body</u>, edited by Rosemarie Garland-Thomson, 158–72. New York: Columbia University Press.

Stockman, Vivian. 2003. <u>Massive Dragline</u>. Photograph. Mountaintop Removal Mining. Ohio Valley Environmental Coalition, October 19. Online.

Taylor, Astra, and Sunaura Taylor. 2006. "Military Waste in Our Drinking Water." <u>AlterNet</u>, August 3. Online.

Taylor, Sunaura. 2011. "Beasts of Burden: Disability Studies and Animal Rights." <u>Qui Parle: Critical Humanities and Social Sciences</u> 19, no. 2: 191–222.

Part 2
New Essays

Section 1   CORPOREAL LEGACIES OF U.S. NATION-BUILDING

8

Blind Indians

Káteri Tekakwí:tha and Joseph Amos's
Visions of Indigenous Resurgence

Siobhan Senier

Káteri Tekakwí:tha (1656–80) was a Mohawk woman who left her home in what is now upstate New York to join a Jesuit mission, where she practiced extreme self-mortification until her death at age twenty-four. Blinded and scarred by smallpox, she has been associated with miracle cures, and in 2012 she became the first Native American woman to be canonized as a saint by the Catholic Church.[1] Often called "the lily of the Mohawks," she is also a patron saint of ecology and the environment.

Almost two centuries later the Wampanoag minister known as Blind Joe Amos was making a more overt defense of his indigenous territory in Mashpee, Massachusetts. Wampanoag people remember Blind Joe preaching under an oak tree because the local minister wouldn't let Mashpee Indians meet in their own church. Amos eventually ousted the scurrilous Rev. Phineas Fish, and in 1833 he led a revolt against settler theft of Mashpee land and timber.

In these two life stories colonial land dispossession and bodily impairment come head to head with indigenous sovereignty and survival. One has been (literally) canonized in Euro-American and popular discourse, the other virtually forgotten outside the indigenous community from which he hailed. One appears (to some indigenous people) a sellout, the other a figure of fierce resistance. But both of these lives challenge us to read disability within indigenous ontologies, which are, in turn, inextricable from indigenous territories, ecologies, and community. Popular histories, biographies, and other media tend to treat these blind Indians like most other blind characters, oscillating between pity and supercripping. But Káteri and Blind Joe can also be read as doing serious ecological and social justice work. Each was a visible part of the fabric of her or his community, and each arguably helped steward tribal environmental and cultural practices. Káteri and Blind Joe embody the toxic legacies of settler colonialism, but they also register the resurgence of indigenous people and their ecological knowledge.

In colonial discourse the representation of these two figures has been eminently predictable. Káteri has been called the most written-about aboriginal person. Almost immediately upon her death two Jesuits who had known her published several biographies, the broad contours of which have been reiterated in more biographies, films as well as paintings, sculptures, coloring books, and Catholic websites. These accounts all hew closely to hagiographic convention.[2] They say that the orphaned Káteri rejected pressure from her relatives to marry young; that she finally fled this family to devote her life to Christ; that she made herself ill by fasting, self-flagellating, and kneeling for prolonged periods in the snow; and that upon her death the smallpox scars miraculously vanished from her face. Her name Tekakwí:tha has been variously translated, but the most popularly invoked version is "She who pushes with her hands."

Blind Joe, conversely, is rarely mentioned by non-Natives. Occasionally a local newspaper will note that the Mashpee Baptist Church (led by Rev. Curtis Frye Jr., Amos's great-great-great-grandson) still celebrates Blind Joe Amos Sunday on July 15.[3] In one report from Massachusetts in 1849, the Commission to

Examine into the Condition of the Indians in the Commonwealth describes Joseph Amos as "tall and manly, with a phrenological development which Spurzheim might have envied, with his face turned to heaven, and his sightless sockets swimming with tears, he seemed the very personification of the loftiest spirit of rapt devotion."[4] This ambivalent (to put it mildly) description reveals the layers of anxiety over the challenge Blind Joe represented to colonial power: the commissioners enlist scientific racism to express simultaneous awe and revulsion for indigenous masculinity and phenotype, and they struggle to contain this power on the grounds of Amos's religious fervor and disability. Like many blind people, then and now, Amos was likely not totally blind; he did wear spectacles. The very phrase "sightless sockets," with its eager insistence on emptiness, belies the state's profound fear that what Amos saw was indeed the limits of its own power. Comparing the image of the veiled lily, so feminine and white, with that of the bespectacled preacher, so visionary and black, it is not surprising that Euro-American and mainstream Christian accounts have preferred the former.

In the emerging conversations among Native American studies, disability studies, and the environmental humanities a thorough reckoning with settler colonialism is the sine qua non. Distinguished from more administrative forms of colonialism (in India, for example, where Britain controlled and colonized a territory from a remote metropolis), settler colonialism is predicated on the expropriation of indigenous lands and the actual removal and replacement of indigenous bodies. Settlers come to exterminate indigenous people or push them out, not simply to exploit or control them. For this reason the historian Patrick Wolfe has famously said that "invasion is a structure not an event": it is not something that happened in 1492 or on any other so-called contact date but is an ongoing process.[5] It continues today in the ransacking of indigenous territories for "natural resources" like oil and minerals and in biopiracy, the theft of indigenous plant knowledge and even indigenous DNA.[6]

Invasion also continues in the production of new disability and illness among Native people. New scholarship on disability in the Global South has begun to articulate the profound connections among disability, colonialism, and ecology. Nirmala Erevelles, Julie Livingston, and the scholars who founded the journal Disability and the Global South are highlighting the different disability politics, disability cultures, and even disability ontologies that emerge outside the Global North and under conditions of neocolonialism, neoliberalism, and transnational capitalism.[7] From this orientation we can see the effects of the colonialism that has never really been "post-" among indigenous people worldwide. These effects appear in the intergenerational trauma that is the legacy of boarding schools from Canada to Australia; in the psychological condition known as "split feathers syndrome," which is a product of the systematic out-adoption of indigenous children away from their home community and culture; and in diabetes, which is only one result of the destruction of indigenous land bases, and thus of traditional foods and dietary practices. The structure of colonialism also appears in blindness and eye disease, which in the twenty-first century continue to occur among indigenous people at much higher rates than among many other groups. Calling Káteri "She who pushes with her hands" depoliticizes her impairment, which was not congenital but caused by disease carried into the Mohawk Valley by French settlers. In a non-Mohawk, colonial context this moniker also tends to make her an object of pity. Many popular Catholic accounts describe her as stumbling around the forest where, they say, she placed small crosses in the ground as a devotional act. The image of a hapless blind Indian—endowed with the spiritual vision lacking

in her heathen compatriots, flagging the earth for the Church—
has obvious use value for settler colonialism. It makes Káteri
what Sarah Jaquette Ray would call an "ecological other," paradoxically romanticizing her "connection with the earth" while
cutting her and her people off from their ongoing political and
territorial claims.[8] Káteri may be a "patron saint of the environment," but that seems to mean little on most Catholic websites
beyond celebrating her as a "child of the forest" who is "close to
nature."[9] The oldest stereotype in the book, this hackneyed image
performs deeply entrenched cultural work, deliberately masking
Native peoples' specific ecological knowledge and land rights.

Káteri was hardly stumbling around in total darkness, any more
than most people labeled "blind." Darren Bonaparte (Mohawk)
has argued that in fact she continued working for her longhouse
by gathering firewood, sewing, and making beaded items. This
last category included wampum belts, the making of which would
have been quite a high-status job because these belts are used
in acts of diplomacy, including the Iroquois Condolence Ceremony. Bonaparte is thus advocating for the Mohawk repatriation
of Káteri's story—the reinterpretation of her life within the horizon
of Mohawk history and community.[10]

The repatriation of Mohawk history more broadly is already
under way by Mohawk scholars and is richly suggestive of new
directions for reading Káteri's life and work. For example, the
Jesuit accounts portray Káteri's move to the mission as a flight
from religious persecution among a barbaric people. And yet she
left at the same time as a mass movement of Mohawk people
from what is now upstate New York to a more northern part of
their territory. The Kahnawake website today has an intriguing
take on this: "In 1667, our people established a community on the
northern part of the Territory at Kentake, now known as Laprairie
Quebec to re-assert Iroquois rights and jurisdiction. It was here

that the first mission was built. In an effort to avoid European contact, the community moved four times [upriver] from 1667 to 1716 to finally settle at its present location, Kahnawake, meaning 'On the rapids.'"[11] In this account the Mohawk move is not for conversion or exile but an act of autonomy and territorial expansion. The Mohawk anthropologist Audra Simpson confirms this interpretation in her important new book Mohawk Interruptus, which clarifies her tribal history as one of refusal of settler colonial domination, not assimilation to it. She acknowledges that Kentake initially attracted a mix of Mohawk and other Iroquoian peoples, but she argues that Mohawk people gradually made the mission more culturally and politically their own, bringing their language, styles of dress, and longhouses and "operationalizing the tenets of a clan system of descent."[12] In this reading Mohawk people are able to embrace Christian practice and belief, intermingle with other groups, and move to different parts of their territory (and even beyond)—all without sacrificing their Mohawkness.

If we intentionally reread Káteri's narrative according to these Mohawk historiographic methods, we can comprehend this blind saint as a full participant in that historic and communal extension of tribal territory—as marking the forest not for the Church but for indigenous communities. The Tuscarora scholar Vera Palmer has gone further, arguing that some of Káteri's documented behaviors are actually extensions of Iroquois condolence ritual, a centuries-old ceremony still of "central importance in Iroquoian spiritual and political identity." If Káteri made wampum belts, it is possible that some of her work was even used in that ceremony. She was certainly, as Palmer emphasizes, no stranger to the community and personal trauma that condolence works to address, as she lost her immediate and much of her extended family to smallpox. But Palmer reads even more deeply in Haudenosaunee symbolic systems to reinterpret, for instance, Káteri's habit of sleeping on a bed of thistles. For the Jesuits this seemed a clear act of piety, but to Palmer

> it also strongly evokes the Iroquoian creation narrative, in which the mother of the originary Sky Woman survives after her brother's fatal illness. . . . In ancient Mohawk tradition [gifted children] are to be kept in seclusion from birth to puberty, in preparation for their roles of service to or healing of the community. Thistles and white down are used to mark the children's fastness and also to serve as a warning if an intruder disturbs the children's seclusion. . . . Rather than a Christian version of ascetic self-abasement, the Iroquoian interpretive register here would be self-defense and spiritual self-identification through the use of thistle and down.[13]

Palmer's reading encourages us to consider other elements of Káteri's practice as reflecting indigenous knowledge, particularly knowledge of the intimate and reciprocal relations among the human and other-than-human—plant, animal, and spirit. Among Káteri's Algonquian people there is a tradition of birchbark mapping, known as awikhiganak, bark maps or other markings left in the forest as a way of communicating hunting territories or whereabouts to family members.[14] Knowing this we can ask whether her placement of crosses in the forest was merely Catholic devotion. Was it instead a way of mapping new space, recalling her familial Algonquian roots while participating in a Mohawk territorial expansion? Or was it a further invocation of indigenous signification systems? Palmer explains that a central symbol for Iroquois communities, in the seventeenth century as today, is the Great Tree of Peace, an image of union and "rootedness in the land" that countermands the Jesuits' narrative of Native displacement and deracination. Was Káteri somehow reconnecting with this vital symbol when she made crosses from twigs and pushed them into the earth or inscribed crosses onto the trees themselves?

It is my belief that the ultimate interpretation of such practices properly belongs to Iroquois people themselves, but that it is incumbent upon all scholars interested in the decolonization of indigenous texts to at least pose the questions and to begin seeking answers in conversation with tribal people, including tribal people's own published scholarship. Similarly the growing conversation at the intersections of disability studies and indigenous studies urges us to consider that indigenous communities also have their own ways of thinking about disability, whether impairment has arrived "naturally" or been produced by colonialism, whether it is construed as "disability" or not. Here again Palmer's reading of the condolence ritual is suggestive, for she explains:

> Loss itself is treated as an illness, with fifteen elements that mark the symptoms of grief and malaise for which Condolence is indicated. The three main focuses of these fifteen elements are the eyes, the ears, and the throat. These three corporeal sites foreground the theme of relationship or communication, which need to be mended throughout the life of the individual or the community in order to regenerate after great loss. The sites respectively correspond to the metaphoric illness of unabated darkness, meaning that one is unable to see matters clearly; the illness of silence or isolation that allows morbid thoughts of self-negation and cuts one off from community with others; and the muteness of choking grief, which isolates a person (or community) and turns that anguish to internal despair or violence and bitterness projected outward.[15]

At first glance this might present disability studies scholars with the familiar specter of narrative prosthesis—the trope of disability as a metaphor for deviance or moral failing, which in turn bolsters the marginalization of disabled people themselves.[16] And yet there is little evidence that Káteri was marginalized because of her impairment(s), or that other Native people—laid flat as they were by smallpox and certainly not unfamiliar with the results of that disease—would have considered her blindness as any kind of personal failing or, really, as all that unusual. On the contrary it has been the hagiographies that have portrayed this saint's blindness as pitiable, exceptional, and traded up for some kind of unique spiritual vision. In Palmer's reading, conversely, Káteri's actions are part of a much larger cultural matrix; her blindness is hardly irrelevant, but it is not entirely her own, and not necessarily something that needs to be "cured" the way collective grief needs to be ritually addressed. This interpretation offers the provocative possibility that, while the Condolence ceremony might use blindness as a metaphor for grief, actual blind people can participate in its administration. That is an entirely different way of thinking about this blind saint, beatified precisely because individual "cripples" could appeal to her for miraculous cures, whose own face was miraculously purged of scars as surely as colonialism hoped to purge the land of indigenous people.[17]

One other Native writer tries to reimagine Káteri's visual impairment, to consider what blindness might have meant for her, and for Mohawk people, both before and after the arrival of colonial settlers. In her novella The Reason for Crows, Diane Glancy (a playwright who identifies as Cherokee) considers Káteri's visual impairment both as the painful product of colonial history and as a sense—not as the absence of sense, nor as the usual ableist metaphor for ignorance or lack of imagination: "My name, Tekakwí:tha, means one-who-walks-groping-her-way. Or moving-all-things-before-her. It means one-who-puts-things-in-order. Or one-who-bumps-into-things. It is a name that can go several ways. It can have several meanings. But they all have to do with seeing what is before me." Glancy's Káteri is lyrically alert to sound: shielding her eyes from the painful sun, she "listened to the forest. The noise of birds as they called to one another . . . to the wind through the leaves, the water in the rivulets and the river. It was sound I saw." She also comprehends through touch: beauty, violence, cultural disruption, and cultural continuity: "[The Father] gave me a rosary. The little beads were wheels. My fingers rolled over them, the way the soldiers' cannons rolled over the land, full of awe and fear. . . . Something was happening when I prayed. They were medicine beads. Wampum beads. They were cherubim wheels." While these passages displace visual sight onto other senses, this is no narrative of mere hypercompensation, for Glancy's Káteri also sees. She sees snow, she sees light, she sees "wisps and swirls of air"; she even sees the shapes of trees on the other side of the river. These, she says, "look like people raising their arms to our God. Yes," she adds, "I would put the new land together with what I remembered of the old."[18]

Glancy thus imagines for Káteri and her people a form of resilience, an ability to adapt to new realities while sustaining older ones. The comparison of trees to "people raising their arms to our God" opens the question, first, of whose or which god. Just as critically it establishes an intimate identification between people and trees, between humans and other-than-humans, and specifically between Mohawk people and their Great Tree of Peace. In Glancy's account this knowledge belongs to Káteri not because she is blind and endowed with mystical vision nor because she is an Indian "at one with the earth." It is because she is a Mohawk woman who has learned practical ecological knowledge in a community that has lived on this land for centuries.

Jesuits seized control of Kâteri's hagiography almost immediately, but the story of Joseph Amos has always been the property of Wampanoag people. Consequently it has done very different cultural work. Blind Joe appears in just about every book written by Mashpee Wampanoag people—and they have written many, especially since their well-known and protracted pursuit of federal recognition.[19] Russell Peters, a prominent tribal leader during that period, published The Wampanoags of Mashpee in 1987 in a clear bid to communicate the inseparability of Mashpee land and Mashpee culture. He presented Amos as the primary community liaison for the writer and activist William Apess (Pequot), who is today better known for his role in the 1833 Woodlot Revolt. At this time Mashpee was a self-governing indigenous community suffering increasing interference from state-appointed overseers and white settlers, who were encroaching on tribal pastures, forests, and fishing grounds. Apess worked with Amos and other tribal leaders to write a petition to the governor of Massachusetts, Levi Lincoln, resolving "that we as a Tribe will rule ourselves" and "that we will not permit any white man to come upon our plantation to cut or carry off wood or hay or any other article without permission after the first of July next." When, on July 1, white settlers began loading up their carts with Mashpee wood, Blind Joe, Apess, and other Mashpee leaders drove them off tribal land. This successful revolt led to the establishment of Mashpee as an independent Indian district the following year.[20]

While the historical recovery of Apess among academic scholars has been more complete, Blind Joe has continued to appear in almost every Mashpee-authored book since 1987.[21] Most of these writers likely owe a debt to Amelia Bingham, one of Amos's direct descendants. Bingham started researching Mashpee's unwritten history in the 1960s, talking with community members and traveling to archives in Plymouth, Boston, Cambridge, and Washington DC. She published much of this research in 1970 on the occasion of Mashpee's centennial. Bingham's pamphlet Mashpee: Land of the Wampanoags gives an entire section to her ancestor, accompanied by the image of him that would become so widely circulated at Mashpee: "Blind Joseph Amos, a Marshpee Indian, was born on the shore of Mashpee-Wakeby Pond in 1805. He lost his sight in early childhood. He was, however, a man of intense intellect, able to memorize whole chapters of the Bible when it was read to him by his mother, and he was a gifted speaker. He had great musical talent. He was, in fact, a natural leader of his people."[22] What is striking is how readily the story of Blind Joe has been retold and amplified, how he is honored as "the common ancestor of almost all present Mashpees."[23] Morgan James Peters, a tribal member who writes under the name Mwalim, has published a humorous retelling called "Turtle and the Oak Tree." In this version Amos appears as "Blind Turtle," who, "in spite of the little pair of pincer glasses that sat on his face . . . couldn't see a thing—at least, not with his eyes." The Harvard-appointed minister who took over the local church, meanwhile, is represented by "a slimy, little water moccasin named Phineas" who preaches "the natural inferiority of turtles, lizards and frogs" and that "all things valuable and beautiful on the earth rightfully belonged to the snakes." Maddened by Joe's renowned ability to hear "the voices of those who went before and those yet to come," Phineas tries to acquire this power for himself, going so far as to replace all the existing meetinghouses with oak structures. He fails, of course, and Blind Turtle and the other animals continue to gather under the oak tree, giving "thanks to the ancestors for their wisdom and guidance, thanks to the trees, bushes and grass for conveying this wisdom, and thanks to the crickets and small birds."[24]

Turtles have spiritual, place-binding significance for Wampanoag and other Native people. Russell Peters was known as "Fast Turtle"; the tribe's beloved medicine man John Peters, who died in 1997, was "Slow Turtle." In an excellent article on indigenous literary animals, Joshua Miner argues that they "express originary non-human presence and kinship," that they "delineate a rhetoric of sovereign rights to land by establishing continuity of time and space." Consequently, he finds, "Native artists and authors have begun reasserting the importance of all human–non-human animal relationships to homemaking for contemporary Native American people."[25] Mwalim's political parable participates in this making of Mashpee homeland. Contravening the stubborn colonial habit of packaging "Native American animal tales" as the cute stuff of children's books ("How Turtle's Back Was Cracked"), the story keeps the history of colonial violence and Wampanoag resistance alive. And it does so not just with a nonhuman animal but with a blind one—and, we might add, with a tree.

Is it a coincidence that trees figure so centrally in the life stories of these two blind Indian spiritual leaders? As shelter for animals and people, as material used by both—and as their own beings, members of a broader human and other-than-human community rooted in the land—trees have been a first line of defense in both Wampanoag and Mohawk territories. In 1990, a century and a half after Mashpee leaders prevented white settlers from stealing their timber, Mohawk people shut down a proposed golf course at Oka, Quebec. The site at issue was both sacred tribal burial ground and a pine forest. In no small irony this land was supposed to be held in trust by the Sulpician Fathers Seminary, a Catholic order that (illegally) had retained the title since 1717.[26]

If the image of blind Káteri putting her crosses in the ground has seemed to endorse such colonial ownership under the most facile kind of environmentalism, the rewriting of Mohawk historiography by Mohawk people and the Mashpee preservation of Blind Joe's story chart paths for new understandings of disability, indigeneity, and ecology. Certainly Blind Joe and possibly Káteri were accepted as spiritual leaders and intellectuals, as pivotal players in their interlocking cultures and land bases. Is there some relationship between their disabilities and this leadership? The disability activist Eli Clare has written a typically beautiful rumination on the relations between ecological diversity and human diversity. In his inimitable, thoughtful way he acknowledges the difficulties with the comparison: "It would be all too convenient and neat to suggest that without disability, humans recreate ourselves as a monoculture." And yet, he ponders, "ecological restoration is one powerful way to repair the damage wrought by monocultures and to resist the forces of eradication. A radical valuing of disabled and chronically-ill bodies—inseparable from black and brown bodies; queer bodies; poor and working-class bodies; transgender, transsexual and gender non-conforming bodies; immigrant bodies; women's bodies; young and old bodies; fat bodies—is another part of the same repair and resistance. . . . Simply put, the bodies of both disabled/chronically ill people and restored prairies resist the impulse toward and the reality of monocultures."[27] Our intersecting fields—indigenous studies, environmental humanities, disability studies—continue to debate how best to conceptualize this kind of "radical valuing"—of bodies and nature, of bodily natures. The term restoration, as Clare shows, is deeply vexed, implying as it does a cure, a return to some ostensibly pristine original state. Many critics nowadays also reject the term sustainability on the grounds that it has been co-opted by corporations invested in greenwashing or by capitalist projects invested in "development." I would like to point out that one benefit of keeping <u>sustainability</u> in the mix is that this term keeps a door open to the growing field of sustainability science, a field only about as old as ecocriticism, which demands community-engaged scholarship and focuses expressly on "coupled human-natural systems." Surely, for the most thoughtful scholars in environmental humanities, disability studies, and indigenous studies <u>systems</u> are critically important. In conversation with sustainability scientists we can attend not only to earth systems, food systems, and cultural systems but to systems of power, domination, and resistance.

Sustainability also keeps a door open to indigenous and global antipoverty movements around the relations between cultural and ecological diversity.[28] One activist, Waziyatawin (Dakota), invokes sustainability as an indigenous value when she observes that, at the very moment of inexorable planetary crisis, we are witnessing the rise of powerful indigenous liberation movements, such as the resistance at Oka and the recent Idle No More movement. "Just when liberation may be within our grasp," she writes, "the ecological destruction may be so complete that Indigenous lifeways may be impossible to practice. In this context there is a simultaneous and urgent need for both the restoration of sustainable Indigenous practices and a serious defense of Indigenous homelands." Waziyatawin calls this "the paradox of indigenous resurgence."[29] She shows that indigenous ecological knowledge is not some primordial, free-floating commodity, ready to be lifted by settler colonials when they feel in crisis, but knowledge utterly intertwined with indigenous sovereignty and self-determination.

What a (re)reading of figures like Káteri and Blind Joe (indigenous, disabled, and culturally and environmentally activist) can show us is that indigenous resurgence is not new and is not happening merely at our current "brink of planetary disaster." Indigenous people have faced disaster at scales that must have seemed planetary for over five hundred years. And yet despite this legacy of unremitting colonial assault, they survive. As Palmer puts it, "Fundamentally and culturally [they] still embrace and endorse the natural world as matrix, mater, and matter—as model and as nourishing substance within which tribal experience inheres, endures, and obtains."[30] In so doing they begin, perhaps, to answer Clare's tender challenge: "How can bodily/ecological loss become an integral conundrum of both the human and non-human world, accepted in a variety of ways, cure/restoration being only a single response among many?"[31]

NOTES

1. In keeping with a good deal of current scholarly practice, I use indigenous, Native, and similar terms interchangeably, as they are all contested. The tribally specific designation is almost always preferred; but when citing scholars who use the term Iroquois to refer to Mohawk and other Confederacy nations, I use that term; I also use Haudenosaunee, sometimes preferred to Iroquois.
2. For a summary of the accounts written by Fathers Pierre Cholonec and Claude Chauchetiere, with an analysis of the "striking consistency of this corpus," see Koppedrayer, "The Making of the First Iroquois Virgin." The most thorough contemporary biography is Greer's Mohawk Saint.
3. See, for instance, Sean Gonsalves, "Blind Joe and the 'Praying Indians,'" Cape Cod Times, July 15, 2012, http://www.capecodtimes .com/article/20120715/News/207150340.
4. Massachusetts, Report of the Commissioners Related to the Condition of the Indians of Massachusetts, 34.
5. Wolfe, Settler Colonialism and the Transformation of Anthropology, 2.
6. These issues are explored further in the special issue of the Journal of Literary & Cultural Disability Studies devoted to disability and indigeneity, edited by Siobhan Senier and Clare Barker.

7. Erevelles, Disability and Difference in Global Contexts; Livingston, Debility and the Moral Imagination in Botswana. See also Grech, "Recolonising Debates or Perpetuated Coloniality?"; Meekosha and Soldatic, "Human Rights and the Global South"; Soldatic, "The Transnational Sphere of Justice."

8. Ray, The Ecological Other.

9. "Saint Kateri Tekakwitha, Model Ecologist."The website of the Kateri Tekakwitha Conservation Center, however, also acknowledges that she continued working for her longhouse after her illness. Káteri's story is so heavily overwritten that it is often shot through with competing voices. Her name likewise has been translated as "She moves things" ("Kateri's Life") and "She who bumps along as she goes." I don't want to overread these representations or specific translations but rather point to the contexts in which they circulate. The latter translation comes from a Haudenosaunee scholar who has also repatriated Káteri, and who describes her not as pitiful but as "a young, hale smallpox survivor" (Palmer, "The Devil in the Details," 276).

10. Bonaparte, A Lily among Thorns. Bonaparte acknowledges that reclaiming Káteri has not always been an easy sell, because while many Mohawk and other indigenous Catholic people do honor her, others have considered her a symbol of conquest and oppression. For a further discussion of Káteri's contentious position in Mohawk history, see Penelope Myrtle Kelsey's reading of the poet Maurice Kenny's tribute in her edited collection, Maurice Kenny: Celebrations of a Mohawk Writer, 20. Additionally Bonaparte calls for the repatriation of Káteri's physical remains, which are currently housed in reliquaries from the Vatican to British Columbia. The saving of saints' body parts or alleged body parts is a subject rich for Native and disability studies, albeit beyond the scope of the essay at hand.

11. "Kahnawake."

12. Simpson, Mohawk Interruptus, 48.

13. Palmer, "The Devil in the Details,"282, 286.

14. Brooks, The Common Pot, 49.

15. Palmer, "The Devil in the Details,"281.

16. Mitchell and Snyder, Narrative Prosthesis.

17. In a further provocation one recipient of such a cure was also Native American. "Lummi Boy Jake Finkbonner Beat a Flesh Eating Disease,

Earns Inspirational Youth Award," <u>Indian Country Today</u>, January 25, 2012, http://indiancountrytodaymedianetwork.com/2012/01/25 /lummi-boy-jake-finkbonner-beat-flesh-eating-disease-earns -inspirational-youth-award-74070.

18. Glancy, <u>The Reason for Crows</u>, 4, 5, 32, 45.

19. The tribe sought federal recognition from 1974 to 2007 in a series of legal decisions so remarkably racist that they became the center-piece of the anthropologist James Clifford's famous essay "Identity in Mashpee," reprinted in <u>The Predicament of Culture</u>.

20. Peters, <u>The Wampanoags of Mashpee</u>, 35.

21. These include Avant, <u>People of the First Light</u>; Mills, <u>Son of Mashpee</u> and <u>Talking with the Elders of Mashpee</u>.

22. Bingham, <u>Mashpee</u>, 43. Bingham has since expanded this history with her own life story in <u>Seaweed's Revelation</u>. Other Wampanoags say that Amos was "born blind" (Mwalim, personal communication, January 7, 2015). To my knowledge nobody has studied the etiologies of blindness, congenital or otherwise, among indigenous people in the Northeast. It is, however, worth noting that another Amos descendant, Curtis Frye, is also losing his sight due to diabetes (Gonsalves, "Blind Joe and the 'Praying Indians'")—just one more bodily index of the ongoing settler colonial invasion.

23. Gonsalves, "Blind Joe and the 'Praying Indians.'"

24. Mwalim, <u>A Mixed Medicine Bag</u>, 37, 38, 42.

25. Miner, "Beasts of Burden," 62, 63.

26. Thanks to Penelope Kelsey (personal conversation, January 7, 2015) for flagging this for me. For more on Oka, see the excellent collection edited by Simpson and Ladner, <u>This Is an Honour Song</u>.

27. Clare, "Natural Worlds, Disabled Bodies, and a Politics of Cure," 215.

28. For a thorough (and often unrecognized) history of sustainability, see Tom Kelly's introduction to Aber et al., <u>The Sustainable Learning Community</u>.

29. Waziyatawin, "The Paradox of Indigenous Resurgence at the End of Empire," 68.

30. Palmer, "The Devil in the Details," 273.

31. Eli Clare, "Natural Worlds, Disabled Bodies, and a Politics of Cure," https://disabilitystudies.wisc.edu/wp-content/uploads/2012/09 /Eli-Clare-Meditations-UW-Madison.pdf.

BIBLIOGRAPHY

Aber, John, Tom Kelly, and Bruce Mallory, eds. The Sustainable Learning Community: One University's Journey to the Future. Hanover: University of New Hampshire Press, 2009.

Avant, Joan Tavares. People of the First Light: Wisdoms of a Mashpee Wampanoag Elder. West Barnstable MA: West Barnstable Press, 2010.

Bingham, Amelia. Mashpee: Land of the Wampanoags. Mashpee MA: Mashpee Historical Commission, 1970.

———. Seaweed's Revelation: A Wampanoag Clan Mother in Contemporary America. San Diego: GGBing, 2012.

Bonaparte, Darren. A Lily among Thorns: The Mohawk Repatriation of Káteri Tekahkwí:tha. Akwesasne NY: BookSurge, 2009.

Brooks, Lisa. The Common Pot: The Recovery of Native Space in the Northeast. Minneapolis: University of Minnesota Press, 2008.

Clare, Eli. "Natural Worlds, Disabled Bodies, and a Politics of Cure." In Material Ecocriticism, edited by Serenella Iovino and Serpil Oppermann, 204–20. Bloomington: Indiana University Press, 2014.

Clifford, James. The Predicament of Culture: Twentieth-Century Ethnography, Literature and Art. Cambridge MA: Harvard University Press, 1988.

Erevelles, Nirmala. Disability and Difference in Global Contexts: Enabling a Transformative Body Politic. New York: Palgrave Macmillan, 2011.

Glancy, Diane. The Reason for Crows: A Story of Káteri Tekakwí:tha. Albany NY: Excelsior Editions, 2009.

Grech, Shaun. "Recolonising Debates or Perpetuated Coloniality? Decentring the Spaces of Disability, Development and Community in the Global South." International Journal of Inclusive Education 15, no. 1 (2011): 87–100.

Greer, Allan. Mohawk Saint: Catherine Tekakwitha and the Jesuits. New York: Oxford University Press, 2005.

"Kahnawake." Lily of the Mohawks: The St. Francis Xavier Mission and Shrine of Kateri Tekakwitha. Accessed January 1, 2015. http://kateri tekakwitha.net/kahnawake/.

"Kateri's Life." Lily of the Mohawks. Accessed January 1, 2015. http://kateritekakwitha.net/kateris-trail/.

Kelsey, Penelope Myrtle. Maurice Kenny: Celebrations of a Mohawk Writer. New York: SUNY Press, 2011.

Koppedrayer, K. I. "The Making of the First Iroquois Virgin: Early Jesuit Biographies of Kateri Tekakwitha." Ethnohistory 40, no. 2 (1993): 277–306.

Livingston, Julie. Debility and the Moral Imagination in Botswana. Bloomington: Indiana University Press, 2005.

Massachusetts. Commission to Examine into the Condition of the Indians in the Commonwealth, F. W. Bird, Whiting Griswold, and Cyrus Weekes. Report of the Commissioners Related to the Condition of the Indians of Massachusetts. House Doc. no. 46, February 1849. https://archive.org/details/reportofcommissi00mass_5.

Meekosha, Helen, and Karen Soldatic. "Human Rights and the Global South: The Case of Disability." Third World Quarterly 32, no. 8 (2011): 1383–97.

Mills, Earl, Sr. Son of Mashpee: Reflections of Chief Flying Eagle, a Wampanoag. North Falmouth MA: Word Studio, 1996.

———. Talking with the Elders of Mashpee: Memories of Earl H. Mills, Sr. Mashpee MA: Mills, 2012.

Miner, Joshua D. "Beasts of Burden: How Literary Animals Remap the Aesthetics of Removal." Decolonization: Indigeneity, Education & Society 3, no. 2 (2014): 60–82.

Mitchell, David T., and Sharon L. Snyder. Narrative Prosthesis: Disability and the Dependencies of Discourse. Ann Arbor: University of Michigan Press, 2000.

Mwalim. A Mixed Medicine Bag: Original Black Wampanoag Folklore. Mashpee MA: Talking Drum Press, Oversoul Theater Collective, 1998.

Palmer, Vera B. "The Devil in the Details: Controverting an American Indian Conversion Narrative." In Theorizing Native Studies, edited by Audra Simpson and Andrea Smith, 266–96. Durham NC: Duke University Press, 2014.

Peters, Russell M. The Wampanoags of Mashpee: An Indian Perspective on American History. Boston: Media Action, 1987.

Ray, Sarah Jaquette. The Ecological Other: Environmental Exclusion in American Culture. Tucson: University of Arizona Press, 2013.

"Saint Kateri Tekakwitha, Model Ecologist." Saint Kateri Tekakwitha Conservation Center. Accessed January 1, 2015. http://www.kateri.org /saint%20kateri.htm.

Senier, Siobhan, and Clare Barker, eds. "Disability and Indigeneity." Special issue, Journal of Literary & Cultural Disability Studies 7, no. 2 (2013).

Simpson, Audra. Mohawk Interruptus: Political Life across the Borders of Settler States. Durham NC: Duke University Press, 2014.

Simpson, Leanne, and Kiera L. Ladner, eds. This Is an Honour Song: Twenty Years since the Blockades. Winnipeg: Arbeiter Ring, 2010.

Soldatic, Karen. "The Transnational Sphere of Justice: Disability Praxis and the Politics of Impairment." Disability & Society 28, no. 6 (2013): 744–55.

Waziyatawin. "The Paradox of Indigenous Resurgence at the End of Empire." Decolonization: Indigeneity, Education & Society 1, no. 1 (2012): 68–85.

Wolfe, Patrick. Settler Colonialism and the Transformation of Anthropology: The Politics and Poetics of an Ethnographic Event. London: Continuum, 1999.

9

Prosthetic Ecologies
(Re)Membering Disability and Rehabilitating Laos's "Secret War"

Cathy J. Schlund-Vials

Ta knew it was dangerous to handle UXOs [unexploded ordnance]. . . . But one day, as Ta studied a corroded bomblet, he slowly convinced himself that it posed little danger. . . . The badly weathered casing was partly open. Ta could clearly see that the bomb's two halves were slightly separated from one another. Bomblets sometimes split as they age and corrode; when they do the bomblet looks as if it is smiling. Of course, from a different angle that smile turns into a scowl or smirk. The cracked case was misleading. It didn't indicate a safe bomblet. With detonator and explosive intact the bomb still possessed the power to maim or kill. . . . When Ta inspected the bombie he envisioned opening the bomb, removing its 90 grams of TNT and using its explosives for fishing. He had seen other men light a fuse, drop a bomb into a pond, wait for the boom, and then skim stunned fish off the surface. Ta just couldn't shake visions of himself proudly carrying a basket of fish into the market. "If I weren't poor, I never would have touched that bombie. It's just that I thought I could sell fish for money."

    —"COPE Patients: Ta's Story"

The contemporary world—tied up in its ecological, demographic, and urban impasses—is incapable of absorbing, in a way that is compatible with the interests of humanity, the extraordinary techno-scientific mutations which shake it. It is locked in a vertiginous race toward ruin or radical renewal. All the bearings—economic, social, political, moral, traditional—break down one after the other. It has become imperative to recast the axes of values, the fundamental finalities of human relations and productive activity. An ecology of the virtual is thus just as pressing as ecologies of the visible world.

—Félix Guattari, Chaosmosis (emphasis added)

Located roughly half a mile from Vientiane's Talat Sao (Morning Market), within sight of the Mekong River and in close proximity to Mahosot Hospital (Lao PDR's primary infectious disease research center and chief medical training site), the Centre of Medical Rehabilitation (CMR) and the Cooperative Orthotic and Prosthetic Visitor Centre sit quietly on Khou Vieng Road, a chief municipal thoroughfare.[1] Known more familiarly by its affectively expressive acronym, COPE, the Cooperative Orthotic and Prosthetic Enterprise was formed in 1997 via a multilateral agreement involving Lao PDR's Ministry of Health and a collective of nongovernmental organizations (NGOs). According to its organizational website, COPE was "created in response to the need to provide UXO survivors with the care and support they required, namely by way of orthotic and prosthetic devices."[2] Presently a local nonprofit organization, COPE shares an intimate partnership with the CMR and other similar entities in the country; accordingly its members work closely with regional rehabilitation centers to "provide access to both orthotic/prosthetic devices and rehabilitation services, including physiotherapy, occupational therapy and pediatric services to people with disabilities."[3]

To better comprehend the precise conditions responsible for bringing COPE into being, one has to necessarily attend to

Lao PDR's distinct bomb history vis-à-vis the "American War in Viet Nam," which as many scholars rightly note was—despite nation-based nomenclature—by no means contained nor by any stretch constrained.[4] Indeed the expansiveness of the U.S. military enterprise in Southeast Asia, along with the excesses of U.S. bombing campaigns, is made overwhelmingly clear in COPE's bellicose characterization of conflict duration and comparative munitions. As revealed on the organization's website, between 1964 and 1973 approximately 580,000 bombing missions were flown over Laos, unloading an estimated 260 million submunitions (known as "bombies") and delivering two million tons of heavy ordnance.[5] Shifting from material reality to militarized temporality, the United States, as Karen Coates evocatively synopsizes, dropped on average a planeload of bombs every eight minutes, twenty-four hours per day, over the course of the nine-year period; U.S. pilots, en route to Thai, Okinawan, and Philippine bases following bombing sorties in North and South Vietnam, were encouraged to unload remaining payloads indiscriminately over Laos, and no province was spared. Set against this collateral backdrop, which involved devastating long-distance campaigns and innumerable large-scale munitions, it is not surprising that Laos has the superlative distinction of being the most bombed country per capita in the world.[6]

Notwithstanding immediate impacts—tragically inclusive of almost thirty thousand wartime casualties and fatalities, profound environmental degradation, and extensive building destruction—it is Lao PDR's postwar imaginary that undergirds this chapter's initial tripartite evaluation of militarized aftermaths, war-driven impairment, and COPE's Visitor Centre. In particular roughly 30 percent of U.S. submunitions dropped failed to detonate, leaving the nation with a peculiarly calamitous militarized legacy: eighty million pieces of unexploded ordnance (inclusive of "bombies" or "bomblets," midsize bombs, and heavy artillery).[7] As is the case with other postconflict regions, specifically the former fronts of mid- and late twentieth-century U.S. warmaking, the country's infrastructure—particularly the ability to provide governmental services—was severely impacted by such wholesale militarized devastation. Predictably perhaps, Lao PDR remains one of the poorest countries in Southeast Asia; among a population of 6.8 million, a third of all Laotians subsist below the international poverty line (living on less than US$1.25 per day).[8] Many Laotians cultivate land (primarily for rice production and domestic consumption), and it is through this labor—which involves manual plowing and physically tilling the soil—that farmers encounter and inadvertently detonate UXOs buried in the soil.

Moreover, as the first epigraph underscores, such ordnance functions as a potential income source (e.g., scrap metal) and work implement (i.e., in fishing). The ubiquity of exploded and unexploded ordnance—large bombs, rockets, grenades, midrange artillery, mortars, landmines, and cluster bombs—is overwhelming apparent in the pervasiveness of munitions and casings in everyday life; explicitly the metal gleaned from discarded U.S. armaments is used in home construction, domestic decoration, and as the basis for cooking utensils. Since 2005 an estimated three hundred new casualties annually have resulted from UXO accidents; since 1973 approximately twenty thousand bomb-related incidents have occurred. The majority of those impacted are children and males, who constitute 50 and 80 percent of victims in the postconflict era, respectively.[9] Admittedly efforts to dispose of cluster bomb munitions have been tragically slow: between 1996 and 2009 the country's unexploded ordnance program, UXO Lao, destroyed 1,090,228 submunitions; this represents only roughly 0.55 percent of the munitions that remain.[10]

These past and present contexts, which involve midcentury U.S. war-making and twenty-first-century NGO humanitarianism, foreground my analysis of disability and the environment in what I term "prosthetic ecologies." Simultaneously suggestive of human-made substitution and reparative embodiment, prosthesis, as defined by the Oxford English Dictionary, refers to "the replacement of defective or absent parts of the body by artificial substitutes." Alternatively the term ecology compresses a subfield of biology primarily concerned with the study of relationships, specifically between organisms and with the physical environment. In common parlance it operates as a convenient synonym for environment and an economical stand-in for preservation movements (e.g., environmentalism).[11] As an adjectival modifier, prosthetic encompasses the postconflict realities of Laos as the most bombed nation particularly in terms of present-day munitions accidents; as significant, the term prosthetic ecologies operates as an analytic upon which to syncretically map the vexed interrelationship between bombed environs, disabled bodies, and the built environment as emblematized by the COPE Visitor Centre, which advocates for those affected by postconflict munitions and promulgates an anti–cluster bomb political agenda.

To be sure, within disability studies prosthetic has historically occupied a prominent position, particularly when situated in the face of unparalleled natural disasters, placed alongside the troubling legacies of distanced warfare, and located in relation to the distressing actualities of violent state conflict. Simultaneously material (e.g., fabricated body parts and artificial devices) and experiential (specifically in terms of daily integration and rehabilitation), the prosthetic has emerged as a significantly flexible analytic upon which to map, as Katherine Ott notes, how "wars, natural disasters, and the application of new technologies to human endeavors such as work, transportation, sports, and entertainment—create large numbers of people in need" of such corporeal enhancements. Not surprisingly, as Ott further explains, "much critical disability studies scholarship examines the enduring relationship between prosthetic technologies and histories of capitalism, empire, and the military industrial complex."[12] Mindful of the interdiscipline's "prosthetic" engagements, which accentuate the complex connections among science, technology, embodiment, and impairment, my ecological focus is undeniably and implicitly indebted to Mel Y. Chen's provocative evaluation of the associations and relationships between humans and non-humans as well as the organic and inorganic (via "animacies").[13]

Correspondingly these prosthetic ecologies—which harness a blended ecological and humanitarian activism born out of mass conflict—cohere with Guattari's assertion of "the extraordinary techno-scientific mutations which shake" the present-day world. I apply these frames to contemporary Lao PDR, a state I maintain is perpetually marked and continually haunted by U.S. militarized excess. Situated within a history of disastrous superfluity and appalling excessiveness, prosthetic ecologies on one level intentionally catalogue the ways U.S. militarization—particularly at the COPE Visitor Centre—is strategically remembered and tactically restaged within a predominantly unreconciled conflict-oriented imaginary. On another level such a frame, which marries the disabled body corpus and the nonreparative body politic, purposefully captures juridical absences (namely the nonpersecution of U.S. military culpability) and rehearses catastrophic topographical realties (during and after 1973). As a closer reading of the COPE Visitor Centre accentuates, these prosthetic ecologies engage a differential model with regard to disability and impairment. To explicate, if COPE's organizational purview is primarily focused on rehabilitation, or a medical model of diagnosis and treatment, its Visitor Centre potently identifies—with a mixed virtual-real imaginary—the long-lasting legacies of militarization, the multigenerational aspects of cluster bomb usage, and pathological dimensions of U.S. imperialism.

Curating Culpability and Disability: The COPE Visitor Centre

Partially obscured by an equal mix of light and dark green foliage, the Centre of Medical Rehabilitation is marked by a gold-lettered sign that bears the telltale emblem of a red cross within a white circle; these medical registers are confirmed by the officious mention of Lao PDR's Ministry of Health. A raised red and white traffic gate is visible from the road; despite regulatory appearances movement within the center is largely unmonitored, especially during the site's public hours (9 a.m.–6 p.m.). Tourists, workers, and those seeking rehabilitation services mingle in an open courtyard organized along a simple square grid. To one's immediate right, prosthetic limbs in assorted states of assemblage and of numerous types (e.g., plastic feet, synthetic legs, fabricated arms, and metal hooks) hang from wooden rafters and rest on makeshift work benches; to the left are COPE's administrative offices, which feature a decidedly modern, architectural veneer of steel, cement, and glass. Likewise contemporary is the COPE Visitor Centre, a white building that occupies the northern part of the organizational compound (figure 9.1); by contrast a traditional Lao housing structure, replete with thatched roof and spare wooden beams, is located perpendicular to the Visitor Centre.

The center's front façade features cluster-bomb casings repurposed as planters along with a statue of a mother and child fashioned from military scrap metal. As one nears the glass door entrance, the individual elements of the COPE sign are much more

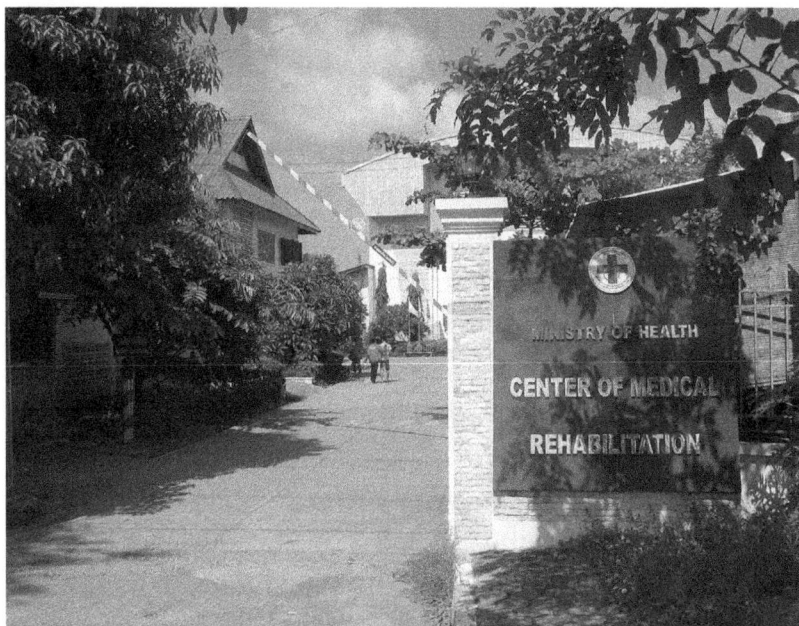

Fig. 9.1. COPE Visitor Centre, front façade, 2014. Photo by Christopher R. Vials.

discernible; in particular the letters have been made using facsimile brown casts of prosthetic limbs. Such architectural collapses, evident in the mix of governmental buildings, open-air structures, on-site artwork, and daily work spaces, are replicated to varying degrees and by divergent ends in the curatorial dimensions and layout of the COPE Visitor Centre, which showcases a free exhibit intended to familiarize sightseers with "the UXO problem in Lao PDR and the work undertaken by COPE and the CMR to provide disability services for people affected by UXOs." Armed with a distinct didactic purpose, the center opened its doors in 2008 with the goal of "increas[ing] awareness about disability in Laos and highlight[ing] the amazing work that is being done to help people with disabilities lead full and productive lives. It also presents the unexploded ordnance (UXO) problem in Laos and how it links in with disability."[14] Open seven days a week, the COPE Visitor Center has become an oft-accessed tourist destination for those vacationing in Lao PDR; this is in part due to its appearance in several travel guides (such as <u>Lonely Planet</u>, Trip Advisor, and individual blogs) and the relative paucity of other museums in Vientiane.[15] This touristic sensibility is furthered by the organization's website, which gives visitors the following practical advice: "While many of the tuk tuk drivers know where we are, it is useful to write the letters COPE on a sheet of paper to show the driver."[16] Visitors are encouraged to borrow bicycles (conveniently housed on site) to tour the surrounding municipality after perusing the museum.

In order to access the multiple exhibits housed in the COPE Visitor Centre, however, one must first go through a crowded, colorful gift shop filled with antiwar T-shirts, tote bags, postcards, homemade crafts, and small dolls with missing and prosthetic limbs. Notwithstanding the plethora of souvenirs available for purchase, the COPE Visitor Centre is very much concentrated on its educational mission; indeed even with its decidedly somber focus on cluster bombs and their dramatic impact, the museum stresses that the exhibits are "suitable for all ages."[17] Furthermore admission is free, though donations are accepted; these monies, along with profits garnered from souvenir sales, are used to fund COPE's rehabilitation project (which, to reiterate, involves occupational therapy and the production of prosthetics and orthotics). Transactions at the close-by Karma Café (also on site) provide another funding source. The use of these monies is implicitly and explicitly evident in the exhibits contained in the museum: testimonials from those who have benefited from COPE's humanitarian work—similar to Ta's opening account— are intermixed with placards describing the center's outreach initiatives (in rural areas and urban sites), sample prostheses, and staff photographs detailing various aspects of prosthetic and orthotic production.

Nevertheless it is the curatorial structure of the museum—particularly as it pertains to the strategic and progressive placement of exhibits—which most clearly demonstrates the center's pedagogical agenda. Although there is no permanent on-site guide, movement through the museum is purposefully directed by the physical and chronological placement of exhibits and the prevalence of informational placards; sightlines vary considerably due to the size and height of exhibits, which simultaneously function as barriers and path markers within the space.[18] However, the interior of the museum is relatively small, comprising a main exhibit space and an adjoining room wherein documentary films about COPE and unexploded ordnance are screened at regular intervals. Upon entering the museum the viewer is shown a red-dotted map of Lao PDR (on the right wall); the dots overwhelm the cartographic space. The viewer is immediately informed by a complementary placard that the dots signify bomb sites, indicating in the process that approximately 85 percent of the nation was bombed during U.S. campaigns in Southeast Asia. Adjacent to the map is a flat-screen television that plays, on a continuous loop, a short animated film focused on the past and present contexts of the nation's cluster munitions crisis. Marked by stark black lines, composed of opaque colors, and featuring a subdued musical score, the film commences with a cartoon drawing of B-52 planes dropping cluster bomb payloads; the movie then shifts to a long-range shot of a small child hoeing in a green field. Slowly the camera shifts to closer range, showing the child's hoe brush against a bomblet in the soil. This precipitates the next scene, which returns to a wide-angle focus on the child, who lies on her back, bleeding, her right leg missing. Narration takes the form of white text that details various facts and figures, such as the amount of munitions dropped, bomb casualties, and remaining unexploded ordnance.

Significantly the short film—by way of mixed camera shots, cluster bomb subject, and data-focused narration—anticipates the types of displays featured in the museum, wherein two-dimensional representations and visual media are presented alongside three-dimensional artillery artifacts and informational placards and posters. What remains most consistent throughout the site is the museum's negotiation of long-distance warfare (e.g., midcentury U.S. bombing campaigns) and the contemplation of intimate victim portrayals (e.g., those adversely impacted by munitions explosions). From the outset the visitor is presented with an overwhelming array of different bombs and munitions (in glass cases and embedded in exhibits), which on one level potently recall what the U.S. military left behind. On another level, at stake in the museum's curation is an equally urgent engagement with these artifacts as disastrously found (in the case of accidental detonation) and necessarily discovered (as a source of economic livelihood) by present-day Laotians. Such collateral impacts—which encompass the legacy of U.S. militarization via the continuation of contemporary Laotian subsistence—are made most immediate in a scaled facsimile of a typical Lao PDR home, which is located in the middle portion of the museum.

As is the case with other exhibits in the museum, the domicile reiterates the exterior of the COPE courtyard, which contains an analogous structure located adjacent to the museum. But whereas the compound affords an exterior visual experience, the museum provides the viewer with an interior perspective through the built representation of living space. Accordingly tourists are able to physically enter the home, which is decorated with a variety of household goods repurposed from found munitions casing; the placards associated with these objects stress the daily dangers facing Laotians, who live in a postconflict, <u>precarious</u> imaginary. As Judith Butler evocatively and provocatively summarizes, such precarity designates a "politically induced condition in which certain populations suffer from failing social and economic networks of support and become differentially exposed to injury, violence, and death. Such populations are at heightened risk of disease, poverty, starvation, displacement, and exposure to violence without protection. Precarity also characterizes that politically induced condition of maximized vulnerability and exposure for populations exposed to arbitrary state violence and to other forms of aggression that are not enacted by states and against which states do not offer adequate protection."[19]

As a "politically induced condition," precarity involves not only those who are at "heightened risk"; such a mode also encapsulates populations that, within a neoliberal, militarized world, incontrovertibly exist within chaotic zones of "maximized vulnerability." Analogously, within the space of the home exhibit visitors are made aware of such maximized vulnerability in relation to a concomitant position as actual sightseer, imagined witness, and virtual victim. Indeed while the visitor enters the home as a tourist, within the domestic interior he or she is prompted to read testimonial accounts, vicariously transforming the individual sightseer into a potential juridical spectator. At the same time the preponderance of munitions within the house exhibit— tactically paired with placards that feature accounts of bomb-focused unpredictability, accident, and injury—renders perceptible a precarious sense that, as Butler asserts, "anything living can be expunged at will or by accident; and its persistence is in no sense guaranteed."[20]

These precarious registers are apparent in exhibits such as the initial animated film and the Laotian house replica; they are also suggested in the crowded placement of exhibits, which creates an uncanny sensation of claustrophobic anxiety that affectively attends to the enormity of the UXO problem in the country. The limited space of the museum is indubitably maximized: in addition to the use of walls (e.g., upon which placards, photographs, and flat-screen televisions are placed), visitors are encouraged to move through larger three-dimensional structures (like the house) and traverse alongside and under exhibits that hang vertically from the ceiling. Two large-scale mobiles are suspended from the ceiling: the first features strings of bombies and bomblets bookended by two halves of a cluster bomb casing (figure 9.2); the second is composed of hanging prosthetic legs (figure 9.3).

Visitors must initially amble alongside the bomb mobile as they make their way into the museum, replicating by way of physical position the wartime history of the U.S. bombing of Lao PDR, which was waged from the air but experienced on the ground. Upon exiting the Laotian domicile, sightseers are prompted to cross a makeshift bridge over which hangs the exhibit of prosthetic legs; this particular path leads the viewer to a workbench and a tower of purposefully assembled prosthetic limbs.

Shifting from curatorial placement to aesthetic form, the use of mobiles tellingly coheres with the overall narrative of the museum, which rehearses and restages a distinct cause-effect relationship between long-range U.S. militarization, munitions-based disability, and COPE's rehabilitation project. As a mechanized, kinetic sculpture, a mobile is designed to highlight equilibrium and balance via a blend of vertical and horizontal placements. On one level these particular exhibits—wherein cluster bomb munitions are placed before prosthetic limbs—makes discernible a corresponding, paired narrative that paradoxically brings into dialogic balance U.S. militarization (as principal cause) and a story of impairment (as catastrophic effect). On another level the balance embedded in the mobile as a particular sculptural mode

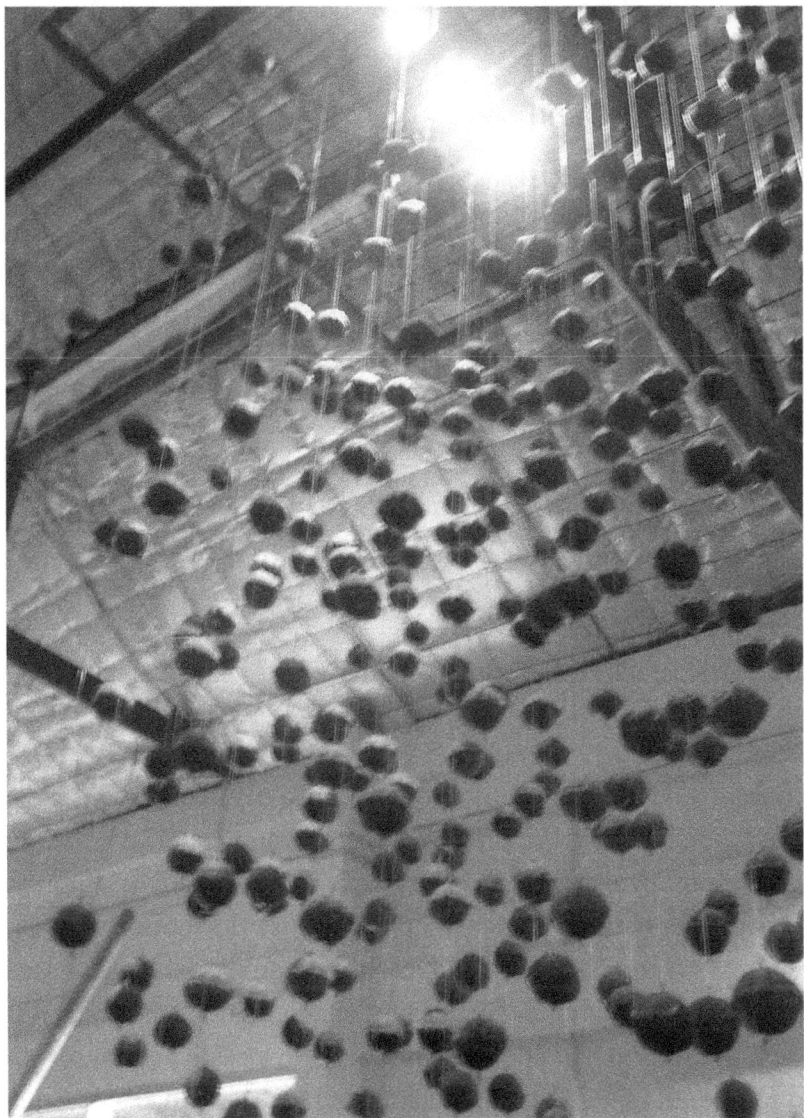

Fig. 9.2. Cluster bomb mobile, 2014. Photo by Christopher R. Vials.

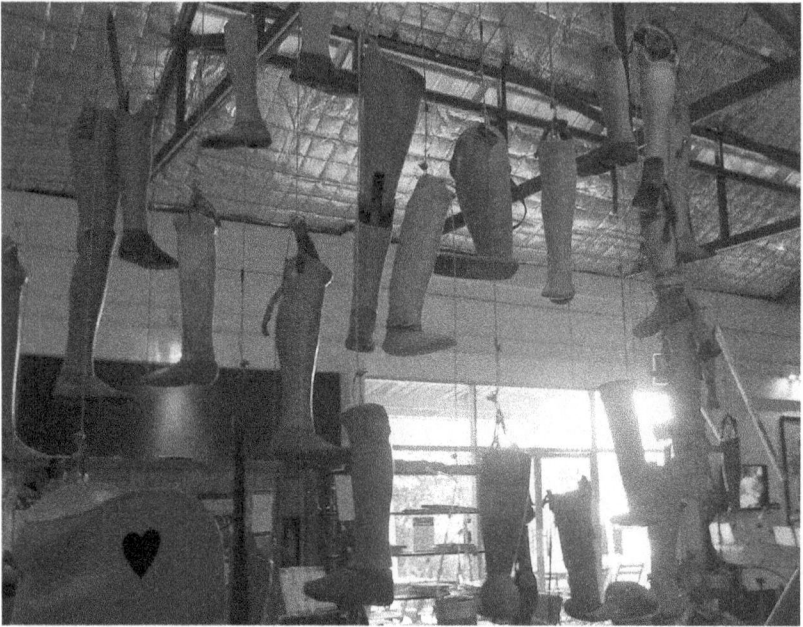

Fig. 9.3. Prosthetic limb sculpture, 2014. Photo by Christopher R. Vials.

mirrors COPE's objective as a rehabilitative medical site. After all, COPE's daily mission of providing humanitarian aid is predicated on a reparative agenda that attempts to "make whole" through prosthesis the present-day victims of past U.S. bombing campaigns.[21] Whereas the first half of the museum's exhibits focuses on the dire conditions responsible for the organization's formation, the second half emphasizes—through smiling patient before and after accounts—an optimism fixed to COPE's local, regional, and national work. Taken as a whole, the museum's curation is unambiguously medical with regard to its diagnostic agenda (U.S. militarization and cluster bombs) and treatment program (prosthetic and orthotic production and postaccident training). Set against these medicalized frames, however, it is the museum's final exhibit, which concerns the Convention on Cluster Munitions, that brings into focus the site's human rights critique of mass militarization and distanced warfare through prosthetic ecologies.

The Convention on Cluster Munitions (CCM) is an international treaty intended to prohibit the use, transfer, and stockpile of cluster bombs. Adopted in Dublin in 2008, the same year COPE's Visitor Centre opened, the CCM would come into force in 2010, when the provision was ratified by thirty member states.[22] Presently 116 states have signed the treaty or assented to its primary provisions, which are outlined in the CCM's Article 1:

1. Each State Party undertakes never under any circumstances to:

   a. Use cluster munitions;

   b. Develop, produce, otherwise acquire, stockpile, retain, or transfer to anyone, directly or indirectly, cluster munitions.

   c. Assist, encourage, or induce anyone to engage in any activity prohibited to a State Party under this Convention.

2. Paragraph 1 of this Article applies, mutatis mutandis, to explosive bomblets that are specifically designed to be dispersed or released from dispensers affixed to aircraft.

3. This Convention does not apply to mines.[23]

Comprising a preamble and twenty-three articles, the CCM defines "cluster munitions victims" as "all persons who have been killed or suffered physical or psychological injury, economic loss, social marginalization or substantial impairment of the realization of their rights caused by the use of cluster munitions. They include those persons directly impacted by cluster munitions as well as their affected families and communities." Notwithstanding widespread international support, the United States—along with China, Russia, India, Israel, Pakistan, and Brazil—has not signed onto the Convention, though it is presently in effect.[24] In 2006 Senator Barack Obama (Illinois), in contrast to his soon-to-be presidential rivals Senator John McCain (Arizona) and Senator Hillary Clinton (New York), supported legislation that would limit the use of cluster bombs; the legislation, which appeared as an amendment to the 2007 Department of Defense Appropriation Act, contained explicit language intended to "protect civilian lives from unexploded munitions." The amendment, however, failed to pass: thirty senators voted for it, but seventy senators voted against it.[25]

To be sure the U.S. resistance to anti–cluster bomb legislation is distressingly part and parcel of contemporary U.S. militarization and "war on terror" strategies that continue to rely on the use of long-range tactics (e.g., drone attacks) and large-scale munitions (particularly with regard to "smart bombs" and depleted uranium shells). Even more distressing is the overt denial of civilian casualty culpability with regard to cluster bomb usage; such disavowals access as a first premise the allegedly humanitarian aspects of distanced warfare. These "humane" justifications are evident in a 2008 Pentagon policy report, which offers the following preemptive assertion: "Because future adversaries will likely use civilian shields for military targets—for example by locating a military target on the roof of an occupied building—use of unitary weapons could result in more civilian casualties and damage than cluster munitions. Blanket elimination of cluster munitions is therefore unacceptable due not only to negative military consequences but also due to potential negative consequences for civilians."[26] Despite the Pentagon's insistence that "blanket elimination of cluster munitions . . . [has] potential negative consequences for civilians," the COPE Visitor Centre's curatorial reiteration of militarized impacts approximately four decades after the U.S. campaign over Lao PDR came to an abrupt end provides a stark counterpoint and legible human rights critique. Set against a backdrop of munitions-based precarity, wherein Laotians must constantly contend with the realities and consequences of unexploded ordnance, the claim of civilian safety disremembers the cluster campaigns that make COPE's rehabilitation mission relevant and urgent.

Conclusion

Such urgency, which is ultimately fixed to a human rights critique of ongoing militarization, presages the final exhibit, which consists of two large, relatively nondescript posters. The first summarizes the scope and briefly details the history of the Convention on Cluster Munitions; the second includes a list of nations that have and have not signed onto the Convention. Bearing the COPE logo (which features a male with a prosthetic right leg raised, smiling and leaning backward), the first poster directly addresses the issue of culpability via the "obligation to assist victims," which, under the auspices of the CCM and according to the exhibit, "requires states to provide medical care, rehabilitation and psychological and economic support to those directly injured, their families and communities living in affected areas."[27] This focus on services, rehabilitation, and support coheres on one level with the mission contexts of the Centre of Medical Rehabilitation and COPE, which seeks to fulfill this obligation via nongovernmental humanitarianism.

Yet on another level it is the final question on the poster that intersects with and engages a distinctly munitions-based human rights critique. The viewer is expressly asked "Has your country signed?" The question intentionally prompts a scan of the second poster, and the viewer is left with the decision to sign an accompanying petition supporting the Convention's adoption by other states. Whereas the mention of the Convention on Cluster Munitions is predicated on state-sanctioned responsibility (to citizens impacted by such large-scale weaponry), the query about signatories concerns international culpability, a point made clear in the poster's insistence that the cluster munitions ban is "binding international law." Thus states that have yet to sign onto the ban—such as the United States—are, as per the logic of the final exhibit, unequivocally cast outside the context and purview of extant human rights law.

If, as Viet Thanh Nguyen maintains, "All wars are fought twice, the first time on the battlefield, the second time in memory," then the U.S. campaign in Laos—as recollected in the COPE Visitor Centre museum—occupies, in the end, a particularly vexed, unreconciled juridical position. The center's memory work, which operates outside the normal confines of state-authorized justice and state-supported reparation, provides a critical means of assessing the extent to which U.S. war-making is undeniably ongoing, ostensibly perpetual, and apparently permanent. Situated in a context wherein state-sanctioned justice is, notwithstanding the munitions convention and global ban, elusive given the fact that the United States has yet to offer any reparations or accountability, the UXO crisis in Lao PDR remains largely open-ended. Hence the museum's insistence on the causes and effects of such large-scale militarization assumes, to varying degrees, the prosecutorial registers of an international tribunal; tourists are correspondingly (albeit temporarily) placed in the position of witnesses and would-be human rights activists. Even more significant, the museum's indefatigable remembrance of U.S. cluster bomb campaigns—which critically juxtaposes its present-day prosthetic mission and the ongoing ecological impact—further underscores a profound nonculpability that implicitly and productively engages a discourse of impunity. Correspondingly and provocatively the United States is cast as both a rogue state (via the ban) and a profound human rights violator (by way of collateral damage).[28]

NOTES

1. The first epigraph is from "COPE Patients: Ta's Story," COPE: Helping People Move On, accessed December 12, 2014, http://www.copelaos .org/ta.php. "Lao PDR" is shorthand for "Lao People's Democratic Republic."

2. These NGOs included POWER, World Vision, and the Cambodian School of Prosthetics and Orthotics.

3. "About COPE," COPE: Helping People Move On, accessed December 12, 2014, http://www.copelaos.org/about.php. According to its website, COPE is charged with four primary functions: "(1) To act as a portal for skills development and training, upgrading clinical skills in physiotherapy, occupational therapy, and P&O [prosthetics and orthotics] within the government rehabilitation services. This is extended to management and administrative skills to ensure that the capacity for COPE to run as a local organization is sustainable. (2) To support expenses of patients who are unable to pay for treatment and associated costs as well as upgrading facilities at the five centres currently supported by COPE. (3) To act as an interface between the donor community and the Lao Government. International donors require a recognized standard of auditing and financial accountability for proposals to be successfully accepted and managed. (4) To facilitate referral between the network of clinical services to provide comprehensive treatment of people living with mobility impairments, ensuring people with disabilities in Lao PDR will have access to the rehabilitation services that can improve their ability to participate in their communities."

4. See Yên Lê Espiritu, Body Counts: The Vietnam War and Militarized Refuge(es) (Berkeley: University of California Press, 2014); Cathy J. Schlund-Vials, War, Genocide, and Justice: Cambodian American Memory Work (Minneapolis: University of Minnesota Press, 2012); Mimi Thi Nguyen, The Gift of Freedom: War, Debt, and Other Refu-

gee Passages (Durham NC: Duke University Press, 2012). As Mariam Lam productively maintains, references to "the American War in Viet Nam" obscure the immense geopolitical scope of the war (which involved Cambodia, Laos, Thailand, and Burma) and elide the complexities of the region vis-à-vis other nation conflicts (e.g., the Cambodian-Vietnamese war). Nevertheless I use this phrase to distinguish the specificities of U.S. involvement from the first Indochina War with France.

5. "Ban Cluster Bombs," COPE: Helping People Move On, accessed November 5, 2014, http://www.copelaos.org/ban_cluster_bombs .php.
6. Coates, Eternal Harvest.
7. "Ban Cluster Bombs."
8. World Bank, "Poverty Headcount Ratio at $1.25 a Day (2011 PPP) (% of Population)," accessed January 13, 2015, http://data.worldbank .org/indicator/si.pov.dday.
9. "Ban Cluster Bombs."
10. "The UXO Problem," National Committee for Rural Development and Poverty Eradication, accessed February 3, 2015, http://www .uxolao.org/index.php/en/the-uxo-problem. UXO Lao has a number of international partners, including Armor Group North America, Japan Mine Action Service, Mines Advisory Group, and the Norwegian People's Aid.
11. OED Online, accessed November 4, 2014, http://dictionary.oed.com/.
12. Ott, "Prosthetics," 140, 143.
13. Chen, Animacies.
14. "About COPE."
15. Other museums include the Lao National Museum, which is in the process (as of August 2014) of being relocated to a renovated site, and the Kaysone Phomvihane Memorial Museum (on the outskirts of the city), which is also the site of the former USAID and CIA compound known as "Six Klicks" (because it was approximately six kilometers outside Vientiane).
16. "About COPE."
17. "About COPE."

18. COPE staff do provide guided tours for groups, NGO personnel, and others who schedule their visits in advance.
19. Butler, "Performativity, Precarity and Sexual Politics," ii.
20. Butler, "Performativity, Precarity, and Sexual Politics," ii.
21. It should be noted that a minority of the testimonials presented by COPE patients involve non-munitions-based accidents (particularly car accidents).
22. The Convention on Cluster Munitions is the first treaty since the ban on antipersonnel landmines was passed in 1997 to attend to the use of large-scale munitions on civilian populations.
23. Convention on Cluster Munitions, "Convention Text," May 30, 2008, http://www.clusterconvention.org/files/2011/01/Convention -ENG.pdf. The following countries have joined the Convention as states: (from Africa) Botswana, Burkina Faso, Burundi, Cameroon, Cape Verde, Chad, Comoros, Congo, Cote d'Ivoire, Ghana, Guinea, Guinea-Bissau, Lesotho, Malawi, Mali, Mauritania, Mozambique, Niger, Senegal, Seychelles, Sierra Leone, Swaziland, Togo, Tunisia, Zambia; (from the Americas) Antigua and Barbuda, Belize, Bolivia, Chile, Costa Rica, Dominican Republic, Ecuador, El Salvador, Grenada, Guatemala, Guyana, Honduras, Mexico, Nicaragua, Panama, Peru, Saint Kitt Nevis, Saint Vincent and the Grenadines, Trinidad and Tobago, and Uruguay; (Asia) Afghanistan, Japan, and Lao PDR; (Europe) Albania, Andorra, Austria, Belgium, Bosnia and Herzegovina, Bulgaria, Croatia, Czech Republic, Denmark, France, Germany, Holy See, Hungary, Ireland, Italy, Liechtenstein, Lithuania, Luxembourg, the FYR of Macedonia, Malta, Moldova, Monaco, Montenegro, Netherlands, Norway, Portugal, San Marino, Slovenia, Spain, Sweden, Switzerland, and the United Kingdom; (Middle East) Iraq, Lebanon, the State of Palestine; (Pacific) Australia, Cook Islands, Fiji, Nauru, New Zealand, and Samoa. Signatories include Angola, Benin Central African Republic, Democratic Republic of Congo, Djibouti, Gambia, Kenya, Liberia, Madagascar, Namibia, Nigeria, Rwanda, Sao Tome and Principe, Somalia, South Africa, Uganda and United Republic of Tanzania, Canada, Colombia, Haiti, Jamaica, Paraguay, Indonesia, the Philippines, Cyprus, Iceland, and Palau.

24. Tellingly these nations represent the primary suppliers and users of cluster bomb munitions.
25. "U.S. Senate Roll Call 109th Congress—2nd Session," accessed January 10, 2015, http://www.senate.gov/legislative/LIS/roll_call_lists/roll_call_vote_cfm.cfm?congress=109&session=2&vote=00232.
26. Quoted in Spencer Ackerman, "U.S. Ducks as Cluster Bomb Ban Takes Effect," Wired, July 29, 2010, http://www.wired.com/2010/07/u-s-ducks-as-cluster-bomb-ban-takes-effect/. "Unitary weapons" refer to chemical weapons such as mustard gas and phosphine gas.
27. COPE Visitor Centre (text derived from author's site visit).
28. Such "critical juxtaposing" accesses Espiritu's important characterization in Body Counts of critical refugee studies as a multivalent site of analysis and critique.

BIBLIOGRAPHY

Butler, Judith. "Performativity, Precarity and Sexual Politics." AIBR: Revista de Antropologia Iberoamerica 4, no. 3 (2009): ii.
Chen, Mel Y. Animacies: Biopolitics, Racial Mattering, and Queer Affect. Durham NC: Duke University Press, 2012.
Coates, Karen. Eternal Harvest: The Legacy of U.S. Bombs in Laos. New York: Things Asian Press, Global Directions, 2013.
Guattari, Félix. Chaosmosis. Indianapolis: Indiana University Press, 1995.
Lam, Mariam. "Presentation: The States of Southeast Asian American Studies." Paper presented at Southeast Asians in the Diaspora Conference, University of Minnesota, Minneapolis, October 4, 2014.
Ott, Katherine. "Prosthetics." In Keywords for Disability Studies, edited by Rachel Adams, Benjamin Reiss, and David Serlin, 140–42. New York: NYU Press, 2015.

10

Reification, Biomedicine, and Bombs
Women's Politicization in Vieques's Social Movement

Víctor M. Torres-Vélez

This ethnography examines Viequense women's intense forms of suffering as triggers for their politicization during the height of the antimilitary struggle in Vieques, Puerto Rico, in the early 2000s.[1] I pay attention to the relationships between environmental degradation, disease prevalence, identity, and social mobilization. I posit that the gendered and intersubjective experience of confronting illness in a complexly rendered sociophysical landscape, such as the Vieques, can impel women to pose new questions and ideas regarding disease etiology. This new embodied language not only renders visible subjugating systems of meaning, such as the biomedical and colonial; it also offers the possibility of rearticulating their own subject position in political terms. In making sense of their experiences with disease, women rearticulate their identity to conquer the public sphere of activism—a traditionally male-encoded space—and break with the institutional reifications subjecting them to passive roles.

In order to understand the emergence of politicized identities we need to recognize the relationship between reification (Taussig 1992) as a process of hiding the negative aspects of capital accumulation and subjection (Foucault 1995; Althusser 1971; Callari and Ruccio 1996) as the process through which institutions constitute disciplined subjects in larger socioeconomic processes and institutions. I argue that women's politicization emerges when they uncover the hidden connections between that which is affecting them and the institutions responsible for their situation.

Ultimately I illustrate the transformation of women's subjectivities in the face of collective health crisis. I reveal how, out of the institutional failure to explain and rectify women's afflictions, women become skeptical of the establishment, their deep frustration propelling them to new forms of meaning-making, and are indelibly politicized. At the intersections of medical anthropology, environmental justice, and disability studies, I conclude that in confronting disease and disability within their own and their family's bodies Viequense women found the strength to fight back against the U.S. Navy. Thus the contribution to this volume and the literature is twofold. This research bridges the gap between the environmental justice literature and disability studies by moving beyond conceptualizing disability as a burden (the way environmental justice literature has done) and instead showing its empowering potential, and by theorizing and bringing to our attention the ways toxic environments—via health crises—can decenter and problematize dominant paradigms of subjection and inequality (such as gender, race, class, and ableness; Johnson 2011; Clare 2014). As Ray and Sibara point out in the introduction to this volume, disability studies needs to pay more attention to the ways toxic environs "disrupt dominant paradigms for recognizing and representing disability."

Mapping the Territory

I begin by briefly discussing the neocolonial condition of Puerto Rico and the U.S. military's toxic legacies in Vieques. A lengthier theoretical framework follows, explaining the relationship between hegemony, reification, and subjection and how women's embodied experiences provided a language to challenge these systems of meaning in order to reframe their own subject positions. The rest of the chapter concentrates on illustrating the phases that women went through in their journey toward politicization. Here I systematically rely on women's oral histories in three main sections. "Dolor: Confronting Life and Death," documents women's experiences with disease and how devastating these experiences are. "Legitimation Crises" illustrates how the inability of governmental, military, and health institutions to explain disease etiology forces women to develop their own embodied explanations. "Rabia: Illness, Identity, and Action" documents how women transform the socially rendered passive experience of disease into an empowering experience through the affective reframing of their challenging circumstances into indignation and action. Thus instead of conceptualizing disease and disability within a toxic environment as disempowering—the way environmental justice does most of the time—I challenge that trope by showing how in such contexts the experience of dis-ablement can sometimes be the catalyst for political action.

Neocolonialism and Toxic Legacies

In the cold war era that lasted into the early 1990s, the number of military bases in Puerto Rico grew, and the island became the largest military complex outside of the continental United States. Vieques became the exclusive training ground for the U.S. Navy from the 1970s on (Wargo 2009). Military activities in Vieques reached an average of 280 days of the year of shooting practice, including air-to-ground and ship-to-shore bombing at close proximity to the civilian population of nine thousand.

Despite the U.S. military's continuous denial between the 1970s and 2000s that it was using its base on Vieques as a missile testing ground, in 2003 it was officially acknowledged that during this time the navy had conducted the most consistent and continuous testing of weapons anywhere in the United States. Wargo

(2009, 96) writes, "Vice Admiral John Shanahan . . . estimated that between 1980 and 2000 the Navy dropped nearly 3 million pounds of ordnance on Vieques every year." If we add up the amount of said ordnance for the total span of military practices on the island, it tops out at a staggering "200 million pounds of weaponry deposited on or near Vieques during the U.S. occupation" (96). These weapons were all detonated within the meager fifty-two square miles of Vieques, and their chemical components were left to degrade and leach into soil, water, and air.

The U.S. Navy tested highly toxic nonconventional weapons on the island (Wargo 2009). Soil and plant samples collected in 2000 revealed evidence of depleted radioactive uranium, a known carcinogen. Moreover in the waters off of Vieques, traditionally heavily relied on for seafood, toxic substances such as inorganic arsenic persist (Mansilla-Rivera et al. 2013).

This profound environmental degradation wrought by U.S. military activity in Vieques between 1970 and 2003 has been well documented (Massol-Deyá and Diaz 2003; Massol-Deyá and Díaz de Osborne 2013; Massol-Deyá et al. 2005). Similarly the articulated roles of environmental degradation and disease in catalyzing public anger and action on Vieques have been discussed by those broadly theorizing the island's mobilizations (Baver 2006; McCaffrey 2002; Wargo 2009). What has been neglected is the documenting and theorizing of how the women who came to spearhead an important arm of the local movement reformulated their quotidian experiences of chronic diseases in toxic landscapes into personal efficacy and social change through affective, embodied manifestations of political consciousness. What has been missing is an analysis of how women's health and environmental activism has the power to bring into focus the contradictions of dominant paradigms of normality (whether gender, race, biomedicine, colonialism, ableness). Thus this research aligns itself with an attempt at merging "feminist disability studies and environmental justice [that] forces us to confront power dynamics that reinforce a narrow view of 'normal'—one that privileges a particular sense of the human body that is constrictive, not expansive" (Johnson 2011, 5).

On Hegemony, Reification, and Subjection

Despite their denial, the U.S. Navy systematically tested highly toxic nonconventional weapons, in addition to conventional weapons, on the island of Vieques beginning in the 1970s (Wargo 2009). Although eventually the navy acknowledged the use of armor-piercing depleted uranium shells, they dismissed the gravity of the finding by arguing that the amounts of ammunition used were negligible. Meanwhile, on the island the cancer incidence had been skyrocketing since the 1990s. Concerns were eventually raised about the relationship between contaminants in the region and the cancer rates.

From a public health perspective, the 1990s marked the beginning of a health crisis in Vieques. However, discourses about health did not become central to collective action until the 2000s. Why did health not become an organizing principle sooner? What kept people from connecting their health issues with their tainted landscape? I argue that a "conspiracy of invisibilities" was responsible for preempting such an understanding, particularly the interplay between hegemony, reification, and subjection in the production of colonial citizens.

The constitution of a hegemonic formation is as much about winning the hearts and minds of people with promises of future gains as it is about underplaying the potential losses of believing such promises. When what is promised overrides the possibility of any other possible path to achieve what's desired, such that the hegemonic "option" becomes common sense, people internalize consent. A hegemonic formation takes place when a political faction is capable of convincing people to tacitly agree about the supremacy of one sociopolitical arrangement over another, even when it might be potentially harmful for some. Hegemony functions without resorting to explicit forms of coercion; in fact it's about achieving consent. It operates in the realm of discourse and practice, that is, the limited repertoire of official stories that frame people's social reality and that people, in turn, use to make sense of their place in the world (Hall 1988; Laclau and Mouffe 1985; Gramsci 1978; Rattansi 1995). Singular attention to militaristic force in Vieques risks missing the equally powerful operation of various forms of hegemony—those articulations of subjugation that appear unacknowledged and unquestioned by the people. In eclipsing the existence of other possible ways of arranging social relations, hegemony depends heavily on reification—the process by which the negative aspects of a given social formation are hidden from view to stem popular protest. The politico-economic system is maintained.

It is the interplay between hegemony and reification that produces what I call "conspiracies of invisibilities." In its traditional Marxist sense, reification refers to the obfuscation of negative aspects of capital accumulation. Here I expand that meaning to include environmental and health factors. Thus conspiracies of invisibility hide the connections between the production of unhealthy environments and unhealthy bodies in the process of capital accumulation. In Vieques, as more generally in Puerto Rico, these processes support the colonial system. Specific instances of reification are fundamental to the constitution of a colonial subjectivity. Reproducing this colonial subjectivity is not just about winning people's hearts and minds but, across time, (re)producing the kinds of subjects who support the social arrangement of their own accord. As long as the different state institutions responsible for this remain within the bounds of legitimation, this type of social reproduction continues. However, when systemic contradictions emerge (as in the case of Vieques's health crises) new opportunities for counterhegemonic action become possible (Althusser 1971; Laclau and Mouffe 1985).

Biomedicine is therefore premised on reification because it undervalues the body as a trustworthy mediator of the environment. Vieques presents an extreme instance of the contradictions of a political-economic system premised upon reification, one in which the colonial body becomes the vessel for and in violent systems of accumulation. Yet the experience of disease in Vieques cannot be understood solely in biomedical terms. As Taussig (1980) explains, disease symptoms and healing technologies are not simple objective realities; they are symbols that disguise social relations, making them appear natural. In other words, Viequenses' health afflictions must be understood as the negative corporeal expression of a political-economic system that does not preoccupy itself with people's well-being. That Viequenses for so many years accepted that cancer, skin diseases, and respiratory problems, as well as other chronic diseases, were the result of "bad habits" (or that certain symptoms of ill health were "in one's head") testifies to the reificatory power of biomedicine on the island.

But like other systems of political legitimation, biomedicine relies on social relations to subject people by persuading them into internalizing an oppressive law (Taussig 1980). Reification is therefore only one part of maintaining a hegemonic formation; subjection is the other. In this framework institutional discourses and practices discipline subjects into being "good" patients and "good" workers, conforming to colonial authority and the particular worldview built around that authority.

For Viequenses the particular interconnections that produce tainted landscapes and wounded bodies have been structurally hidden by an atomistic perception of reality—that of a medical regime, a government, and etiological models on the part of the U.S. Navy that place the blame and responsibility for illness on individuals. Via self-discipline such institutional discourses and practices socialize people into accepting as natural both the social order and their place in it. Biomedicine persuades people into distrusting their senses, into distrusting their body (Amarasingham Rhodes 1990; Csordas 2002; DiGiacomo 1987; Good 1994). Once experts diagnose a disease, one's identity is reduced to it. One is rendered disabled and passive. This negation of the validity of individuals' perception and sense-making precludes them from making the phenomenological connections between environmental conditions and health or illness. In the process of becoming colonial citizens Viequenses tacitly inscribed into their flesh the wounds of the dominant politico-economic order.

Despite the powerful operation of the twin forces of reification and subjection, the explosion of health crises in Vieques did finally propel Viequenses to question the institutions in charge of framing their health afflictions in a manner that coincided with their embodied experiences. Neither persuasive institutional discourses nor institutional disciplining could deter people from beginning to interrogate the roots of their environmental and health crises. The former hegemonic discourses of disease causation were laid bare during this health crisis. Environmentally situated experiences of disease, coupled with institutional failure on the part of both the U.S. military and biomedicine on the island to produce satisfactory explanations, prompted people to unearth the hidden connections of their health crises. From this epistemological clash between two different perceptions of reality—atomistic and embodied—it became evident that people's health crises were not their fault, as many had believed, but the result of an unjust political system that allowed for the degradation of the environment and its people in Vieques. In the process of making sense of a world seriously disrupted by disease, people began to see the causal roots of their health problems. Clarifying these obscure health-environment connections was not the only thing they achieved: the very process of searching for an answer proved to be emancipatory for many, in that it forced them into a process of self-reevaluation that resulted in action. Women were in the front lines of this process.

Viequenses' lived experiences with health contribute to the anthropological literature on how, out of collectively created understandings, an oppositional subjectivity emerges. In other words, this ethnographic work addresses a question that Foucault left unanswered: What happens to the subject when the institutional power of subjection is exposed and weakened? In the context of subjection weakening through institutional legitimation crises, individuals' search for meaning becomes life-asserting in front of institutional failure. People's skepticism toward the establishment, in this case the colonial regime, and the institutional inability to give satisfactory answers opens up spaces in which people more readily negotiate and rearticulate available discursive repertoires and modes of action. In the collective process of searching for meaning, people re-create meaning, and in doing so they also rearticulate their own positioning in relation to their oppressive reality.

Dolor: Confronting Life and Death

My daughter was a juvenile diabetic since she was eleven, but she was never hospitalized for this. One day, on April 16, 1995, two days after my oldest son got married, my daughter woke up with abdominal pain. We spent the whole day at the local clinic trying to figure out what was wrong with her. At 6:00 p.m., with some labs in hand, the doctor sent us to the mainland. After taking the ferry, three hours later, we were at the pediatric doctor in [the coastal town of] Fajardo. They were also unable to diagnose her, so they referred us to the Pediatric Hospital of Centro Médico in San Juan. At 3:00 a.m. the oncologists and hematologists told me that it was not leukemia. Two days later a battery of labs proved them wrong. It was leukemia. We went to three different hospitals just to have a diagnosis. We started radiation and chemo treatment that same day. We put up a fight for two years, going to Centro Médico every two weeks. In March 1997, after quitting my job to keep her alive, she died. I was devastated. This tragedy happens too often in Vieques.

—Mónica, 2003

Like those of many other women in Vieques, Mónica's narrative underscores the fact that women, particularly mothers, constitute the front line in dealing with these horrible chronic diseases. Considering the fact that this community has the highest incidences of cancer and other chronic diseases in Puerto Rico, this is not a small challenge (Ortiz-Roque et al. 2000). At the same time what is remarkable about Mónica's experience of frustration, death, and loss is that it is not an isolated experience but a painfully rampant and unbelievably prevalent one. As Mónica points out, many other people in Vieques are experiencing similar kinds of tragedies. In fact none of the people I interviewed was exempt from having a family member or close friend affected by chronic diseases. That is, in my more than fifty in-depth interviews and countless conversations with people on the island, a story of illness or loss always emerged. Adding insult to injury, the inaccessibility of health care on the island is particularly problematic. With limited resources people have to travel to the Puerto Rican mainland for treatment. For cancer patients this is particularly traumatic: "They have to receive treatment in [mainland] Puerto Rico. How is that? They have to take the ferry before dawn. Once in Fajardo, they take a public bus to get to Centro Médico in Río Piedras [San Juan]. Then they get their radiation and chemotherapy, throw up three or four times, and catch the bus back to Fajardo. Often they don't get back on time to catch the last evening ferry. What do they do? They don't go. . . . It's terrible" (Jésica, 2003).

Inaccessibility of health care highlights the fact that, in Vieques, no aspect of people's lives escapes the experience of being sick; Jésica emphasizes the practical, economic, and social implications of having limited access to care. Women's caregiving under these already stressful circumstances is heroic for they are under the same kind of traumatic stress situation that military personnel experience in combat. That is, every day they are under constant fear for their lives. They might be the next person to fall due to another five-hundred-pound bomb missing the target or because cancer finally catches up with them, due to the military exercises and rampant pollutants. Either way the fear of falling ill is all too real, all too stressful.

As the environmental justice literature has shown (Bevington 1998; Di Chiro 1998; Epstein 1997; Mellor 1994; Moore and Head 1993; Sze 2007), and these narratives so powerfully convey, environmental devastation disproportionately affects women, for they tend to be the health care seekers and tenders of their family and community. In Vieques too women disproportionately carry the brunt of providing care for others and confronting the negative consequences of their toxic environs. Ana describes this, noting both the physical and the psychological effects of living near a military zone:

How can you explain the majority of my husband's coworkers dying from cancer? You know, if maybe one or two died from cancer, but all of them! We were traumatized because we even belong to a pro-Navy organization. We were psychologically affected, you know, not having the money for health expenses. I was sitting right there when I heard on television that it was true; people were getting sick [from the pollution] with heavy metals. I called [my husband]; I screamed, "Pepo!" Because until that moment I never thought that all our health problems, including those of our four daughters and our nine grandchildren, were results of [heavy] metals [poisoning]. (Ana, 2003)

Ana's case is particularly salient because her family depended on her husband's work for the military. Even though her husband was ill, and many of her family members were falling ill—and Ana was aware that something about this was terribly wrong—she could not believe activists' counterinstitutional model of disease causation. It was not until activists' views about disease etiology garnered mass media attention, and when a separate, institutionally sanctioned route (in this case a class action lawsuit) appeared to deal with their problem, that her views changed. In Ana's account, like those of many other women in Vieques, despite the many encounters with health care providers, they neither acknowledged nor entertained activists' explanatory model of disease causation; hence Ana's surprise at the news. However frequent these encounters with medical experts were, it seems clear that biomedical models were incapable of expanding their perspective to include social and environmental factors. Moreover these experts' etiological models reified connections that people had been educated to believe, thus keeping the colonial and military status quo in place. This is why most of the health practitioners who interacted with Viequenses were, at a discursive level, part of the conspiracy of invisibilities that maintained Vieques as a tainted landscape.

Biomedical models have become an integral part of how the people of Vieques understand not only health and disease but other realms of life and work as well. In a sense biomedicine mediates everyday life in Vieques. Vieques's health crises have forced people to inhabit the kingdom of medical institutions. As Taussig (1980) explains, the doctor-patient relationship can powerfully reinforce a culture's basic premises for patients. The anxious state of a sick person serves as an easy point of entry into the patient's psyche, thus facilitating the structuration of the patient's conventional understanding. However, whereas in most contexts chronic illness produces a "biographical disruption" that challenges people's identity in disempowering ways, confronting chronic diseases in Vieques enabled people—especially women—to rearticulate both their traditional role and their identity in surprising ways. The experiential world of disabled bodies (their own and others') enabled women in Vieques to recognize the limits of biomedicine, thus creating a legitimation crisis. Consequently women came to the forefront in challenging common biomedical roles that assign people to be passive patients or victims. People comply with institutional requirements for individual behavior and definitions of morality (good and evil) only if they understand that such requirements are perceived to be legitimate; in the case of Vieques this acceptance was beginning to wear thin.

Legitimation Crises

Social mobilization in Vieques demonstrated that the explanations offered by the U.S. Navy and governmental scientists have not satisfied the health concerns of the inhabitants of the island, bringing about legitimation crises of the state and its institutions. The contradiction between a government's responsibility for public health and the Puerto Rican government's encouragement of military practices—permitted for the sake of maintaining nonconflictive relations with the U.S. government—provided the grounds for this crisis of legitimation. In other words, those who were experiencing environmental degradation and the devastating results of military practices on their health were increasingly suspicious of claims and assurances from the authorities.

The case of Vieques has generated a great deal of debate, never seen before in Puerto Rico, with regard to whether military practices (particularly the use of heavy metals) are the cause of the health crises in the island. What's new is the widespread involvement of the public in the etiology debates; at stake is the power to define. Official governmental, military, and biomedical definitions of disease etiology, while justifying the order of things, disregard people's everyday life experiences with disease. Moreover, as feminist authors in other places have observed, expert knowledge often underplays women's knowledge about their own situation (Brown and Ferguson 1995; Di Chiro 1998; Epstein 1997; Gilbert 1994; Krause 1993). A fundamental part of coping with disease is searching for meaning (Hahn 1995; Mattingly and Garro 2000; Scheper-Hughes 1992); as we have seen, conflict arises when biomedical institutions fail to address embodied experiences. In Vieques, where there is a public health crisis and biomedical institutions are unable to provide satisfactory answers of meaning and causality, women especially become skeptical of experts and their corresponding institutions. In the narratives that follow we hear not only women's expressions of skepticism but, most important, their sharp cultural critiques of biomedical and "expert" knowledge—critiques that stem from their situated experience.

In an interview with members of La Alianza de Mujeres, a local women's coalition whose purpose was to advocate for women's health on Vieques, the following narrative, among many others, captured women's clear correlation of environmental degradation with communal disease: "The navy does a thousand scientific studies. . . . But we have it right in our sight: our own family, our own people are dealing with disease in our everyday life. This cannot be hidden. [Vieques] is too small and everybody knows each other and we know when somebody gets sick. If you go to a bigger place, maybe you could hide, but maybe not. Here we are like a big family" (Milagros, 2003). Women's emerging disease etiologic model is thus attentive to the health-environment inter-section. It is a social model rooted in women's experiences, and therefore it is informed by physically being-in-the-world. What's important about these narratives is that in confronting the health crises women developed what amounts to a bottom-up critique of the dominant way of understanding disease causality. In doing so they have reinvented their place in the world as agents of social change rather than passive victims.

Common sense tells you that if a place like Vieques has been used for testing all kinds of destructive military weapons for sixty years—weapons like uranium and napalm—and if you also see the impacted areas totally devoid of life, then you know that the navy's military practices are responsible for the pollution. We know that pollution is carried by the wind; we know that all of those particles get to our residential areas; we know that we are still breathing them. When you see that everybody getting tested has heavy metals in them, tons of heavy elements such as aluminum, uranium, and cadmium, then you know that metals are not only in the environment or in the air. These heavy metals are in people's bodies. These contaminants make your body more susceptible to illness.

When normalizing institutions fail to address people's experi-ences, spaces are opened in which inscriptions other than the institutional ones acquire greater relevance in people's articulation of their positions. In these cases the power that biomedical and sociopolitical institutions have over people to normalize certain ways of seeing and being becomes less effective. In the process of making sense of illness people start to develop collective ways of understanding the world and their place in it; in Vieques women's participation in different activist organizations made possible the rebuilding of an altered world and an altered self—a world and sense of self that was transformed by suffering and disease.

Rabia: Illness, Identity, and Collective Action

> My son's condition, the suffering, the pain, gave me the courage to act. This rage gave me more energy to put into the protests.
> —Jésica, 2003

While experiences of illness are often debilitating, sometimes the shared experience of illness can be empowering. Critical medical anthropology, political ecology, and social movement literature seldom examine this issue of sociocultural empowerment connected with disease. The emergent public health crises in Vieques, as well as people's dissatisfaction with institutional responses to their issues and experiences with disease, has forced them to develop collective ways of understanding and of acting. The collective endeavor of confronting disease has allowed women to rework not only their understandings but, most important, their very selves.

> Believe it or not, my first trip abroad was to Washington as a representative of the people of Vieques. I had never before left Vieques. That's how you can see how things changed around

here, how [Vieques's] circumstances took me to unexpected places. Having to go there and see that many people didn't even know what Vieques was, God, gave me a stronger desire to keep the struggle. I also went to Philadelphia to speak about Vieques, and guess what? I had never spoken in public before, much less in English. . . . . Circumstances force you to do the unexpected, things you didn't know you were capable of. (Mónica, 2003)

Mónica's story of politicization through suffering illustrates how Viequense women moved from a state of internalizing and accepting patriarchal roles of submission and passivity into actively challenging the political, social, and medical status quo that silenced their voices. Jésica added:

Recognizing our bodies has liberated all of us because we grow up in a culture where knowing and taking care of our bodies is not well seen. Five years ago I wouldn't have dared, but now I have to take care of myself, I have to know my body. Five years ago I wouldn't have dared to develop a girls' program on how to manage their sexuality. Now I feel the strength, the energy, the social compromise, and the support to do so. We have decided that if these girls are going to be the future of Vieques, they need to grow up healthy in physical, emotional, and spiritual terms. We are putting all of our energy so that these girls don't have to pass through what we passed through.

Within a biomedical system that denies women's embodied knowledge and that undervalues their perspectives, this reinscribing of their bodies becomes a fundamental way to engage and confront expert abstract knowledge, particularly as women are at the front lines of their community's health. Through their interactions in protests, in women's groups, in hospitals—essentially through the collective process of making sense of endemic illness—women have connected narratively "the cause and effects of their illness to their ongoing lives convert[ing] the liminality of [disease] into a social resource. In a process of inversion weakness becomes power" (Hunt 2000, 88–89). In this process of inversion women in Vieques have challenged biomedicine's distrust of their senses, and by doing so they have reaffirmed their own embodied knowledge. Women's bodies have become their center of awareness of a politicized identity and of political action.

Women challenging the status quo through their body has meant putting themselves at odds with doctors and governmental representatives, but it has also often placed them at odds with their husbands, other activist groups, and community members in general. Jésica explains:

> I have had to confront things here head on. For instance, the other day I was sharing a situation I had with a guy with Father Andrés. Father Andrés told me, "That's odd, because he didn't tell me anything about it." I told Father Andrés, "Well, you are Father Andrés, but I'm young, black, and a woman. It is okay to yell at me, but it is not so to yell at you." Of course I don't allow anybody to do that to me. In that sense, in emotional and mental health terms, I have had to work with myself. I remember this time when I had to stop, go to my place, and stay there trying to relax. I had to look for professional help, because after that incident it became harder to continue the struggle. After that it was heavy to continue. To be able to be here telling you this is not easy either. For many women it is not easy. It is not easy to deal with issues of health, participation, and many other things of which everybody has an opinion. (2003)

While women's activism is at times particularly trying, Vieques's women activists confronted adversity by building and maintaining different kinds of social networks. Part of their success can be attributed to the fact that Viequense women were the first ones to successfully articulate the U.S. Navy's offenses in terms of the (presumably apolitical) body rather than political or economic terms, focusing their organizing around health concerns. Because of the apparently nonthreatening character of health discourse (generally considered a "private" concern) and women's assumption of this discourse as a presumably natural extension of their role as caregivers within the broader cultural matrix, women were able to enlist a variety of allies to their pleas and also at times to invert the cultural expectations that frequently prevented them from connecting with one another. Paradoxically women's self-assertion within these women's groups opened the doors to their collaboration with men from the community. Jésica explains:

> We also have some male partners that openly say, "I am from La Alianza de Mujeres." When other activist groups organize something, these groups of male partners always volunteer to work with us. They say, "We are going to be with el grupo de La Alianza." In other words they feel they belong to our women's group; they support us. Even in front of the worst criticisms, they have been the first ones defending us. Of course, they always say, "[These women] know how to take care of themselves alone." But just in case, they are there to help us. (2003)

Finally, owning and asserting their situated worldview as women from Vieques, these women were able to reach beyond health and environmental concerns to share with the larger community their feminist perspectives:

[This process of liberation] has allowed me to develop a number of health projects that are going to help improve Vieques's women's health and quality of life. [This process of liberation] has allowed me to free myself of all those taboos and fears that didn't allow me before to speak of certain things. [Our alternative medicine explorations] emerged not only out of our deception by a government that does not respond [to our health issues], but it also emerged from not wanting to die, from the fact that I have to do something. It emerged out of our desire to live and from not wanting any other of our women dying. . . . Our activism [also] stems out of our desire to live in a Vieques without the navy. (Jésica, 2003)

This sense of liberation propelled women, after more than sixty years of collective actions, to take center stage in the struggle by broadening the field of what was considered action. This new gendered space and their articulation of powerful narratives of suffering, loss, and indignation allowed the introduction and validation of a new discursive language that placed women's embodied and affective experiences at the head of the social movement.

Conclusion

I have attempted to theorize how women became politically active within a toxic and health crisis context. I offered this case study as a possible bridge between the environmental justice and disability literature. Implicitly I equated women's condition of marginality (colonial, gendered, class-based, racial) with the marginality that disabled people experience within a context of ableness as social normativity. This shared condition of marginality stems from a patriarchal (also biomedical) and ableness normative paradigm that places both at the bottom of the social hierarchy.

Within toxic environments such as Vieques chronic diseases run rampant. Women disproportionately carry the burden of disease. However, conceptualizing toxic-induced chronic diseases as a burden in no way implies that people debilitated by these health conditions (the dis-abled) are also conceptualized as a burden and thus as passive recipients of power.[2] On the contrary women's activism illustrates that embodying this new altered state of being (as a dis-abled person) was necessary for political action. Dis-ability, as the literature points out, is not in the individual but in the social and spatial conditions that limit social inclusion. In theorizing the destabilizing effects that toxic environs have, mostly via health crises, on normative paradigms of subjection (gender, race, class, ableness), this research connects with the disability literature (Johnson 2011; Clare 2014). In sum, Viequense women bore the brunt of environmental problems by coping with their own afflictions and taking care of unwell family members. During a politically pivotal time in the island's history, Viequense women transformed their unenviable position on the front lines of disease into a vanguard of collective contestation (see Velez-Velez 2010; McCaffrey 2008). The women's rich oral histories showed what it was like to confront chronic diseases such as cancer in a militarized Vieques. Women conquered the public space of activism, which was a traditionally male-encoded space, to break away from passively constructed gender roles. Their everyday meaning-making struggle with disease, far from being disempowering, became the eventual catalyst for their politicization, which opened up new spaces of action and in doing so undermined the reificatory power of institutions that for too long blamed them as victims.

NOTES

1. The narratives explored in this chapter are a subset of over fifty in-depth interviews I conducted between 2001 and 2003 with Viequenses, the majority of whom were women.
2. For instance Ray and Sibara explain in the introduction to this volume: "Work in environmental justice, in both the humanities and social sciences, has made some motion in the direction of disability studies by emphasizing toxicity and 'body burdens,' but it rarely draws on the insights of disability studies scholars, who assert that disability not be understood as a 'burden.'"

REFERENCES

Althusser, Louis. 1971. Lenin and Philosophy and Other Essays. New York: Monthly Review Press.

Amarasingham Rhodes, Lorna. 1990. "Studying Biomedicine as a Cultural System." In Medical Anthropology: Contemporary Theory and Method, edited by Carolyn F. Sargent and Thomas M. Johnson, 165–80. New York: Praeger.

Baver, Sherrie L. 2006. "'Peace Is More Than the End of Bombing': The Second Stage of the Vieques Struggle." Latin American Perspectives 33: 102–15.

Bevington, Douglas. 1998. "Earth First! In Northern California: An Interview with Judi Bari." In The Struggle for Ecological Democracy: Environmental Justice Movements in the United States, edited by D. Faber, 248–71. New York: Guilford.

Braidotti, Rosi, et al. 1994. Women, the Environment and Sustainable Development: Towards a Theoretical Synthesis. London: Zed Books in association with INSTRAW.

Brown, Phil, and Faith Ferguson. 1995. "'Making a Big Stink': Women's Work, Women's Relationship and Toxic Waste Activism." Gender and Society 9, no. 2: 145–72.

Callari, Antonio, and David F. Ruccio. 1996. Postmodern Materialism and the Future of Marxist Theory: Essays in the Althusserian Tradition. Hanover NH: Wesleyan University Press.

Clare, Eli. 2014. "Meditations on Natural Worlds, Disabled Bodies, and a Politics of Cure." In Material Ecocriticism, edited by Serenella Iovino and Serpil Oppermann, 204–18. Bloomington: Indiana University Press.

Csordas, Thomas J. 2002. Body / Meaning / Healing. New York: Palgrave.

Di Chiro, Giovanna. 1998. Environmental Justice from the Grassroots: Reflections on History, Gender and Expertise. New York: Guilford Press.

DiGiacomo, Susan M. 1987. "Biomedicine as a Cultural System: An Anthropologist in the Kingdom of the Sick." In Encounters with Biomedicine: Case Studies in Medical Anthropology, edited by H. A. Bear, 315–46. New York: Gordon and Breach.

Epstein, Barbara. 1997. "The Environmental Justice/Toxic Movement: Politics of Race and Gender." Capitalism Nature Socialism 8, no. 3: 63–87.

Foucault, Michel. 1995. Discipline and Punish: The Birth of the Prison. New York: Vintage Books.

Gilbert, Alan. 1994. "Third World Cities: Poverty, Employment, Gender Roles and Environment During a Time of Restructuring." Urban Studies 31, nos. 4–5: 605–33.

Good, Byron. 1994. "The Body, Illness Experience, and the Lifeworld: A Phenomenological Account of Chronic Pain." In Medicine, Rationality, and Experience: An Anthropological Perspective, 116–34. Cambridge, UK: Cambridge University Press.

Gramsci, Antonio. 1978. Selections from the Prison Notebooks. New York: International.

Hahn, Robert A. 1995. Sickness and Healing: An Anthropological Perspective. New Haven CT: Yale University Press.

Hall, Stuart. 1988. "The Toad in the Garden: Thatcherism among the Theorists." In Marxism and the Interpretation of Culture, 58–74. Urbana: University of Illinois Press.

Harding, Sandra. 1991. Whose Science? Whose Knowledge? Thinking from Women's Lives. Ithaca NY: Cornell University Press.

Hunt, Linda. 2000. "Strategic Suffering: Illness Narratives as Social Empowerment among Mexican Cancer Patients." In Narrative and the Cultural Construction of Illness and Healing, edited by C. Mattingly and L. Garro, 88–107. Berkeley: University of California Press.

Johnson, Valerie Ann. 2011. "Bringing Together Feminist Disability Studies and Environmental Justice." Washington DC: Barbara Faye

Waxman Fiduccia Papers on Women and Girls with Disabilities and Center for Women Policy Studies.

Krause, Celene. 1993. "Women and Toxic Waste Protests: Race, Class and Gender as Resources of Resistance." Qualitative Sociology 16, no. 3: 247–62.

Laclau, Ernesto, and Chantal Mouffe. 1985. Hegemony and Socialist Strategy: Towards a Radical Democratic Politics. London: Verso.

Mansilla-Rivera, Imar, Cruz M. Nazario, Farah A. Ramírez-Marrero, and Carlos J. Crespo. 2013. "Assessing Arsenic Exposure from Consumption of Seafood from Vieques-Puerto Rico: A Pilot Biomonitoring Study Using Different Biomarkers." Archives of Environmental Contamination and Toxicology, November. Online.

Massol-Deyá, Arturo, and Elba Diaz. 2003. "Trace Elements Composition in Forage Samples from Various Anthropogenically Impacted Areas in Puerto Rico." Caribbean Journal of Science 29: 215–20.

Massol-Deyá, Arturo, and Elba Díaz de Osborne. 2013. Vieques en Crisis Ambiental: Ciencia y Ecologia. Adjuntas, Puerto Rico: Terranova Editores.

Massol-Deyá, Arturo, Dustin Pérez, Ernie Pérez, Manuel Berrios, and Elba Diaz. 2005. "Trace Elements Analysis in Forage Samples from a US Navy Bombing Range (Vieques, Puerto Rico)." International Journal of Environmental Research and Public Health 2:263–66.

Mattingly, Cheryl, and Linda C. Garro. 2000. Narrative and the Cultural Construction of Illness and Healing. Berkeley: University of California Press.

McCaffrey, Katherine T. 2002. Military Power and Popular Protest: The U.S. Navy in Vieques, Puerto Rico. New Brunswick NJ: Rutgers University Press.

———. 2008. "Security Disarmed Critical Perspectives on Gender, Because Vieques Is Our Home: Defend It!" In Security Disarmed: Critical Perspectives on Gender, Race and Militarization, 157–76. New Brunswick NJ: Rutgers University Press.

Mellor, Mary. 1994. "Building a New Vision: Feminist Green Socialism." In Toxic Struggles: The Theory and Practice of Environmental Justice, 36–46. Gabriola Island, Canada: New Society.

Merchant, Carolyn. 1995. "Gaia: Ecofeminism and the Earth." In Earthcare: Women and the Environment, 3–26. New York: Routledge.

Moore, Richard, and Louis Head. 1993. "Acknowledging the Past, Confronting the Present: Environmental Justice in the 1990s." In <u>Toxic Struggles: The Theory and Practice of Environmental Justice</u>, edited by R. Hofrichter, 118–27. Gabriola Island, Canada: New Society.

Ortiz-Roque, Carmen, José Ortiz-Roque, and Dulce Albandoz-Ortiz. 2000. "Exposición a Contaminantes y Enfermedad en Vieques: Un Trabajo en Progreso." Report. Río Piedras: Departamento de Farmacología Recinto de Ciencias de la Universidad de Puerto Rico.

Rattansi, Ali. 1995. "Just Framing: Ethnicities and Racisms in a 'Postmodern' Framework." In <u>Social Postmodernism: Beyond Identity Politics</u>, edited by L. Nichols, 250–86. Cambridge, UK: Cambridge University Press.

Scheper-Hughes, Nancy. 1992. <u>Death without Weeping: The Violence of Everyday Life in Brazil</u>. Berkeley: University of California Press.

Sze, Julie. 2007. <u>Noxious New York: The Racial Politics of Urban Health and Environmental Justice</u>. Cambridge MA: MIT Press.

Taussig, Michael. 1980. "Reification and the Consciousness of the Patient." <u>Social Science and Medicine</u> 14: 3–13.

———. 1992. "Reification and the Consciousness of the Patient." In <u>The Nervous System</u>, edited by Michael Taussig, 83–110. New York: Routledge.

Velez-Velez, Roberto. 2010. "Reflexivity in Mobilization: Gender and Memory as Cultural Features of Women's Mobilization in Vieques, 1999–2003." <u>Mobilization: An International Journal</u> 15, no. 1: 81–97.

Wargo, John. 2009. <u>Green Intelligence: Creating Environments That Protect Human Health</u>. New Haven CT: Yale University Press.

11

War Contaminants and Environmental Justice

The Case of Congenital Heart Defects in Iraq

Julie Sadler

In the twelve years since the invasion, Iraq has seen the decimation of its health care system and a marked rise in children born with congenital birth anomalies due to environmental exposure to war contaminants. These children often go without medical care and remain largely unaccounted for in both statistical and media coverage, and thus represent a disappeared, marginalized population. When these children do appear in official documentation and media coverage, they are understood as the inevitable result of an essentialized Third World violence and poverty. This narrative functions to strip these children of agency and personhood and to obscure the material production of these birth anomalies through a history of colonial violence. This colonial violence is both the outright violence of war and the slow violence of environmental destruction and economic impoverishment, which work together to create transgenerational disablement of children. Rather than being the natural consequence of Third World instability and violence, these birth anomalies are the material result of imperialist foreign policy and its attendant environmental destruction, and thus present urgent questions to our understanding of environmental justice in the context of ongoing imperialist violence.

How are environments shaped by neocolonialism, which environments are targeted, and how do places of violence become environments of violence through the ongoing environmental destruction of war? What are the long-term effects on populations and their struggles for justice? Disability politics and theory demand we take seriously the lives of those disabled by war and regard them as more than simply tragic emblems of violence. To understand these children as already dead in the context of environmental justice is to replicate the imperialist schema that disabled them in the first place. Theories of toxicity and animacy offer a way to understand the ongoing effect of neocolonialism and racism on the environments and bodies of the Iraqi people, while also opening up a space to respect and center the subjectivities and personhood of the children disabled by this violence. An understanding of toxicity and war contaminants, their role in colonization, and their participation in the production of transgenerational disablement may offer a way to reconceptualize the matrix of biopower-necropower that has shaped the emergence and persistence of birth anomalies in Iraq.

I focus on congenital heart disease (CHD) as a case study in the material and discursive production of disability in the postwar Iraqi context. The affective symbolism of the heart gestures to the social meanings of bodies and their relation to violence, a resonance that deeply informs the neocolonial discourse that surrounds NGO fundraising. There is highly developed treatment available for CHD in the Global North; this is a sharp contrast to the lack of resources that characterizes Iraq's health care system, and this difference denaturalizes the presence and so-called disease burden of CHD in Iraq.

In the United States children with congenital heart disease who are uninsured or are using Medicaid benefits frequently receive initial repairs in infancy and then go without follow-up. However, the practices of the two major congenital heart centers in Toronto regarding people with complex lesions indicate the need for yearly follow-up, especially during rapid developmental periods, with additional follow-up during periods of functional change or in pre- and postsurgery stages. In the absence of follow-up from a specialist cardiologist, people with CHD are given misinformation about their chances of survival or experience functional decline or worsening of symptoms that go untreated until they can no longer be ignored—often to the point where people are already in heart failure when they do seek treatment. This can seriously affect recovery time, time off from work or school, time off for careers, physical and emotional distress, and chances of survival. Heart failure can also lead to the need for a transplant, which comes with yet another set of financial, social, emotional, and medical challenges. Lack of access to timely and appropriate treatment creates and perpetuates functional decline, ill health, and emotional distress for people with CHD and their families.

Heart Disease and Birth Anomalies in Iraq

In a global context a lack of access to resources is complicated by not only the financial component of complex medical care but also by war, imperialism, and violence. Iraq has seen a radical increase in birth anomalies since 1991. In Basra birth anomalies increased after the 1991 Gulf War; this was linked to the use of depleted uranium in that conflict.[1] Birth anomalies jumped again in Basra in 2003, from 1.37/1,000 live births to 23/1,000.[2] There has been a similar increase recorded in Fallujah, where 15 percent of all children are born with congenital birth anomalies.[3] Many of these birth anomalies are so complex and systemic that they do not exist in the scientific literature.[4] Of the congenital birth anomalies that can be identified and medically categorized,

Fallujah has a high incidence of CHD and neural tube defects; the rate of CHD in particular far exceeds the global average.[5] It is extremely difficult to be precise about the numbers given that there is only one physician in Fallujah recording these cases; this physician has reported that she works without formal support from the government. Due to the widespread systemic problems in the Iraqi health care system, many of these children with birth anomalies never even enter the care of a physician and so remain uncounted.[6]

This rise in birth anomalies fits within a pattern of violence that has marked the country for the past thirty years. The use of chemical agents in the genocide against the Kurds in northern Iraq has been linked to the spike in CHD in particular.[7] This may give some indication as to possible causes for the birth anomalies that arose after the U.S. invasion. Currently no published information on birth anomalies in general or CHD in particular is available for northern Iraq.[8] Rather than positing single causes, which is difficult to do given the lack of information, it may be helpful to consider a web of causes and events that have created almost thirty years of violence.

The biological mechanism of the production of birth anomalies is unclear, particularly as it relates to depleted uranium. This, combined with unreliable statistics on birth anomalies in Iraq prior to the 1980s, has led some scientists to the conclusion that causality cannot be established.[9] There is some debate over consanguineous marriage as a possible root cause of heart defects in particular.[10] But these claims are specious, imperialist, and racist; they posit genetic causes ("inbreeding") over and above the extreme social and environmental factors to which the Iraqi population has been subject. A recent study on polygamous families with children with heart defects explicitly addresses consanguineous marriage through its study design. The authors strongly emphasize environmental factors and contact with "war contaminants" as likely causes of birth anomalies; they cite specifically long-term exposure rather than acute exposure as a likely cause.[11] The location and timing of these incidents point to the relationship between military action in Iraq and the continuing cost to the Iraqi people in the form of, among other things, the generational harm to children.

I am particularly concerned with the incidence of congenital heart disease in Iraq. Though it is not as dramatic as some of the birth anomalies that have been recorded in the country, it is a medically recognized diagnostic category with a significant body of research; this makes it easier to examine the difference in outcomes between North American children and those born in Iraq. Seventy years of funded medical research, specialization, and surgical development have increased the forty-year survival rate for cyanotic birth from 5 percent to 90 percent in North America.[12]

Even given the spike in congenital heart disease in Iraq, these children would not necessarily experience a serious threat to life due to the condition if they had access to timely and appropriate medical care. Children who have access to specialist care and receive appropriate surgery generally do quite well; a Toronto hospital is currently experiencing an overload of adult CHD patients because when the clinic was founded children did not survive to adulthood at the same rate they currently do.[13] The decimation of the Iraqi medical system due to sanctions and violence has created a significant backlog of children awaiting surgery or dying from lack of medical treatment for all kinds of illnesses, CHD included.[14] Structural and physical violence rather than the defects of individual bodies are what endanger the lives of these children.

The structural and physical violence in Iraq has rendered it a Third World "space of terror": a place where "the conditions of global capitalism produce spaces of extreme exploitation and oppression," which is explicitly linked to neocolonialism and colonialism and imperialist violence.[15] To call Iraq "Third World" is to bring forward the violence that has created these conditions and to denaturalize them. This violence is not only physical; it is structural as well. Prior to the invasion in 2003 by the United States and its allies, Iraq had a publicly funded health care system, but economic sanctions and physical violence have decimated that system. Reconstruction efforts are complicated by an unstable government; conflicting priorities among doctors, administrators, and UN officials; ongoing violence; and a severe shortage of health care professionals.[16] Iraq has an internally displaced population of 1.3 million people, while another 1.4 million are refugees in neighboring states.[17] The lack of a viable health care system and the displaced population are not the natural state of a savage and backward country; these conditions are the direct result of imperialist violence.

In this Third World place of terror we find Mbembe's necropolitical deathworld: "Colonies are the location par excellence where the controls and guarantees of judicial order can be suspended—the zone where the violence of the state of exception is deemed to operate in the service of 'civilization.'" The rhetoric of civilization and democratization was instrumental to the 2003 invasion of Iraq and continues to be the banner under which that intervention is legitimized in its more benevolent-seeming forms. Like Palestine in Mbembe's analysis, Iraq is ruled by "a concatenation of multiple powers: disciplinary, biopolitical, and necropolitical."[18] These powers are particularly heightened around issues of disability, illness, and access to health care.

Disabled people in the Third World are at risk of becoming invisible in global media and within their own societies through the erosion of social services; this invisibility engenders further dehumanization.[19] Within the context of heart disease in Iraq, this is evident in the relative paucity of available statistics. A lack of resources dedicated to understanding the scope of the problem leads to the illusion that the problem does not exist, creating further institutional neglect. Congenital heart disease in Iraqi children is produced by physical and environmental violence, and then rendered invisible by structural violence. In the case of CHD the lack of structural acknowledgment and support confines these children to domestic spaces invisible to social services; it also negatively affects their health outcomes. This is a population that is effectively already dead from a statistical and structural point of view.

This statistical invisibility is contrasted with a kind of hypervisibility that naturalizes these disabilities as the result of violence.[20] When birth anomalies in Iraq do enter public consciousness, they are steeped in metaphoric references, particularly with regard to congenital heart disease. CHD awareness in the Global North trades heavily on the metaphorical connotations of the heart as the seat of emotion and selfhood. In an Iraqi context this is heightened by violence while simultaneously serving to erase the roots of that violence.

Broken Hearts and Signature Wounds

The Preemptive Love Coalition (PLC) is a charity based in the United States whose stated mission is to provide "lifesaving heart surgeries for Iraqi children in pursuit of peace between communities at odds."[21] Their promotional material stresses the prevalence of congenital heart disease over and above other birth anomalies like neural tube defects, even though some regions have equal rates of both. PLC is an administrative and brokerage body that coordinates other services in Iraq and internationally to perform CHD repair and to train Iraqi doctors and nurses in those surgeries. In their promotional material they stress the action of chemical weapons deployed by Saddam Hussein against Iraqi Kurds as a possible cause of the spike in birth anomalies.[22] They neglect to mention the role of the United States in that conflict and do not address the role of the United States in decimating the Iraqi health care system through sanctions. Likewise the discussion of depleted uranium is limited to the harm caused by depleted uranium to U.S. and British soldiers in the Gulf War and the potential contribution of depleted uranium to CHD; neglected is the issue of who was bombing whom and why. It is heavily implied that the communities at odds are the Kurds and Arab Iraqis, thus furthering the imperialist fantasy of bringing democratized peace to the region through U.S. intervention. By stressing the role of Hussein's genocide and use of chemical weapons, PLC implicitly bolsters the imperialist military action that has made their presence in the region possible. Heart surgery trades on the metaphorical resonance of the heart—particularly the "broken heart" as an image of injured affect—in order to discursively create and then heal a signature wound of a specific conflict. Signature wounds are "a means through which to construct a history of armed combat that foregrounds the wounding capacities of new weapons systems and the damage they can do."[23] In the case of congenital heart disease in Iraq, the PLC emphasizes the role of depleted uranium and chemical weapons in creating CHD, particularly as they were used in the Gulf War and the Kurdish genocide. In PLC's promotional material the metaphorical associations of the broken heart are brought forward through an emphasis on social suffering in Iraq that simultaneously obscures the imperialist roots of such suffering.

Congenital heart defects become broken hearts, implying that the injury of the war is not only to bodies but also an injury of affect. Affect operates both as an emotional faculty and as "the capacity to affect and be affected,"[24] so the image of injured affect in the broken heart trope is both an image of emotional suffering and of limited efficacy, that is, disability. While the broken heart trope is common in North American CHD fundraising and patient support, here the broken heart gestures to the emotional outcomes of violence through the image of the body. These broken hearts are identified with weapons of war in their creation, while the continued distress of these children is identified with the failures of the Iraqi state to respond to them. Healing the heart defects through surgery is identified with the healing of injured affect and social suffering. The broken heart of Iraqi children is made to stand in for the broken state and is then healed through benevolent U.S. intervention.

This fantasy of healing the broken heart is not only imperialist; it is physiologically inaccurate and misleading. Congenital heart defects can be surgically ameliorated, but they cannot be eradicated. A person born with CHD will always have a heart that is defective because the defect is structural. Surgery can significantly improve health outcomes—in some cases to the point where the person with CHD will not experience what the medical professions understand to be functional or clinical limitations—but the structure of the muscle itself will always be abnormal. Improved health outcomes are highly dependent on continued, reliable, and barrier-free access to medical expertise and technology. Individual surgeries are not sufficient to produce good health outcomes for the population of Iraqi children with CHD; this is an individualized response to an illness that requires systemic reform. The signature wound and its healing obscures the material reality of violence by substituting a metaphorical healing for the actual structural reform. Disability and illness as they are produced in a Third World place of terror are thus individualized and naturalized by obscuring the role that the colonial foreign policy of the United States and its allies has played in shaping the current landscape in Iraq.[25] This movement obscures the broader dynamics of imperialism that have shaped both the violence and its aftermath in an Iraqi context by using the signature wound as an emblem of the conflict.

The construction of the signature wound also reifies the designation of Iraq as a Third World place of terror.[26] In their promotional material the Preemptive Love Coalition frames Iraqi hospitals as impoverished in staff and expertise; in particular they speak of children being "turned away" from hospitals or surgeries.[27] Absent is a consideration of the historical strength of the Iraqi medical system or of the dynamics between the U.S.-supported government and Iraqi doctors: consider the physician in Fallujah who tracks birth anomalies without support from the government. When sanctions are discussed it is as a possible culprit for the spike in CHD; the role these same sanctions have played in decimating the Iraqi medical system and its ability to respond to these children is submerged, as is the relation of imperialism and neocolonialism to the imposition of sanctions. In the Preemptive Love Coalition narrative the Third World produces broken hearts that are physiologically aberrant and emotionally injured as a consequence of its status as a place of terror. Iraq becomes essentially injurious in character, and the children born there require U.S. medical intervention before they can become potential citizens rather than statistical ciphers. The complexity of the political and economic situation in Iraq is thus disappeared, as is the role of U.S.-initiated economic and physical violence in producing both the place of terror and the current wave of disabled and ill children. In PLC's narrative children are "saved," and doctors—especially white Western expert doctors—are exalted. Medicalization combines with imperialism to dehumanize even the children who are supposedly saved. All surgeries are filmed, and the names and pictures of all children who have received services from PLC are posted on their website.[28] Some of the filmed surgeries are used as promotional videos, which reinforces the "broken heart," personal tragedy, and salvation narrative. The question of consent and coercion is profound in this situation. The disabled racialized body is on display for an implicitly white North American audience for either evaluation, in the case of medical professionals, or for emotional edification, as in the case of the potential donor. A few children are lifted out of the invisible mass of those born with birth anomalies to be given faces, names, and heart surgery—which, in the logic of the broken heart metaphor, is implicitly a reparation of injured affect. These children are not only made visible; they are discursively presented as more human because of this repaired affect. They have become recognizable individuals with normative bodily boundaries (unlike infants born with their organs external to their bodies) and repaired affect. The children marked for life through surgery become potential productive citizens under the auspices of U.S. intervention.

While this process individualizes and names these children—to the point of transgressing North American norms of medical confidentiality—it is actually a process of profound dehumanization. The aliveness of these children is acknowledged and reinforced through a medical and colonial gaze according to the priorities of the U.S. interveners. U.S. sanctions decimated the Iraqi health care system, then the use of depleted uranium and phosphorous weapons created a population in need of access to specialized medical care. Within this context the U.S. organization offering surgeries has almost complete control over who lives and who dies.

Children are evaluated for surgery based on the organization's "risk tolerance"—meaning that children who have complex heart defects requiring risky surgeries or already in heart failure (and therefore more likely to die while under the Preemptive Love Coalition's jurisdiction) are declined.[29] The children who fail the organization's test of risk tolerance are understood as being in some ways already dead. Normative citizenship is not possible for these children; surgical treatment is held to be a waste of effort and resources that could be spent on less complex or risky surgeries. These children recede back into the invisible mass of children who, statistically speaking, do not exist. The process of selecting individual children for salvific surgery while rejecting others creates potential normative citizens from those most able to be normalized while those deemed too disabled or too near death are once again excluded and disappeared. The process of marking certain people as near death or too likely to die excludes them from resources, thus producing the deaths that were already assumed. The necropolitical impulse of war to target and destroy populations allows for a more benevolent-seeming biopolitics that nonetheless continues to order the lives and deaths of Iraqis.[30]

Toxicity and War Contaminants

How do we speak of the atrocities of chemical warfare without speaking of those affected by it as if they are already dead? And equally important, how do we value the lives of children disabled by war without appearing to excuse systemic economic and physical violence? An understanding of toxicity may help to undo the knot of imperialist bio- and necropolitics.

Mel Y. Chen approaches toxicity as a space of queer productivity that troubles a biopolitical exceptionalism through the animacy of toxins.[31] Toxicity troubles the notions of object and subject, for the nonliving toxin acts on the human body in ways that trouble its designation as nonliving or lifeless. Valuing toxic subjectivities and expanding the notion of subject disrupts the idea that some lives are worthwhile and worthy of resources and others are not.

In the context of war contaminants in Iraq the toxins animated and deployed as weapons during the war were white phosphorous and depleted uranium. The U.S. military has defended its use of these weapons: white phosphorous is classed not as a chemical weapon but as an "incendiary" weapon; it was deployed against insurgents, not civilians, and was used to provide smoke cover.[32] Likewise the depleted uranium bombs deployed by the U.S. military and its allies are not classed as weapons of indiscriminate effect or as poisonous weapons, so their use is legal under international conventions of war.[33] These toxins were deployed initially as explosive and incendiary agents of war against targets identified as enemies or insurgents.

These toxins have lives beyond their initial deployment and continue to affect the population beyond their initial targets. Particles of these toxins inhabit the environment and work on the bodies of the humans (and animals) that inhabit it. War contaminants, like the domestic toxins Chen discusses, have "the capacity to poison definitively animate beings, and as such achieve [their] own animacy as an agent of harm."[34] Depleted uranium and phosphorous act on the bodies of the living in their initial deployment and secondarily on those living in the environment, as well as on those who are not yet born. The toxins act on the bodies of adults to produce future disablement in children, or they act upon the liminally alive fetus, thus further troubling the distinctions between life and nonlife.

These toxins are in some sense a material emblem of colonization, a microscopic continuance of the colonial war that writes power on the bodies of those who are not yet born. These toxins make the death world microscopic. Chen writes, "A 'normal' world order is lost when, for instance, things that can harm you are not even visible to the naked eye." Likewise a "normal" world order is uprooted in the process of creating the colonial death world. "Toxins participate vividly in the racial mattering of locations, human and nonhuman bodies, living and inert entities, and events such as disease threats."[35] War contaminants were initially animated by racist and colonial practices and policies, and their effects are used to continue to justify these policies. These toxins are instrumental to the creation and maintenance of the death world. This microscopic death world is both dependent on and gives rise to the matrix of imperialist bio- and necropower that shapes the lives and deaths of disabled and ill Iraqi children.

Chen's work is valuable for illuminating toxicity and for offering a way forward to value toxic subjectivities. The current schema values those less severely affected by toxins: children who are more likely to survive surgery and need less follow-up care. The people most disabled and threatened by the microscopic colonialism of war contaminants are further excluded from resources and from the realm of the living: "When biopolitics builds itself upon 'life' or 'death' . . . it risks missing the cosubstantiating contingencies in which not only dead have died for life, but the inanimate and animate are both subject to the biopolitical hand."[36] Taking toxic subjectivity seriously may offer a way to disrupt the biopolitics that devalues toxic bodies without occluding the colonialist violence that has produced them. Chen's toxic subjectivity is not always able to engage in normative modes of sociality, communication, or health; the toxic body is held to be less alive in a normative biopolitical scheme, even as the very fact of toxicity speaks to the murkiness of what we consider to be alive or agentive.

Congenital heart disease in Iraq is a subjectivity or bodily configuration produced by toxins. The way some Iraqi children with
CHD are valued more than others (through institutional access
to resources) is consistent with a biopolitical scheme that values
those who are deemed to be more alive, agentive, and appropriate for citizenship over those who are ill and deemed to be
closer to death and more passive. Just because these children are
ill does not mean they are necessarily less alive: Chen stresses
repeatedly that the very ill toxic subjectivity can be understood as
a subjectivity that orients itself toward other kinds of socialities.
This valuing of a life within illness resists the tendency to value
those children who can be "saved" over those who presumably
cannot.

The toxic body is a body with porous boundaries that speaks to
intercorporeality against the fantasy of self-contained wholeness.
These porous boundaries are literalized in some children, who are
born with their organs external to their body. This contravention
of normal bodily arrangements and boundaries gestures to intercorporeality; the toxic invasion alters not only national boundaries
but bodily ones. Likewise congenital heart disease is a condition
of flexible bodily boundaries, of medical technology that visual-
izes the occult workings of the body and of the literal opening of
the chest cavity. The porosity of bodily boundaries to which toxicity gestures become literalized. These bodies inspire a reflexive
looking away because they speak unnervingly to intercorporeality
and the attendant widespread implications of violence.

Talking about toxic subjectivities is a way of drawing attention
to the far-reaching issues of power and violence implicated in
the use of war contaminants without consigning those affected
by it to mere victimhood. It speaks to the value of multiple ways
of being alive; in valuing these different kinds of lives we can

question the legitimacy of the colonial biopolitical violence that shapes these lives.

The surge of birth anomalies in Iraq is not the natural consequence of Third World poverty and instability; it is not an incomprehensible horror that has grown out of the essential character of the country. Rather it is the production of a colonial set of policies and actions that began with economic sanctions and has continued through invasion and into reconstruction. Iraq has been reordered as a necropolitical colonial state, with U.S. and coalition interests first producing disability and then dictating who may have access to resources and who is excluded. War contaminants, animated by imperialism and racism, act upon the bodies of Iraqis to produce disabled toxic subjectivities and bodies. These bodies are then evaluated based on the colonial bio-necropolitical scheme that finds them wanting, and then further excluded from resources and from meaningful humanness as being too close to death. Though these subjectivities are the production of violence, valuing them as toxic subjectivities may provide a way to speak to the ongoing violence of war contaminants without consigning those affected by them to the realm of the already dead.

NOTES

1. Al-Hadithi et al., "Birth Defects in Iraq and the Plausibility of Environmental Exposure," 3.
2. Al-Sabbak et al., "Metal Contamination and the Epidemic of Congenital Birth Defects in Iraqi Cities."
3. Alaani et al., "Uranium and Other Contaminants in Hair from the Parents of Children with Congenital Defects in Fallujah, Iraq."
4. Goodman, "Ten Years Later, U.S. Has Left Iraq with Mass Displacement and Epidemic of Birth Defects, Cancers.

5. Alaani et al., "Uranium and Other Contaminants in Hair from the Parents of Children with Congenital Defects in Fallujah, Iraq."

6. Goodman, "Ten Years Later, U.S. Has Left Iraq with Mass Displacement and Epidemic of Birth Defects, Cancers."

7. Abolghasemi et al., "Childhood Physical Abnormalities Following Paternal Exposure to Sulfur Mustard Gas in Iran," 13.

8. Al-Hadithi et al., "Birth Defects in Iraq and the Plausibility of Environmental Exposure."

9. Al-Hadithi et al., "Birth Defects in Iraq and the Plausibility of Environmental Exposure."

10. Khalid et al., "Consanguineous Marriage and Congenital Heart Defects"; Nabulsi et al., "Parental Consanguinity and Congenital Heart Malformations in a Developing Country."

11. Alaani et al., "Four Polygamous Families with Congenital Birth Defects from Fallujah, Iraq," 94.

12. Moons et al., "Temporal Trends in Survival to Adulthood among Patients Born with Congenital Heart Disease from 1970 to 1992 in Belgium."

13. This information was obtained from personal communications with several staff members and from patient education presentations given by this clinic.

14. Jamail, "Iraq"; Savabieasfahani, "Epidemic of Birth Defects in Iraq and Our Duty as Public Health Researchers."

15. Erevelles, Disability and Difference in Global Contexts, 122.

16. Skelton, "Health and Health Care Decline in Iraq"; Crawford, "Civilian Death and Injury in the Iraq War"; Webster, "Roots of Iraq's Maternal and Child Health Crisis Run Deep."

17. Watson Institute, "Iraq's Population Flight."

18. Mbembe, "Necropolitics," 24, 29.

19. Erevelles, Disability and Difference in Global Contexts.

20. Erevelles, Disability and Difference in Global Contexts.

21. Preemptive Love Coalition, "Preemptive Love Coalition."

22. ICARE Charity, "Reconciliation through Healing."

23. Terry, "Significant Injury."

24. Chen, Animacies, 11.

25. Erevelles, Disability and Difference in Global Contexts.

26. Erevelles, Disability and Difference in Global Contexts.

27. Preemptive Love Coalition, "Backlog of Children Dying from Heart Defects in Iraq."
28. Preemptive Love Coalition, "About Our Kids."
29. Preemptive Love Coalition, Annual Report 2011.
30. Mbembe, "Necropolitics."
31. Chen, Animacies.
32. BBC News, "U.S. Used White Phosphorus in Iraq." White phosphorous was used in Fallujah in 2004. Given the creeping redefinition of insurgent to include any male of military age, we should perhaps be cautious about assuming that these weapons were not deployed against people who might have considered themselves civilians at the time. It is worth noting too that the U.S. government has denied the use of white phosphorous on a number of occasions and has provided a variety of explanations for its use when confronted.
33. International Criminal Tribunal for the Former Yugoslavia, "Final Report to the Prosecutor by the Committee Established to Review the NATO Bombing Campaign against the Federal Republic of Yugoslavia."
34. Chen, Animacies, 187.
35. Chen, Animacies, 203, 10.
36. Chen, Animacies, 193.

BIBLIOGRAPHY

Abolghasemi, H., M. H. Radfar, M. Rambod, P. Salehi, H. Ghofrani, M. R. Soroush, and E. J. Mills. "Childhood Physical Abnormalities Following Paternal Exposure to Sulfur Mustard Gas in Iran: A Case-Control Study." Conflict and Health 4, no. 1 (2010): 13.

Alaani, S., M. Savabieasfahani, M. Tafash, and P. Manduca. "Four Polygamous Families with Congenital Birth Defects from Fallujah, Iraq." International Journal of Environmental Research and Public Health 8, no. 1 (2010): 89–96.

Alaani, S., M. Tafash, C. Busby, M. Hamdan, and E. Blaurock-Busch. "Uranium and Other Contaminants in Hair from the Parents of Children with Congenital Defects in Fallujah, Iraq." Conflict and Health 2 (2011): 5–15.

Al-Hadithi T., et al. "Birth Defects in Iraq and the Plausibility of Environmental Exposure: A Review." Conflict and Health 6, no. 1 (2012): 3.

Al-Sabbak, M., S. Sadik Ali, O. Savabi, G. Savabi, S. Dastgiri, and M. Savabieasfahani. "Metal Contamination and the Epidemic of Congenital Birth Defects in Iraqi Cities." Bulletin of Environmental Contamination and Toxicology (2012): 1–8.

BBC News. "U.S. Used White Phosphorus in Iraq." November 16, 2005. http://news.bbc.co.uk/2/hi/middle_east/4440664.stm.

Chen, Mel Y. Animacies: Biopolitics, Racial Mattering, and Queer Affect. Durham NC: Duke University Press Books, 2012.

Crawford, Neta. "Civilian Death and Injury in the Iraq War, 2003–2013." Costs of War, March 2013. http://watson.brown.edu/costsofwar/files/cow/imce/papers/2013/Civilian%20Death%20and%20Injury%20in%20the%20Iraq%20War%2C%202003-2013.pdf.

Erevelles, Nirmala. Disability and Difference in Global Contexts: Enabling a Transformative Body Politic. New York: Palgrave Macmillan, 2011.

Goodman, Amy. "Ten Years Later, U.S. Has Left Iraq with Mass Displacement and Epidemic of Birth Defects, Cancers." Democracy Now, March 20, 2013. http://www.democracynow.org/2013/3/20/ten_years_later_us_has_left.html.

ICARE Charity. "Reconciliation through Healing: Preemptive Love." YouTube, August 21, 2011. https://www.youtube.com/watch?v=J7RxWyFBwkA.

International Criminal Tribunal for the Former Yugoslavia. "Final Report to the Prosecutor by the Committee Established to Review the NATO Bombing Campaign against the Federal Republic of Yugoslavia." 2000. http://www.icty.org/sid/10052.

Jamail, Dahr. "Iraq: War's Legacy of Cancer." Al Jazeera, March 15, 2013. http://www.aljazeera.com/indepth/features/2013/03/2013315171951838638.html.

Khalid, Y., M. Ghina, B. Fadi, C. Fadi, K. May, R. Joseph, G. Makhoul, and T. Hala. "Consanguineous Marriage and Congenital Heart Defects: A Case Control Study in the Neonatal Period." American Journal of Medical Genetics Part A 140, no. 14 (2006): 1524–30.

Mbembe, J.-A. "Necropolitics." Translated by Libby Meintjes. Public Culture 15, no. 1 (2003): 11–40.

Moons, P., L. Bovijn, W. Budts, A. Belmans, and M. Gewillig. "Temporal Trends in Survival to Adulthood among Patients Born with Congenital Heart Disease from 1970 to 1992 in Belgium: Clinical Perspective." Circulation 122, no. 22 (2010): 2264–72.

Morrison, D. R., and M. J. Casper. "Intersections of Disability Studies and Critical Trauma Studies: A Provocation." Disability Studies Quarterly 32, no. 2 (2012).

Nabulsi, M. M., H. Tamim, M. Sabbagh, M. Y. Obeid, K. A. Yunis, and F. F. Bitar. "Parental Consanguinity and Congenital Heart Malformations in a Developing Country." American Journal of Medical Genetics Part A 116, no. 4 (2001): 342–47.

Preemptive Love Coalition. "About Our Kids." Accessed April 2013. http://preemptivelove.org/about/our-kids.

———. Annual Report, 2011. Accessed February 2013. http://www.preemptivelove.org/annual_report_2011.

———. "Backlog of Children Dying from Heart Defects in Iraq." Accessed April 2013. http://www.preemptivelove.org.

———. "Preemptive Love Coalition." Accessed April 2013. http://www.preemptivelove.org.

Savabieasfahani, Mozhgan. "Epidemic of Birth Defects in Iraq and Our Duty as Public Health Researchers." Al Jazeera, March 15, 2013. http://www.aljazeera.com/indepth/opinion/2013/03/2013312175857532741.html.

Skelton, Mac. "Health and Health Care Decline in Iraq: The Example of Cancer and Oncology." Costs of War, 2013. Accessed May 2013. http://costsofwar.org/sites/default/files/Health_and_HealthCare1.pdf.

Terry, Jennifer. "Significant Injury: War, Medicine, and Empire in Claudia's Case." WSQ: Women's Studies Quarterly 37, no. 1 (2009): 200–225.

Watson Institute. "Iraq's Population Flight." Accessed June 2013. http://costsofwar.org/article/refugees-and-health.

Webster, P. C. "Roots of Iraq's Maternal and Child Health Crisis Run Deep." Lancet 381, no. 9870 (2013): 891–94.

Section 2   (RE)PRODUCING TOXICITY

12

Toxic Pregnancies

Speculative Futures, Disabling Environments, and Neoliberal Biocapital

Kelly Fritsch

News headlines sounded alarm bells in early 2014: "Scientists Name 6 More Toxins Affecting Developing Brains"; "Growing Number of Chemicals Linked with Brain Disorders in Children"; "Putting the Next Generation of Brains in Danger"; "Researchers Warn of Chemical Impacts on Children"; "Toxic Chemicals Blamed for 'Silent Pandemic' of Brain Disorders in Children"; "Doctors Fear Kids' Brain Disorders Tied to Industrial Chemicals"; "Number of Chemicals Linked to Autism and Other Disorders Doubled in Past 7 Years, Study Shows."[1] Philippe Grandjean, a professor of environmental health at the Harvard School of Public Health, and Phillip Landrigan, an American epidemiologist and pediatrician, link chemical exposure to what they call "neurodevelopmental disabilities, including autism, attention-deficit hyperactivity disorder, dyslexia, and other cognitive impairments."[2] Based on Grandjean and Landrigan's research, all these media representations warn that "we are endangering the brains of the future" by exposing fetuses to chemicals in the everyday spaces we move through and the objects we touch.[3] According to Grandjean and Landrigan's research, which these media stories were citing, these disabilities "can have severe consequences—they diminish quality of life, reduce academic achievement, and disturb behaviour, with profound consequences for the welfare and productivity of entire societies."[4]

In this chapter I examine the discourses surrounding Grandjean and Landrigan's 2006 and 2014 studies that highlight the dangers of exposing fetuses in utero to toxic chemicals that are commonly present in our environment. In examining their analysis of neurodevelopmental toxicity and the effects of such toxicity on the economy, I argue that the material-discursive production of disability is intimately linked to forms of neoliberal biocapitalism that have consequences for how we think toxicity and disability together. Grandjean and Landrigan's studies draw attention to the sorely lacking standards and laws regulating chemical production and distribution in the United States and how everyday environmental exposure to particular toxic chemicals can debilitate certain populations more than others. However, the emphasis of their studies and the resulting media attention have focused not solely on lax regulations but also on the economic impact that arguably results from toxic chemical exposure to the developing fetal brain. The production of disability as economically unviable in their studies is comprehensible precisely because of the ways disability is entrenched in neoliberal biocapitalism and speculative futurity. This speculative future demands disabled entrepreneurs to capacitate themselves and to overcome their individualized debilities so as to contribute to the present and future profitability of neoliberal biocapitalism.[5] Using Grandjean and Landrigan's studies as a starting point, I develop a critical disability studies response to the material-discursive production of toxic, disabling environments by placing disability studies in conversation with feminist science studies. As such I critique the relationship between toxic environments and neoliberal biocapitalism to attend to its forms of producing particular speculative futures of disability. In doing so I emphasize the importance of reproducing disabled lives—future lives—worth living while still critiquing neoliberal economies that produce disability.

The Silent Neurotoxic Pandemic

Enacted in 1976 the U.S. Toxic Substances Control Act (TSCA) regulates the introduction of new or already existing chemicals and mandates the Environmental Protection Agency (EPA) to protect the public from "unreasonable risk of injury to health or the environment."[6] The TSCA was formed to oversee the creation of a list of safe and approved chemicals and to regulate the use of any chemicals determined to be harmful by limiting or banning their use in products for commercial or public consumption. However, the TSCA's effectiveness in creating safe environments remains questionable. Indeed because some sixty-two thousand chemicals in use prior to the TSCA have never been systemically tested by the EPA but were grandfathered in as "safe," fewer than 20 percent of the eighty-four thousand chemicals registered with the EPA by 2008 have had any substantial safety testing.[7]

In 2006 Grandjean and Landrigan published a review in the Lancet calling for new precautionary approaches to be taken in recognition of the dangers of exposing untested chemicals to "the unique vulnerability of the developing brain."[8] Their study compiled lists of industrial chemicals that are known to cause neurotoxic effects in humans by drawing on information from the hazardous substances databank of the U.S. National Library of Medicine, fact sheets created by the U.S. Agency for Toxic Substances and Disease Registry, and information provided by the EPA. With a list of 202 known neurotoxic substances, the authors searched a number of databases for these chemicals, identifying all available published data in English. In reviewing and collating the publicly available data and literature on the human neurotoxicity of industrial chemicals, the authors characterize the ways in which the developing nervous system of the fetus is particularly vulnerable to chemical toxicity, highlighting a number of substances that could have detrimental effects on fetal and early childhood neurological development that warrant further study. These include lead, methylmercury, arsenic, polychlorinated biphenyls, solvents, pesticides, manganese, fluoride, and perchlorate.

Grandjean and Landrigan note that while most chemical toxicity testing is done in relation to adult humans, neurotoxicity is a much greater risk for the developing brain. This susceptibility stems from the fact that during pregnancy the brain of a fetus expands from a single strip of cells into a complex organ consisting of billions of highly interconnected specialized cells. For the brain to optimally develop, neurons must move precisely along pathways to establish connections and communication with other cells within "a tightly controlled time frame" and within "the correct sequence." As such, "windows of unique susceptibility to toxic interference arise that have no counterpart in the mature brain, or in any other organ. If a developmental process in the brain is halted or inhibited, there is little potential for later repair, and the consequences can therefore be permanent."[9]

The authors found that while the placenta acts as a protective barrier against some chemical exposure, "many metals easily cross the placenta, and the mercury concentration in umbilical cord blood can be substantially higher than in maternal blood." Further, "the blood-brain barrier, which protects the adult brain from many toxic chemicals, is not completely formed until about 6 months after birth." Because the brain continues to grow into early childhood, Grandjean and Landrigan conclude that the "susceptibility of infants and children to industrial chemicals is further enhanced by their increased exposures, augmented absorption rates, and diminished ability to detoxify many exogenous compounds, relative to that of adults."[10]

With these toxins already present in our environment, the problem is not that the effects of exposure are not felt but that these environmental pollutants can exert a range of adverse effects that are not usually tracked by doctors and other officials. Referred to as "subclinical toxicity," the effects of chemical toxicity are often not made readily apparent through a standard medical examination.

The concept of subclinical toxicity emerged from research showing that children exposed to lead could have significant reductions in intelligence levels and changes in their behavior "even in the absence of clinically visible symptoms of lead toxicity." Grandjean and Landrigan warn that "there is a dose-dependent continuum of toxic effects, in which clinically obvious effects have subclinical counterparts," leading to a "silent pandemic" of neurotoxicity that is "not apparent from standard health statistics." Global health statistics do not reflect actual exposure levels because the effects of exposure are often not obvious or cannot be clearly linked to a particular toxin. This "silent pandemic" might be responsible for "impaired brain development in millions of children worldwide."[11]

The authors conclude that testing protocols for potentially toxic chemicals need to be expanded to include examination of neurobehavioral functions affecting children. Present test protocols rely mainly on more obvious physical attributes, such as brain weight and general body formation. The authors argue that the lack of long-term research done on many chemicals significantly puts fetal and postnatal brain development at risk, and they suggest that the number of chemicals that could cause neurotoxicity "probably exceeds 1000, which is far more than the estimated 200 that have caused documented human neurotoxicity." However, without systematic testing "the true extent of the neurotoxic potential of industrial chemicals is unknown. . . . The few substances proven to be toxic to human neurodevelopment should therefore be viewed as the tip of a very large iceberg."[12]

In 2014 Grandjean and Landrigan released a follow-up to their 2006 review, noting that since 2006 further evidence had given credence to their claims that industrial chemicals contribute to "the global, silent pandemic of neurodevelopmental toxicity." Updating the list of recognized human neurotoxins and increasing the number of such chemicals from 202 to 214, their 2014 study details the ways exposure to toxins like lead, tetrachloroethylene, and phthalates can lead to IQ deficits, reduced school performance, delinquent behavior later in life, deficient neurological function, increased risk of psychiatric diagnoses, shortened attention span, and impaired social interactions. Grandjean and Landrigan argue that more than two hundred foreign chemicals have been detected in umbilical cord blood and that many environmental chemicals are transferred to infants through human breast milk. Throughout their review they cite evidence that lead exposure in early childhood reduces school performance and increases delinquent behavior; that prenatal and early postnatal exposure to arsenic is associated with cognitive deficits that are apparent at school age and can lead to a higher risk of neurological disease during adult life; that exposure to manganese reduces schoolchildren's mathematics scores, diminishes intellectual function, reduces olfactory function, impairs motor skills, and increases hyperactivity; that maternal occupational solvent exposure during pregnancy can be linked to increased risks for hyperactivity and aggressive behavior; that prenatal and early childhood exposure to the solvent tetrachloroethylene (also called perchloroethylene) in drinking water increases the risk of psychiatric diagnoses; that prenatal exposure to phthalates shortens attention span and impairs social interactions, particularly in boys; and that both exposure to air pollution and phthalates is linked to behaviors that resemble components of autism spectrum disorder. They conclude, "Industrial chemicals known or suspected to be neurotoxic to adults are also likely to present risks to the developing brain."[13] As Grandjean summed it up for a CNN reporter, "We are putting the next generation of brains in danger."[14]

Within days of publishing their 2014 review in the Lancet news headlines created a stir among other scientists, the EPA, and among families with disabled children. Mothers with disabled children wondered in blog posts and in comments following online news stories if they were to blame for their child's condition; others called for increased institutional accountability or emphasized the importance of eating organic foods. The attention garnered by Grandjean and Landrigan's studies tapped into cultural preoccupations with problematizing where disability originates and how to stop its reproduction, which is deeply embedded in notions of speculative futurity underwritten by neoliberal political economy and governance.

That is, not only do Grandjean and Landrigan believe that the next generation of brains is at risk of becoming disabled as a result of inadequate testing and regulation, but they also emphasize that neurodevelopmental disabilities have deep and dire economic consequences. While their 2006 review made some reference to the economic impact of this "silent pandemic," their 2014 review specifically calls attention to and emphasizes the economic impact of neurotoxic disability. As I will argue, the invisible nature of these chemical risks are embedded in the emergence of neoliberal biocapitalism and are both biological and economic, marking the present and the speculative future. This has some troubling consequences for how ableism and environmental activism come together against disability, particularly when disability is framed as an individual health problem resulting from a toxic environment.

Sounding the Alarm Bells

Grandjean and Landrigan's 2006 and 2014 reviews draw attention to the sorely lacking standards and laws regulating chemical production and distribution in the United States and how everyday environmental exposure to particular toxic chemicals can affect fetal and postnatal neurodevelopment. However, the studies and resulting media attention have focused not solely on lax regulations but also on the economic impact toxic chemicals have on the developing fetal brain. Rather than marking how exposure to toxins can result in changes in IQ or modes of social interaction that we are collectively responsible for engaging, the issue becomes what kind of "human capital" is being reproduced with fetal exposure to toxic chemicals.

For example, in their 2006 study Grandjean and Landrigan explain that nearly all children born in industrialized countries between 1960 and 1980 were exposed to petrol containing high levels of lead. During this period the aggregate number of children at risk of exposure to airborne lead was about 100 million, and such exposure "could have reduced the number of children with far above average intelligence (IQ scores above 130 points) by over 50 percent and might likewise have increased the number with IQ scores below 70.95," resulting in "diminished economic productivity" with costs ranging from US$110 billion to $319 billion in each year's birth cohort. They further argue that the contemporary costs of lead poisoning "are estimated to be $43 billion in each birth cohort in the USA, whereas the costs of prenatal methylmercury toxicity are estimated to amount to $8.7 billion yearly."[15] In their 2014 review Grandjean and Landrigan cite evidence linking average national IQ scores with gross domestic product (GDP), a correlation "that might be causal in both directions": "Poverty can cause low IQ, but the opposite is also true. In view of the widespread exposures to lead, pesticides, and other neurotoxicants in developing countries, where chemical controls might be ineffective compared with those in more developed countries, developmental exposures to industrial chemicals could contribute substantially to the recorded correlation between IQ and GDP."[16]

Grandjean and Landrigan's estimate that each IQ point lost due to exposure or other causes decreases average lifetime earnings capacity by about $18,000 is consistent with figures presented by other researchers.[17] For example, in a 2012 study David Bellinger determined that Americans have collectively forfeited forty-one million IQ points as a result of exposure to lead, mercury, and organophosphate pesticides. The economist Elise Gould argues that a loss of one IQ point corresponds to a loss of $17,815 in lifetime earnings. Based on this figure "the combined current levels of pesticides, mercury, and lead cause IQ losses amounting to around $120 billion annually—or about three percent of the annual budget of the U.S. government."[18] Grandjean and Landrigan note, "Since IQ losses represent only one aspect of developmental neurotoxicity, the total costs are surely even higher" because the treatment of the various conditions arising from neurodevelopmental toxicity "is difficult, and the disabilities they cause can be permanent; they are therefore very costly to families and to society."[19]

The future painted by Grandjean and Landrigan gets even bleaker. The costs to "families and to society" relate to "antisocial behaviour, criminal behaviour, violence, and substance abuse that seem to result from early-life exposures to some neurotoxic chemicals." This can "result in increased needs for special educational services, institutionalisation, and even incarceration." Grandjean and Landrigan posit that phasing out or banning particular toxic chemicals can reduce these costs; they point out that the phasing-out of lead additives in petrol in the United States "generated an economic benefit of $200 billion in each annual birth cohort since 1980, an aggregate benefit in the past 30 years of over $3 trillion," figures that do not even take into account the economic benefits resulting from the "prevention of degenerative brain disorders," which "could be very substantial."[20] The benefit of preventing disability is thus substantial: not only does healthy brain development mean a better economy, but it also points to a speculative future of brain cells that are economically optimized. The problem, then, as marked by Grandjean, Landrigan, and the resultant media stir, is not just that disability is an abnormality that should be prevented but also that all forms of embodiment are entrenched in neoliberal speculative futures in dangerous ways.

Neoliberal Biocapitalism and Toxic Futures

Grandjean and Landrigan's studies encourage a neoliberal biocapitalist logic that economizes life, individualizes disability, and promotes a speculative futurity that does not include disability, or can include disability only if disability can be capacitated or enhanced.

Biocapitalism and the economization of life marks a way of talking about more and less valuable lives in economic terms rather than solely in biological terms. The economic viability of disability in Landrigan and Grandjean's studies is comprehensible precisely because of the ways disability has been entrenched in neoliberal biocapitalism. Neoliberalism as a social and economic reorganization of capitalism and governance intervenes extensively and invasively in every area of social life, including life itself, or what Michelle Murphy terms "the economization of life," which centers on the profitability of future-oriented human biocapital. Neoliberalism is the economization of life such that the future of life is intimately tied to profitability and productivity. Life is made to live—have a future—if it is profitable, while unprofitable life has no future and is made to wither. Neoliberal biocapitalism, in its orientation to multiplicity and differentiation, seizes on the economization of life to govern all forms of living "for the sake of fostering economic development and enhancing national GDP."[21] As such, capitalism becomes neoliberal biocapitalism, which has particular consequences for how we critically pair disability and toxicity together.

Murphy argues that neoliberal notions of "human capital" depend upon "the embodied capacities of a person that can produce future economic benefits for that person, her employer, and even her national economy."[22] Murphy's work on the economization of life argues that as neoliberalism developed throughout the mid- to late twentieth century it became increasingly common to render and govern lives in purely economic terms (e.g., as more or less valuable) rather than solely in biological terms. In the economization of life, normal and abnormal biology are less important than how different forms of life can be made profitable.

In capitalizing on the life of the nation neoliberalism imposes "not so much the generalized commodification of daily life . . . as its financialization." While Keynesian economic approaches attempt to "safeguard the productive economy against the fluctuations of financial capital, neoliberalism installs speculation at the very core of production."[23] Murphy, drawing on Foucault's formula of the racial state, notes that practices of population control have been tied to GDP and GDP per capita, resulting in a "eugenic necropolitics" that "declared that some must die so that others may live more healthfully . . . some must not be born so that future others might live more abundantly."[24]

While embodying "human capital" means mitigating any risks to our embodied capacities as a population, neoliberalism is a system of individualization that "'privatizes' the risks and capacities of populations onto individuals, encouraging them to take charge of their own exposure to risk or opportunity in relative isolation or independence." Laura Hengehold explains, "The privatization or individualization of risk was a change in governmental technique, implemented by cutting back on many of the social insurance programs and legal protection programs of the welfare state. It was designed to extract a little more profit and self-care from citizens' embodied subjectivity, and to reduce the state's obligations to mediate between the rich and poor. But it did so by moralizing the act of work, by valorizing entrepreneurial risk-taking when employment was lacking, and by evaluating communities and affinities based on how well they promoted such activity."[25] As quality of life measures, selective abortion, prenatal screening, and other invasive reproductive medical practices highlight, in the contemporary economic and social moment the economic devaluation of a disabled life transforms it into a less viable life and the source of preventable economic costs in the future.

However, individual risk is not limited to the individual but to the future life that individual produces or has the potential to produce. Economization affects the present, but it is also speculative: embodiment becomes a value that is future-oriented. As Hengehold notes, the rise of neoliberal governmentality encourages competitive behavior and gives individuals the responsibility "for preventing or surmounting risks."[26] Furthermore, as Murphy argues, such risks are not limited to one generation, as research looks at the way exposure to chemicals can affect the future reproductive capacities of fetuses. Specifically Murphy notes that research done on pregnant mice exposed to the estrogenic chemical bisphenol A "has found that the significant effects occur not so much for the fetus in utero, but for the eggs being formed inside that fetus, and hence effects are manifest for the potential grandchildren."[27] This kind of research precisely marks the ways economization affects the present and also creates future-oriented speculative value.

Part of this economization of life is a result of the clinical gaze being supplanted by the molecular gaze, so much so that many living in neoliberal economies have come to experience themselves and their individualized risks in highly profitable biomedical terms. This is reflected in Grandjean and Landrigan's message across various media interviews encouraging pregnant women to "eat organic," to remove wall-to-wall carpeting which can trap chemicals, and to ensure that grass and sports fields where children play have not been sprayed with pesticides.[28]

With normalizing discourses representing disability as the failure of the body to meet some normative standards, toxicity acts as a potentially polluting element that must be prevented, fixed, eliminated, tolerated, or overcome, all of which are costly. The speculative futurity ingrained within neoliberal biocapitalism emphasizes hopeful progress narratives, mobilized in the originating moment of bodily failing (be it by accident, illness, or, increasingly, in probing human genetics), in order to facilitate progress (optimism for cure, or miraculous medical intervention as the solution to the problematic deficient body, finding ways to integrate disabled bodies into the economy).[29] Normative discourses of disability have not disappeared; people still want "a healthy baby" to such an extent that disability deeply disturbs this desire. There is an important relationship between the desire for a healthy baby and health cast as an economic argument. However, there are further tensions in that disabled bodies can also be a source of revenue and a site of investment. As opposed to seeing disability exclusively as the basis for exclusion and disabled bodies as objects to be normalized, Jasbir Puar has come to question how economies of disability that capacitate some disabled bodies while leaving other unproductive disabled lives to wither produce differential forms of disability in neoliberal economies.[30] The silent pandemic of toxic exposure–related disabilities is not outside of this economy.

This is because, while Grandjean and Landrigan warn of the costs associated with toxic exposure–related disabilities, these expenses are also key to economic profitability. This is to say, disability as an expense is also key to the functioning of the neoliberal biocapitalist economy. The question of human capital is a question of how individualized entrepreneurs can be capacitated or debilitated or made to overcome their debilities so as to contribute to the profitability of neoliberal biocapital. As disabled life has become economized, the biological difference of impairment has come to matter less in some cases than the potential of making disabled bodies productive through therapies, drug regimens, and assistive devices, and thus profitable for private companies developing drugs and producing body-modifying equipment. Joseph Dumit turns to this in his review of the pharmaceuticalization of American life as companies capitalize on new cultural health paradigms that mark our everyday lives as risky and bodies as inherently ill and in need of chronic treatment, through continual growth in disease categories and risk factors that can be met with medications. Dumit remarks, "Health is not simply a cost to the nation to be reduced; contradictorily, it is also a market to be grown." Grandjean and Landrigan's "silent pandemic" of "subclinical toxicity" marks what Dumit has described as "a new mass health model in which you often have no experience of being ill and no symptoms your doctor can detect," where "the facts imply that we are not doing enough screening and treating."[31]

Disability is not just about being abnormal or embodying an absolutely oppressed identity; it is also about charting the gradations of debility and capacity that are written through, across, within, and between all bodies in neoliberal biocapitalism. This is made clear when considering the ways disability intersects with other marginalized and marked populations. Importantly many marginalized populations have long felt the gradations of debility and capacity that underwrite neoliberal biocapitalism and toxicity. Mel Chen, for example, states that black bodies in America have always already been presented as "mentally deficient, impulsive and spastic." But, as Chen points out, studies similar to Grandjean and Landrigan's resonate so strongly with the public not because their studies challenge systems that reinforce structural environmental racism but rather because present and future generations of white children are at risk. Grandjean and Landrigan's studies break down the barriers that assume certain populations are always already toxic while others are "safe" and draw attention to the fact that there is no absolutely safe toxic-free zone for anyone. This is to say, while black children are "assumed to be toxic," the threat of toxic exposure to "white children is not only that they risk becoming dull, or cognitively defective, but also that they lose their class-elaborated white racial cerebrality and become suited to living in the ghettos." As environmental hazards "encroach on zones of privilege," marking the ways disability is differentially capacitated and debilitated becomes pressing for how to respond to the differential ableism and racism of toxicity as it is embedded in transnational neoliberal biocapital. Chen writes:

There are those who find themselves on the underside of industrial "development"—women hand-painting vaporous toys by the hundreds daily without protection; agricultural workers with little access to health care picking fruit in a cloud of pesticides, methane, and fertilizer that is breathable only in a strictly mechanical sense; people living adjacent to pollution-spewing factories or downwind of a refinery installed by a distant neo-colonial metropolis, or in the abjected periphery of a gentrified urban "center"; those living in walls fortified with lead that peel inward in a false embrace; domestic workers laboring in toxic conditions, taking into their bodies what their better-vested employers can then avoid.[32]

While these chemicals continue to circulate and affect populations unevenly, both of Grandjean and Landrigan's reviews seek to show that "better-vested employers" also cannot avoid toxicity. As with disability, toxicity is not to be found elsewhere, whether that be in black bodies or the bodies of farm workers or those working in factories. Toxicity, like disability, is not contained in individually bounded bodies; it circulates, altering the life chances of future generations, as Murphy points to in her look at bisphenol A. This circulation is entrenched in social, political, economic, and environmental regulations and policies. In the next section I grapple with the circulation of toxicity and disability outside of the individualized lens provided by neoliberal biocapitalism. While Landrigan and Grandjean's study provides a clear example of the ways in which disability cannot be separated from, and indeed has emerged through, neoliberal biocapitalism, I push against this individualized accounting.

Toxic Circulations and Desirable Disabilities

Chen poignantly remarks, "Toxins are not so very containable or quarantinable; they are better thought of as conditions with effects, bringing their own affects and animacies to bear on lives and nonlives."[33] Toxins "as conditions with effects" mark the environment not just as the background but as what Stacy Alaimo describes as "always as close as one's own skin—perhaps even closer." The environment is not out there; it "is the very substance of ourselves," making both disability and health not a static status that one is or isn't but rather a relation with effects.[34]

The point is that if toxins, health, and disability are deeply embedded in the environment that is social, economic, cultural, and political, then what we are left to grapple with is how to not simply reduce toxic exposures to a "natural" healthfulness gone astray, which reaffirms what Eliza Chandler calls "an understanding of disability as individually located, with a static, singular meaning as a problem in need of a solution."[35] Another way of suggesting this circulation of toxins and disability is put forward by Eula Biss: "If we do not yet know exactly what the presence of a vast range of chemicals in umbilical cord blood and breast milk might mean for the future of our children's health, we do at least know that we are no cleaner, even at birth, than our environment at large. We are all already polluted. We have more microorganisms in our guts than we have cells in our bodies—we are crawling with bacteria and we are full of chemicals. We are, in other words, continuous with everything here on earth. Including, and especially, each other."[36] Indeed if toxins and disability are not individual health problems of bodies or environments gone astray but rather shared continuities of each other—what I have elsewhere referred to as intracorporeal emergences—then these relations with effects can be held accountable to their differential, multiple, and changing sites of emergence.[37]

This is to agree with Grandjean and Landrigan in their desire for more intensive chemical regulation and stricter systematic long-term testing that takes into account the effects of chemicals on adults and also on developing life forms, both human and nonhuman. While I am in favor of increased and stronger regulation, I also want to be able to desire disability differently, to open up desire for precisely what disability disrupts, marking the particular ways in which disability is both capacitated and debilitated at once and multiply across neoliberal biocapitalism. The production of disability as an abnormality and as economically unviable and unlivable must be held to account in our positing of futures yet to come. Toxins and disability are all around us and in us and of us, and we of them. If problems get the solutions they deserve, then the problem is not toxicity or disability but rather our continued emphasis on disability as an individually economically quantifiable toxic condition. Can we desire our animate and inanimate lives and nonlives of our toxic environmentally situated selves in a way that takes seriously regimes of capacitation and debilitation that unevenly affect populations, species, and affects? To put it another way: the challenge is to speculate on different kinds of futures that welcome the black baby, the autistic baby, and the insect with three legs as a reflection of our shared and circulating toxic and disabled world, all the while working to undo the very logics of neoliberal biocapitalism that are deeply invested in the economization of life.

NOTES

1. Each of these articles can be found in the bibliography.
2. Grandjean and Landrigan, "Neurobehavioural Effects of Developmental Toxicity," 330.
3. Gordon, "Doctors Fear Kids' Brain Disorders Tied to Industrial Chemicals."
4. Grandjean and Landrigan "Neurobehavioural Effects of Developmental Toxicity," 330.
5. Fritsch, "Gradations of Debility and Capacity."
6. Schierow, "The Toxic Substances Control Act (TSCA)."

7. Grandjean and Landrigan. "Developmental Neurotoxicity of Industrial Chemicals"; Hamblin, "The Toxins That Threaten Our Brains"; Schierow, "The Toxic Substances Control Act (TSCA)."
8. Grandjean and Landrigan, "Developmental Neurotoxicity of Industrial Chemicals," 2167.
9. Grandjean and Landrigan, "Developmental Neurotoxicity of Industrial Chemicals," 2167–68.
10. Grandjean and Landrigan, "Developmental Neurotoxicity of Industrial Chemicals," 2168.
11. Grandjean and Landrigan, "Developmental Neurotoxicity of Industrial Chemicals," 2174.
12. Grandjean and Landrigan, "Developmental Neurotoxicity of Industrial Chemicals," 2175.
13. Grandjean and Landrigan, "Neurobehavioural Effects of Developmental Toxicity," 330, 331–33.
14. Young, "Putting the Next Generation of Brains in Danger."
15. Grandjean and Landrigan, "Developmental Neurotoxicity of Industrial Chemicals," 2167, 2174.
16. Grandjean and Landrigan, "Neurobehavioural Effects of Developmental Toxicity," 334.
17. Grandjean and Landrigan, "Neurobehavioural Effects of Developmental Toxicity," 334.
18. Hamblin, "The Toxins That Threaten Our Brains."
19. Grandjean and Landrigan, "Neurobehavioural Effects of Developmental Toxicity," 334; Grandjean and Landrigan, "Developmental Neurotoxicity of Industrial Chemicals," 2167.
20. Grandjean and Landrigan, "Neurobehavioural Effects of Developmental Toxicity," 334, 335.
21. Murphy, "Distributed Reproduction," 29.
22. Murphy, "The Girl."
23. Cooper, Life as Surplus, 10.
24. Murphy, "Distributed Reproduction," 30.
25. Hengehold, The Body Problematic, 16, 274.
26. Hengehold, The Body Problematic, 13.
27. Murphy, "Distributed Reproduction," 33–34.

28. Weintraub, "Researchers Warn of Chemical Impacts on Children"; Hamblin, "The Toxins That Threaten Our Brains"; Woerner, "Number of Chemicals Linked to Autism and Other Disorders Doubled in the Past 7 Years, Study Shows."
29. Fritsch, "Gradations of Debility and Capacity."
30. Puar, "Coda."
31. Dumit, Drugs for Life, 8, 9.
32. Chen, "Toxic Animacies, Inanimate Affections," 270–71, 272, 276.
33. Chen, "Toxic Animacies, Inanimate Affections," 281–82.
34. Alaimo, Bodily Natures, 2, 4.
35. Chandler, "Mapping Difference," 49.
36. Biss, On Immunity, 76.
37. Fritsch, "Desiring Disability Differently."

BIBLIOGRAPHY

Alaimo, Stacy. Bodily Natures: Science, Environment, and the Material Self. Bloomington: Indiana University Press, 2010.
Berman, Jessica. "Toxic Chemicals Blamed for 'Silent Pandemic' of Brain Disorders in Children." Voice of America, February 15, 2014. http://www.voanews.com/content/toxic-chemicals-blamed-for-silent-pandemic-of-brain-disorders-in-children/1852000.html.
Biss, Eula. On Immunity: An Inoculation. Minneapolis: Greywolf Press, 2014.
Chandler, Eliza. "Mapping Difference: Critical Connections between Crip and Diaspora Communities." Critical Disability Discourse 5 (2013): 39–66.
Chen, Mel Y. "Toxic Animacies, Inanimate Affections." GLQ: A Journal of Lesbian and Gay Studies 17, no. 2 (2011): 265–86.
Cooper, Melinda. Life as Surplus: Biotechnology and Capitalism in the Neoliberal Era. Seattle: University of Washington Press, 2008.
Dumit, Joseph. Drugs for Life: How Pharmaceutical Companies Define Our Health. Durham NC: Duke University Press, 2012.
Fritsch, Kelly. "Desiring Disability Differently: Neoliberalism, Heterotopic Imagination and Intracorporeal Reconfigurations." Foucault Studies 19 (2015): 43–66.

————. "Gradations of Debility and Capacity: Biocapitalism and the Neo-liberalization of Disability Relations." Canadian Journal of Disability Studies 4, no. 2 (2015): 12–48.

Gordon, Andrea. "Doctors Fear Kids' Brain Disorders Tied to Industrial Chemicals." Toronto Star, February 14, 2014. http://www.thestar.com/life/2014/02/14/doctors_fear_kids_brain_disorders_tied_to_industrial_chemicals.html.

Grandjean, Philippe, and Philip J. Landrigan. "Developmental Neurotoxicity of Industrial Chemicals." Lancet 368 (December 2006): 2167–78.

Grandjean, Philippe, and Philip J. Landrigan. "Neurobehavioural Effects of Developmental Toxicity." Lancet Neurology 13 (February 10, 2014): 330–38.

Hamblin, James. "The Toxins That Threaten Our Brains." Atlantic, March 18, 2014. http://www.theatlantic.com/features/archive/2014/03/the-toxins-that-threaten-our-brains/284466/.

Harvard School of Public Health. "Growing Number of Chemicals Linked with Brain Disorders in Children." February 14, 2014. http://www.hsph.harvard.edu/news/press-releases/chemicals-linked-with-brain-disorders-in-children/.

Hengehold, Laura. The Body Problematic: Political Imagination in Kant and Foucault. State College: Pennsylvania State University Press, 2007.

Murphy, Michelle. "Distributed Reproduction." In Corpus: Bodies of Knowledge, edited by Paisley Currah and Monica Casper, 21–38. New York: Palgrave Macmillan, 2011.

————. "The Girl: Mergers of Feminism and Finance in Neoliberal Times." Scholar and Feminist Online 11, no. 2 (2013). http://sfonline.barnard.edu/gender-justice-and-neoliberal-transformations/the-girl-mergers-of-feminism-and-finance-in-neoliberal-times/.

Puar, Jasbir. "Coda: The Cost of Getting Better. Suicide, Sensation, Switch-points." GLQ 18, no. 1 (2012): 149–58.

Ricks, Delthia. "Scientists Name 6 More Toxins Affecting Developing Brains." Newsday, February 14, 2014. http://www.newsday.com/news/health/scientists-name-6-more-toxins-affecting-developing-brains-1.7084963.

Schierow, Linda-Jo. "The Toxic Substances Control Act (TSCA): Implementation and New Challenges." Congressional Research Service Report for Congress, July 28, 2009. https://www.acs.org/content/dam/acsorg/policy/acsonthehill/briefings/toxicitytesting/crs-rl34118.pdf.

Weintraub, Karen. "Researchers Warn of Chemical Impacts on Children." USA Today, February 14, 2014. http://www.usatoday.com/story/news/nation/2014/02/14/chemicals-adhd-autism/5494649/.

Woerner, Amanda. "Number of Chemicals Linked to Autism and Other Disorders Doubled in the Past 7 Years, Study Shows." Fox News, February 15, 2014. http://www.foxnews.com/health/2014/02/15/number-chemicals-linked-to-autism-and-other-disorders-doubled-in-past-7-years/.

Young, Saundra. "Putting the Next Generation of Brains in Danger." CNN, February 17, 2014. http://www.cnn.com/2014/02/14/health/chemicals-children-brains/.

13

"That Night"

Seeing Bhopal through the Lens of Disability and Environmental Justice Studies

Anita Mannur

The struggle of man against power is the struggle
of memory against forgetting.

—Milan Kundera, The Book of Laughter and Forgetting

In her painting Bhopal Looking Back the Indian American artist Chitra Ganesh presents a group of five children clad in mourning white and colorful clothing. They each meet the viewer's gaze and their unsmiling faces implore the viewer to look at them. In the foreground is a young girl wearing a long-sleeved red and white dress. Her hair, swept up into pigtails with colorful baubles, bespeaks her youth. And yet in a jarring contrast her unsmiling visage, rendered in color, contrasts with what is in her hands. She holds a copy of the iconic photograph taken in 1984 by Pablo Bartholomew. Titled Bhopal Gas Disaster Girl, Bartholomew's color photograph, taken in the immediate aftermath of the Bhopal disaster, is remarkably similar to Raghu Rai's black-and-white photograph Burial of an Unknown Child. Both photographs sent shock waves across the world for their stark and unadorned simplicity that also horrified many. Of the thousands who died that day in 1984, both photographers were drawn to a single child. In an interview Rai notes that he was drawn to a child whose blinded eyes, as the journalist Elizabeth Day puts it, were "staring blankly out of the rubble." The strange beauty of Rai's piece speaks to the power of being a witness to history. Rai notes, "It is important to be a witness and at times it's very painful. At times, you feel very inadequate that you can only do so much and no more." He also comments, "This unknown child has become the icon of the world's worst industrial disaster, caused by the U.S. chemical company, Union Carbide. No one knows his parents, and no one has ever come forward to 'claim' this photograph" (Day 2010).

In Ganesh's painting (which cites Bartholomew's photo) photography of the immediate aftermath of Bhopal is an important intertextual narrative that unearths a crucial story about the Union Carbide disaster. The children in Ganesh's painting, though less iconic than the child in Rai's or Bartholomew's photograph, are no less unsettling. Even though the children are unnamed, much as the child in the photos is unnamed, they are collectively the inheritors of the Union Carbide disaster. The painting refuses the viewer the choice of looking away, for in not meeting the children's gaze the viewer must confront the image of Bartholomew's photograph, also looking out at them. Though the child, silent in death and blinded by the harshness of the chemicals, cannot see, her face is not silent. Indeed the bodies in Ganesh's painting and Bartholomew's photograph tell a different kind of story. In their eyes is the weight of a stare that will haunt and will look back. There is no reprieve from the suffering here, nor, Ganesh's painting suggests, should there be a refuge from the stares of the dead who, though blinded by industrial greed and environmental negligence, must not remain unseen or voiceless.

Ganesh's painting helps to set the stage for this essay. In the varied stories that have emerged in response to the Union Carbide disaster, the figure of the child functions as the device that unrelentingly refuses to let viewers or audiences to be passive observers. Moreover a narrative of disability often figures into

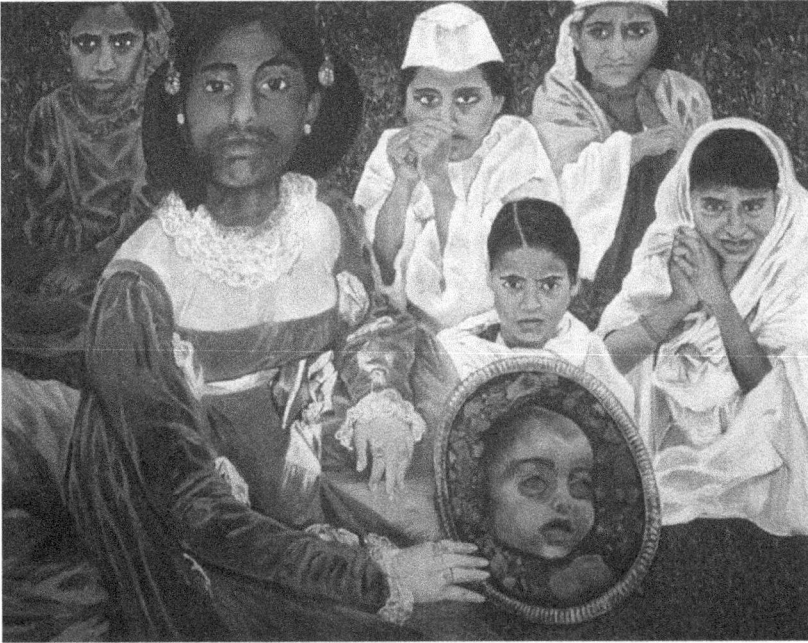

Fig. 13.1. Chitra Ganesh, Bhopal Looking Back, 2001, acrylic on fabric.

narratives about the Union Carbide disaster. Paradoxically the surfeit of attention on the way the chemical gas leak killed and severely crippled, blinded, and disfigured so many has not meant that disability studies perspectives have been brought to bear in significant ways to think about the Bhopal disaster.[1] Pursuing an analysis of the disaster by considering where and how the discourse of disability studies should enter the discussion necessarily complicates and makes more complex the construction of the disaster, thus allowing for an analysis that negotiates the intricacies of telling stories. In particular, a critical hinge for this essay is how we might approach the legacy and effects of Bhopal by examining the literary and cultural responses to the event that simultaneously told a story the world did not want to hear while also attending to the question of who has the power to tell stories.

Ous Raat, उस रात: Historical Context

For the residents of Bhopal, the phrase <u>that night</u> in Hindi, ous raat, उस रात, has one overarching meaning: <u>that night</u> is always the night of December 3, 1984. <u>That night</u> is always the night that life as Bhopalis knew it unalterably changed. That night the Union Carbide factory in Bhopal was responsible for unleashing the world's worst chemical disaster on the residents of the city. That night, while residents were sleeping, water entered a tank containing forty-two tons of the gas methyl isocyanate. A resulting exothermic reaction inside the tank led internal temperatures to rise well above 200°C (392°F), thereby raising the pressure to dangerously unstable levels. Unable to sustain the pressure, the tank developed a leak, releasing toxic gases into the air. During the early morning hours of that night the deadly chemical gas swept through the city, destroying flora, fauna, and human life that came its path. Bano Bi, a thirty-five-year-old mother and wife, recalls the event from a sensory perspective. While she sat sewing clothes, waiting her husband's return from a poetry reading, she thought she smelled the acrid odor of burning chilies. When the choking fumes did not relent she began coughing and experienced loss of breath. As she made her way to the door to see what was happening around her, she recalls, "some gas had leaked. Outside there were people shouting, 'Run, run, run for your lives'" (Hanna et al. 2005, 5). In the next few days more than 20 percent of the city's population died; the immediate death toll was in the thousands. A further sixty thousand were injured in the subsequent days, months, even years. The damage to the human and animal world, the natural and built environment, was almost impossible to quantify and continues to be immeasurable in large part because of the refusal of Union Carbide—now owned by the global conglomerate Dow Chemicals—to be accountable for its reckless actions.

On the occasion of the twenty-fifth anniversary of the Bhopal disaster, the Indian American writer Suketu Mehta (2009) exhorted Americans to remember that night. In a moving description published in the New York Times Mehta writes:

Methyl isocyanate is a deadly chemical used to kill insects. The night that 40 tons of it wafted out of the factory is, for the survivors, a fulcrum in time, marking the before and after in their lives. They still talk about "the gas" as if it were an organism they know well—how it killed buffalo and pigs, but spared chickens; how it traveled toward Jahangirabad and Hamidia Road, while ignoring other parts of the city; how it clung to the wet earth in some places but hovered at waist level in others; how it blackened all the leaves of a peepul tree; how they could watch it move down the other side of the road, like a rain cloud seen from a sunny spot.

Of note in Mehta's narrative is the idea that as the gas meandered through the city it acquired a larger-than-life status. Unfurling a kind of damage never before seen in Bhopal, methyl isocyanate unleashed such a degree of fury on the streets of the crowded metropolis that so many stories proliferated that night—and on subsequent nights—about the villain in this tragic tale of death, loss, and suffering. Mehta's description evokes a quiet landscape devastated in this one instant of time. The image of a place destroyed so suddenly and without warning is striking, but equally resonant in his description of the wafting gas is the idea that the gas inhabited a far more devastating temporality. The gas did not stop traveling but continued to insinuate itself into nooks and crannies of the physical and human environment far beyond the scope of that night. Thus while it is compelling to think about the big picture in which that night becomes the primary referent, much is to be gained from also attending to what Rob Nixon (2011, 2) usefully names "the long dyings—the staggered and staggeringly discounted casualties, both human and ecological that result from toxic aftermaths." Nixon's concept of slow violence in the context of environmental (in)justice attempts to complicate how disasters like Bhopal and Chernobyl are understood. Rather than understanding their effect as immediate, Nixon suggests that it is more productive and ethically resonant to understand violence as a form of "long dying"; the effects of violence are never contained by a single spatiotemporal moment. As he puts it, "violence is neither spectacular nor instantaneous, but rather incremental and accretive" (2).

Despite having shocked the world in 1984 the story of Bhopal remains unknown to many. Pointedly it has also not garnered much interest or empathy. Other chemical disasters, notably the Chernobyl chemical disaster that took place two years later, in 1986, have been much more widely discussed and theorized. Although there is a large corpus of literary and cultural work about the Bhopal disaster, little of it is in English. The literary scholar Upamanyu Mukherjee (2007, 135) notes, "There has been some very popular street theater, poetry and at least one play—all written and performed in Hindi and other non-English Indian languages, but it is the non-literary media—sculpture, photography and film documentaries—that have tended to respond best to the Bhopal tragedy and its aftermath." What, then, is the relationship between the vernacular and the absence of this story in the Anglophone literatures of India and its diaspora? In light of the limited attention Bhopal has received on the international stage one can also conceivably describe the stories of the event as embodying traces of the excessively foreign. Attending to the critical lacunae of this particular moment, I undertake a comparative analysis of this cultural work, focusing on novels that consider how the aftermath of the Bhopal environmental disaster become more complex when read through a disabilities studies perspective. Moreover in attending to the literary equivalent of Ganesh's painting—the long stares of the children—I examine those works that tell a different kind of story about environmental injustice. Rather than focusing purely on the tragedy of one night, the works I consider collectively recast the story of Bhopal as the story of long stares and long dyings.

To this end I examine two markedly different narratives. The first is a widely acclaimed novel, nominated for the prestigious Man Booker Prize, Animal's People. Authored by a longtime activist for Bhopal justice, Indra Sinha (2007), the novel unsettles the narrative privileging of that night in order to attend to the slow violence of the story. Juxtaposing this novel with a chick-lit novel, Amulya Malladi's (2007) A Breath of Fresh Air, in which the Bhopal disaster serves as a critical catalyst, I look for ways we can think of these stories as ones that simultaneously narrate the tragedy of that night while also anchoring the critical aftermath of Bhopal, to evoke Nixon's helpful terms, within a narrative of slow dyings. In Sinha's novel the character known as Animal walks on all fours due to a severely twisted spine, a result of the environmental disaster that destroyed the fictional town of Khaufpur. In Malladi's novel Bhopal provides an occasion to tell a story about a more privatized form of tragedy, the story of a woman who devotes her life to making life better for a child who is the second-generation inheritor of the Bhopal disaster. Though the bulk of my analysis focuses on Sinha's novel, I suggest that Animal's People and A Breath of Fresh Air create fictionalized spaces for understanding how disability studies and environmental studies can be put into conversation in order to better understand the ramifications of considering the disabled as a metaphor for the disabled nation. Julie Avril Minich (2011, 38) argues that the use of disability merely as a metaphor is inherently problematic: "Certainly, literary and critical tendencies to treat both the disabled body and the U.S.-Mexico border as mere metaphor rob both of their sociopolitical specificity and erase, misappropriate, or misrepresent the lived experiences of people with disabilities." Taking this critique of the dissolution of disability into mere metaphor as its starting point is one way to delve further into the strategic ways these novels both use and deconstruct what it means to describe Bhopal as a city crippled by devastation, a disabled city, and the strategic focus on the central character for whom disability is not a metaphor. Exposing the limitations of disability as metaphor in telling the story of Bhopal's chemical disaster thus propels the critical thrust of this essay.

Not Human, Not Accessible: Animal's People

In Sinha's (2007) novel Union Carbide is referred to only as "the Kampani," and the city of Bhopal is rendered by its fictional renaming as Khaufpur. Though subsequent work by Sinha (2009) would suggest that Khaufpur is not Bhopal but another city that has suffered intolerably from the reckless actions of multinational corporations, the relationship between Khaufpur and Bhopal remains radically unstable. Khaufpur cannot not be Bhopal, at the same time that it is not Bhopal. Key to understanding this point is a figure of classical rhetoric, the litote, that figuration of language that deploys the double negative in order to affirm. Allan Punzalan Isaac (2007) argues that the figuration of the double negative in the trope of the litote "subverts an easy opposition between a set of proximate terms connected by the double negative while also uncomfortably blur[ring] the boundaries between them. Absent texts are marked before and after the utterance, but also in the widening gap between the terms used."

Khaufpur is thus not Bhopal, but it is also not not Bhopal. At the center of this tale about this Indian city that has been devastated by a lethal explosion of chemicals is Animal, a child orphaned on the night of December 3, 1984. Much like the dead child memorialized in Rai's photo, Animal is a child with no accessible history. By way of explanation of his vague and uncertain origins he muses, "Whose was I? nobody knew. Mother, father, neighbors, all must have died for no living soul came to claim me. Was I Hindu or Muslim? How did it matter? I was not expected to live" (Sinha 2007, 14). Like the child in Rai's photograph, Animal has a story to tell: about a profound act of environmental injustice in which those who bear the burden of telling the story are also those who are least likely to be granted an audience. With no one who has claimed him, as no one has ever claimed the child in Rai's photo, Animal forges his own identity, establishing his own kinship networks with individuals who in one way or another care deeply for Bhopal. Phoenix-like he is reborn from the chemical flames that engulf the city. This rebirth results in his choosing to remain nameless and to disaffiliate from the human world. His opening words intimate his nonhuman status: "I used to be human once. So I'm told. I don't remember it myself, but people who knew me when I was small say I walked on two feet just like a human being" (1). Though the novel's protagonist is Animal it is very much invested in modes of storytelling. Throughout the reader accesses Animal's story via a series of transcribed cassette-tape interviews. Animal's story, we learn, has been commissioned by an Australian journalist, known only as "jarnalis," interested in telling the Khaufpuris' story to the world. Astutely Animal asks why Khaufpur is of interest to the media only in terms of one particular story. "You have turned us Khaufpuris into storytellers," he says, "but always of the same story. Ous raat, cette nuit, that night, always that fucking night" (95).

From the outset of the novel Animal is positioned as a story-teller and occasionally an empathetic figure who is reminded every day, physically and psychically, of what he so aptly calls "that night." So often the narrative about Bhopal in the media has been obliquely centered on the "monstrosity" of Union Carbide's actions. So much of the focus on this event has been about Union Carbide's refusal to extend a basic form of humanity to the residents of Bhopal—denial of health care, denial of any kind of compensation or support. And indeed there is a strong case to be made about how and why this environmental disaster also violates basic human rights—access to potable water being per-haps one of the central issues. And yet consider how this narrative does not fully recognize the import of thinking about disability outside of a representational matrix. In particular might disability studies offer an important way to sort through the messy cul-tural and ethical politics of the events in Bhopal? Because the central character possesses an extraordinary ability to speak about his disability the novel is perhaps unique in setting itself up as one that will seriously undertake the problem of under-standing disability instead of merely presenting disability solely as a discourse to create empathy for wronged persons through a lens of pity. Though it would be accurate to suggest that the events of December 3, 1984, created innocent victims—especially given the number of children who were affected—few of these narratives have developed a cogent way to ascribe agency to the disabled body. As Rosemarie Garland-Thompson (1996, 9) notes, "disabled literary characters usually remain on the margins of fiction as uncomplicated figures or exotic aliens whose bodily configurations operate as spectacles, eliciting response from other characters or producing rhetorical effects that depend on disability's cultural resonance. Indeed, main characters almost never have physical disabilities." With the character of Animal,

Sinha creates an unsettling narrative precisely because of the novel's refusal to see Animal as a hapless victim or an empowered subject who wishes to hide his disability in order to guarantee the comfort of others around him.

With his foul mouth and generally unpleasant demeanor, Animal is a marked departure from the "noble savage" ideal attached to the disabled body. There is little about his character, on the surface at least, that is likeable. It is also apparent that people around him often poke fun at his disability rather than express sympathy. Only the idealist socialist activist Zafar declares that "he dislikes teasing of the disabled." Suggesting that he prefers to think of Animal as "especially abled" Zafar also objects to Animal's choice of name: "You should not allow yourself to be called Animal. You are a human being, entitled to dignity and respect" (23). Rather unyielding on this point, Animal repeatedly declares, "My name is Animal. I'm not a fucking human being. I've no wish to be one" (23). Straddling the line between the human and nonhuman, Animal willfully disaffiliates with the human, repeatedly insists he is not a human being, and rejects being understood by the categories that ableist discourse provides. To allow people in would be to expose his vulnerability, something he refuses at all costs. Not unlike disabled individuals who have been dehumanized and ridiculed, Animal is cognizant that his disability is what makes him interesting to the journalistic eye. In terms of telling a pathos-laden tale of suffering, what could be a better embodiment of environmental injustice than an orphan who walks on all fours and whose best friend is a dog? Early in the novel Animal is quick to recognize how little his story itself matters to the journalist; it is the story of the wronged individuals that moves the journalist, not the particulars of any one individual story. Animal wonders, "What? Does he think he's the first outsider ever to visit this fucking city? People bend to touch his feet, sir, please sir, your help sir, sir my son, sir my wife, sir my wretched life. Oh how the prick loves this! Sultan among slaves he's, listens with what lofty pity, pretends to give a fuck but the truth is he'll go away and forget them, every last one. For his sort we are not really people. We don't have names. We flit in crowds at the corner of his eye. Extras we're, in his movie" (9). Being cognizant that he is an extra in the journalist's story is a startlingly revealing indictment of the journalist's motives in narrating this story. In this environmental and humanitarian crisis characters like Animal are prized for the dramatic value they bring to stories about human suffering. People like Animal are photographed for magazines and news stories, but there is no deep transformative understanding of what this disability means. Rather there is a perverse kind of visual pleasure and pain in seeing the horror of the disabled children.

Jarnalis's dogged pursuit of Animal's story can also be compared to the Boasian strategy of recording voices and salvaging testimonies and artifacts of an assumed disappearing past. For jarnalis recording the memory of this disaster condemns Animal to repeat a single story forever, just as "salvage ethnography sought to record memories of an assumed disappearing past in the face of disaster."[2] In identifying that he is a nameless entity, an extra in this movie, so to speak, Animal seizes on an important issue, pointing out that Khaufpuris are part of a longer chain of exploitation. They are mistreated first by the Kampani's reckless actions and now by the desires of journalists looking to put a unique spin on their reports about the city before they move on to the next important social issue of the day. The larger narrative that emerges about Bhopal is how easily the residents of that city have been forgotten. And yet is it enough to merely be remembered when actual forms of social justice have been slow to prevail? At the time the novel was published the Union

Carbide trial was ongoing. The novel itself imagines that the trial takes place, with Khaufpuris demanding that the Kampani be accountable for its actions.

What is it, then, that foreign journalists like the character in the novel wish to remember? What is it they wish to access, and where or what are the places they cannot or refuse to go? I deliberately use the word access here to signal the issues of mobility that are central to understanding this issue from a disability studies perspective. McRuer (2006) notes that accessibility cannot be understood simply in terms of physical mobility, though it is certainly an important aspect of understanding the myriad significations of what disability means. Rather "an accessible society, according to the best, critically disabled perspectives, is not simply one with ramps and Braille signs on 'public' buildings, but one in which our ways of relating to, and depending on, each other have been reconfigured" (94). So much of Animal's narrative is presented as inaccessible. He is limited in his mobility—and it is precisely this aspect of his difference that draws the journalist's attention—but he also refuses to allow the journalist, the inquisitive eye of the West, to penetrate the spaces most intimate to him: his heart and his home. Through the course of the novel Animal spins a marvelous tale about that night, bringing attention to the places, psychic and physical, that he inhabits, but without sharing the most intimate details. Home for Animal, we learn, is the most unlikely and perhaps most likely space. He explains, "Ever since that night the Kampani's factory has been locked up and abandoned. No one goes there, people say it's haunted by those who died. It's a shunned place, where better for an animal to make its lair?" (29). Amid the decaying walls and the corroding platforms and railings he makes a home. "This is my kingdom," he states. " In here I am the boss" (30). In the dangerous grasses choking the walls of the factory he sleeps, and for warmth he lies against the Kampani papers that form a thick quilt. Because he feels he has nothing more to lose and because he rejects the easy human/animal binary imposed on him, he does not fear and arguably even embraces the spaces where only feral creatures and stray animals would go.

In this world, an abandoned world that is off the grid, Animal ventures into a part of the built environment that has merged with the natural world. His interaction with this space is, as Alison Kafer (2013, 135) might suggest, a narrative of a person whose body and mind cause him "to interact with nature in nonnormative ways." This is a space that is "off the main trail," much like Bhopal itself is not yet part of the trail of disaster tourism and remains inaccessible to all but Animal. And yet, compelling as this story about living among the ruins of the chemical factory might be, it is a story he refuses to share with jarnalis. In a gesture that refuses empathy or pity, he denies others access to this space, thus preventing his home from becoming a mere sideshow attraction. His home, though dangerous to his health, is the only space he imagines he can be free. His world has become defined by the Kampani and the factory—it is one he seeks refuge from. And yet the irony is that his only refuge from the world created by the factory is within the walls of the old factory.

The element of risk and apparent recklessness is difficult to overlook in this instance. As Sarah Jaquette Ray (2013, 40) notes, oftentimes "the myth of an inaccessible wilderness lends risk culture its appeal and meaning [but] can be redefined by a different sensibility, one that values an array of bodies and a wider spectrum of positive ways to interact with nature." Living inside the factory, I would submit, is a form of risk in the terms Ray suggests; I would also argue that Animal's movement within the factory coupled with the desire not to create a public for this particular part of his life is a significant way he resists being cast as the ecological other, a mere curiosity or sideshow.

Privatized Trauma and Chick Lit

While a novel like Animal's People is categorically praised for tackling a story of crucial political and social importance, a novel like A Breath of Fresh Air succumbs to the kinds of critiques that are roundly levied against the larger genre of chick lit. The rise of the genre in North American and global markets has put it under larger scrutiny. While some critics have castigated chick lit for its emphasis on consumerist values within a neoliberal economy, others have noted the potential for the genre to subtly shift the focus onto issues relevant to women of color. Jigna Desai and Pamela Butler (2008, 4) ask, "Might women of color chick lit illuminate relations of power in the U.S., or address multiple social and economic formations?" To take a more expansive view of chick lit, particularly women of color chick lit, would complicate the view that stories about empowerment are necessarily wedded to a consumerist ethos. Malladi's (2007) A Breath of Fresh Air is interesting precisely because it is a different kind of chick lit novel. Attentive to social inequities it is pointedly disinterested in an ethos of consumerist excess and seeks instead to consider where and how the tentacles of global capitalism reach into the private sphere of women's lives.

Malladi presents a disabled child, but unlike in Sinha's novel, the child's role is to serve as a foil to understanding the central drama of the novel. The novel tells the story of Anjali, a woman whose body and subsequent life come to bear the symbolic freight of the Bhopal gas tragedy. On the evening of December 3, 1984, Anjali waits for her husband, Prakash (who has forgotten about her imminent return), to meet her incoming train. On the platform of the Bhopal train station Anjali is on the front lines of the gas leak. We learn that the exposure to the gas damages her uterus to the point that she cannot bear a child who would be considered "normal" by normative mainstream discourse. When Anjali learns that her husband's infidelity is what led to her being forgotten at the train station, she divorces him. Some years later she remarries and gives birth to a child, Amar, who has a degenerative disease. Though Prakash had been out of Anjali's world following their divorce, circumstances unfold in such a manner that the former couple find themselves in each other's lives once again. When Prakash returns to the scene, Anjali confronts him for being the root cause behind her "damaged son." Amar dies in due course, but this detail is ornamental, much like Amar is an ornamental detail in the novel. Part of the reason I cannot accurately describe Amar's disability is because it is not fleshed out in the novel; it is reduced to a plot point. So in a sense this novel is a prefect rendering of the problem Garland-Thomson (1996) identifies for disabled characters: they are not the central character, though they might add to the overall intrigue of the novel. Amar's character is important insofar as it reveals something about the failure of the traditional structure of heterosexuality to reproduce able-bodied citizens of the nation. Moreover the tragedy of Bhopal becomes embodied in Anjali's broken womb and Amar's disability.

One telling point is the notion that causality can tell the story of Bhopal. If Anjali had not been made to wait at the railway station, she would have been saved. Her failure is personal rather than a larger collective response. The burden is on the individual and the realm of the private—the philandering and negligent husband. Heteronormative domesticity's failure is castigated rather the corporation's failure to attend to the public health and safety of the larger environment. Moreover the solution to the problem is acts of individual reparation, in this case Prakash's effort to make amends for creating the conditions that led to Amar's death. Further, the only way to create empathy for those impacted by environmental injustice is to imagine its effects on the body of a child.

Conclusion

In 2009, on the twenty-fifth anniversary of the Bhopal disaster, Indra Sinha resurrected Animal's story for the South Asian diasporic magazine Himal. In the short story "Animal in Bhopal" the eponymous character is now somewhat of a celebrity on the transnational celebrity circuit. As he travels with Zafar, leaving Khaufpur for the first time in his life, he learns of other places that are not unlike Khaufpur. In the following exchange he learns about Bhopal, Khaufpur's litotetic other:

> "Bhopal. It's a city not very far from Khaufpur," says Zafar. . . .
> "How come I've never heard of it?"
> "You and ninety-nine percent of the world," says he, "either have not heard, or have forgotten. It's a city where a horrible disaster happened twenty-five years ago."
> He begins to tell me about Bhopal, where a chemical factory owned by a giant Amrikan kampani had exploded, releasing a cloud of poison gases over the sleeping city. Eight thousand died in a night. Hundreds of thousands were injured. After twenty-five years there are one hundred thousand souls in the city who cannot draw a breath without pain. Every day someone else dies. . . .
> But this is just like Khaufpur! I exclaim. "Incredible. A city close to ours where the exact same thing has happened, how come you've never talked about? Full of suspicion, I'm. Tales' too preposterous to be true."
> "There are many places like Khaufpur," says Zafar. "Some look much like our city, others quite different, but in each

the suffering of people, the diseases, and the causes, are the same." He rattles off a list of names I've often enough heard before—Minamata, Seveso, Chernobyl, Halabja, Vietnam, Hiroshima, Nagasaki, Toulouse, Falluja.

This story directly tackles the issue of where to position Khaufpur as not Bhopal and not not Bhopal and links to other global cities also impacted by environmental injustice. That 99 percent of the world remain ignorant, willfully or otherwise, suggests a systemic lack of empathy and care for the dimensions of human suffering that are brought about by chemical and industrial disasters.

Animal's People is a remarkable novel that sets into motion a complex debate about how empathy figures into the ways of thinking about the effects of this environmental disaster. With so many disabled by the deadly explosion of methyl isocyanate, the predominant image is of disability. But to return to the images discussed at the beginning of this chapter, recall how the figure of the innocent child becomes the most salient way to tell a story of moral outrage at the hands of corporations with a complete disregard for the ethics of existence. The image of the innocent suffering child, after all, is a compelling one. And when that child is blind or otherwise disabled, that image becomes all the more heart-wrenching. Certainly this is the primary emotional and affective plane on which A Breath of Fresh Air operates: without the figure of the child, the narrative is merely sad; with the addition of his story it becomes a moving and horrific tragedy. One can think about how the image of the wide-eyed suffering child, often with tears trickling down his or her face, is used to evoke sympathy from the West for an impoverished Third World. Yet Sinha's novel deliberately and strategically navigates away from this particular kind of narrative wherein the child is an innocent whose symbolic existence is meant to elicit sympathy. Animal's

disability is rendered in such a way that his boorish and obnox-
ious demeanor complicates a simple outpouring of sympathy for
what he is going through. Disability in his case becomes a social
location from which he can resist being defined by the probing
eye of Western journalism as a one-dimensional disabled human
who evokes sympathy because of his bodily suffering.

As Minich (2014, 195) argues, "The prevailing critical assumption has . . . been that on the rare occasions when images of
disability are used to represent the national collective, they
signal national failure or decay. The alignment of the national
with this socially dominant body and its corollary . . . has had
deleterious consequences for those whose embodiment differs
from this norm."

For at least two decades disability has been a defining mode for
representing what has happened to Bhopal. And for good reason.
But as my reading of these novels suggests, we must more fully
attend to the work of this form of representation and rethink the
role of metaphor in telling a story of global capitalism's reckless
disregard for humanity and the concomitant devaluing of the
lives of the poor and impoverished. If disability is the prevailing
metaphor for understanding this act of environmental injustice,
what are the further injustices that are perpetrated? Instead we
might consider disability not as a "metaphor for the failure of
nationalism . . . but as a social location from which to imagine
forms of political community that might fulfill the nation's democratic obligation to its citizens" (Minich 2014, 24). I have gestured
to how a disability studies perspective can allow us to understand
how the issues of environmental injustice have been brought into
the public eye. One must also attend to the way the discourse of
disability tells stories about environmental disaster in the Global
South that have been largely obscured by the interests of global
capitalism in an era of neoliberalism. Above all, I hope to see this

as the beginning of a conversation that will more fully attend to the inherent complexities of understanding how we see, think about, and reflect on the modes of transmission about narratives about environmental genocide.

NOTES

1. One exception is Jina Kim's "'People of the Apokalis': Spatial Disability and the Bhopal Disaster," Disability Studies Quarterly 34, no. 3 (2014), http://dsq-sds.org/article/view/3795/3271.
2. I am grateful to Mark Minch for sharing this insight about the novel with me (personal communication, March 30, 2015).

REFERENCES

Barker, Clare, and Stuart Murray. 2010. "Disabling Postcolonialism: Global Disability Cultures and Democratic Criticism." Journal of Literary and Cultural Disability 4, no. 3: 219–36.

Day, Elizabeth. 2010. "Raghu Rai: An Interview." Guardian, January 16. http://www.theguardian.com/artanddesign/2010/jan/17/raghu-rai-photography-exhibitions-london.

Desai, Jigna, and Pamela Butler. 2008. "Manolos, Marriage and Mantras: Chick Lit Criticism and Transnational Feminism." Meridians 8, no. 2: 1–31.

Garland-Thompson, Rosemarie. 1996. Extraordinary Bodies: Figuring Physical Disability in American Culture and Literature. New York: Columbia University Press.

Hanna, Bridget, Ward Morehouse, and Satinath Sarangi, eds. 2005. "Bano Bi's Story 1990." In The Bhopal Reader, 5–7. Goa: The Other India Press.

Isaac, Allan Punzalan. 2007. "Negation and Asian Racialization in Ozawa (1922) and Thind (1922)." Paper presented at Modern Language Association Convention, Philadelphia, December 2009.

Kafer, Alison. 2013. Feminist, Queer, Crip. Bloomington: Indiana University Press. Kindle.

Kundera, Milan. 1996. The Book of Laughter and Forgetting. London: Faber and Faber.

Malladi, Amulya. 2007. A Breath of Fresh Air. New York: Ballantine.

McRuer, Robert. 2006. Crip Theory: Cultural Signs of Queerness and Disability. New York: NYU Press.

Mehta, Suketu. 2009. "A Cloud Still Hangs over Bhopal." New York Times, December 2.

Minich, Julie Avril. 2011. "Disabling La Frontera: Disability, Border Subjectivity and Masculinity in 'Big Jesse, Little Jesse' by Oscar Casares." MELUS 57, no. 4: 35–52.

———. 2014. Accessible Citizenships: Disability, Nation and the Cultural Politics of Greater Mexico. Philadelphia: Temple University Press.

Mukherjee, Upamanyu. 2007. Postcolonial Environments: Nature, Culture and the Contemporary Indian Novel in English. London: Palgrave Macmillan.

Nixon, Rob. 2011. Slow Violence and the Environmentalism of the Poor. Cambridge MA: Harvard University Press.

Ray, Sarah Jaquette. 2013. The Ecological Other: Environmental Exclusion in American Culture. Tucson: University of Arizona Press.

Sinha, Indra. 2007. Animal's People. New York: Simon and Schuster.

———. 2009. "Animal in Bhopal." Himal South Asian: A Review Magazine of Politics and Culture, December. http://old.himalmag.com /component/content/article/687-animal-in-bhopal.html.

Section 3 FOOD JUSTICE

14

Disabling Justice?

The Exclusion of People with Disabilities from the Food Justice Movement

Natasha Simpson

What, <u>exactly</u>, is the connection between disability and food justice? Despite rampant food insecurity among people with disabilities, the food justice movement has yet to significantly acknowledge the barriers for disabled people in achieving food justice that is based in an understanding of ableism, or disability oppression.[1] <u>Ableism</u>, or the oppression of disabled people, operates in part through "deeply rooted beliefs about health, productivity, beauty, and the value of human life, perpetuated by the public and private media, [which] combine to create an environment that is hostile to those whose abilities fall outside of the scope of what is currently defined as socially acceptable" (Rauscher and McClintock 1996, 198). Although there is overlap between the food justice and disability justice movements, which I will illuminate, a disability justice framework is necessary to deepen the food justice movement's intersectional analysis of oppression. Ableism is not only pervasive; it is also bound to other systems of domination. Infusing food justice organizing with this understanding means that nuances of oppression within the food system become clearer, as do more possibilities for mobilization. Both the food justice and disability justice movements arose from the realities and priorities of people of color and both implement intersectional praxis; this leads me to articulate the potential for more explicit connections between them.

Disability justice, named in the vein of other justice-based social movements, was developed by Patricia Berne initially with other disabled queer women of color and later joined by other disabled people like Leroy Moore, is defined as a movement-building framework that emphasizes the leadership of disabled people of color and disabled queer and gender-nonconforming people. Disability justice includes people with chronic illnesses or who identify as sick as well as others not traditionally recognized as disabled (Allen 2013; Lamm et al. 2015; Berne 2015). This movement distinguishes itself from the disability rights movement in intentional and specific ways.[2] Berne points out that while disability rights undoubtedly have had positive impacts on the lives of people with disabilities, they fail to include many people with disabilities who are marginalized in multiple ways, and also fail to address structural oppression, instead mainly emphasizing the attainment of rights through legislative means rather than through a broader social movement (Allen 2013; Lamm et al. 2015). It is this specific framework that I am referring to when I refer to disability justice throughout this essay.

The radical Black origins of food justice also illustrate the importance of widespread cultural and political shifts and building across social movements. The Black Panther Party understood Black struggles for food access both as a manifestation of the structural oppressions Black people face in the United States and as a site where many of these structural oppressions converge. Government interference and, later, co-optation of the Free Breakfast for School Children Program, run by the Black Panthers, effectively ended it (Potorti 2014), and the most popular representations of the movement have continued shifting toward reform rather than revolution. For instance, unfortunately, "structural critiques of capitalism and racism that were integral to the Black Panther's political work" are less visible in food justice today (Holt-

Gimenéz and Wang 2011, 89). My aim in revisiting these origins is to honor this historical and continuing vein of food justice and to imagine the liberatory potential of food justice for disabled people, especially those who are multiply oppressed.

The food justice movement is rightfully meant to center the experiences of poor Black communities and other communities of color; however, it also often centers specific notions of health, which can erase food access struggles experienced by disabled people, including disabled people of color, as being an expression of ableism. Conceptions of food access can be expanded within the context of ableism. I believe this recognition and, further, the potential for more mobilization around this is particularly vital. Most importantly, the food justice movement has the potential for transforming society beyond increasing food access; through a disability justice politic, food justice is a site where ideals privileging "normal," "healthy" bodyminds can be challenged.

Methods

In 2015 I analyzed the online mission statements of four food justice organizations based in Oakland, California, that explicitly articulated race and class as dimensions of food access struggles, and I have traced their discourses regarding health, illness, and disability to ableist ideologies that have potentially harmful impacts on food access for people with disabilities. As I stated above, ableism is pervasive, and it is for this reason, and because of the potential for food justice organizations and the movement more broadly to be receptive to this analysis, that I do not find it useful to single out the organizations by name.

Ableist discourse within the food justice movement is often centered around chronic illnesses, which I also refer to here as nonapparent disabilities; for this reason I conducted interviews regarding experiences of ableism with chronically ill people/

people with primarily nonapparent disabilities. I received four responses to my posts on social media from potential interview participants, and I interviewed those who responded: four cisgender women with nonapparent disabilities. Three of the four women identify as white; one identifies as a mixed-race Latina. Two of the women openly identify as queer. The interviews conducted were semistructured. I draw only on themes of the interviews here due to space considerations. The women articulated experiencing intense pressures to perform abledness as well as lack of recognition of access needs (a term I learned from Sins Invalid) that, they feel, stem from their disabilities presenting as nonapparent. The reach of ableism, especially through notions of "healthy," "normal" bodyminds, affects many people, not only those who "look" disabled to the abled.[3] Although I am examining discourses and their underlying ideologies, this essay is very much rooted in furthering the understanding of their <u>material</u> implications, illustrated by the struggles in food access that disabled people experience.

Why Disability?

A wealth of information has been gathered regarding the impacts of race, class, and, to a lesser extent, immigration and migration status in the food system, which has led to the common acknowledgment that "certain populations of bodies are structurally recognized as less worthy of sustenance" (Slocum and Saldanha 2013, 1). Judith Carney (2013, 74) echoes this, stating, "The right to a meal has been used in specific historical periods to deny some people their fundamental humanity." It is surprising in this context that questions about the role of disability in the food system have, until relatively recently, been absent. The USDA reports that not only are households that include an adult with a disability considered "food insecure" at rates alarmingly higher than households without, but also experience more severe food insecurity; the utilization of disability assistance programs and food and nutrition programs were found not to be wholly effective in ensuring food security for disabled people (Coleman-Jensen and Nord 2013).[4] Additionally, higher rates of food insecurity are the case even for moderate-income households that include an adult with a disability (Coleman-Jensen and Nord 2013).

These conditions, however, have not stimulated an ableism-informed analysis within the food justice movement. While the movement's primary food access concerns are proximity to food, affordability of food, and knowledge about food (Oakland Food Policy Council n.d.)—all also relevant to disabled people—this conception of food access is not enough to encompass additional barriers to food access that people with disabilities experience. There is a range of potential additional considerations for disabled people in accessing food, such as experiencing social isolation and being homebound; inaccessibility of transportation options and inaccessibility of grocers; difficulties transporting groceries and preparing and cooking food (Webber et al. 2007; Coleman-Jensen and Nord 2013). While these barriers are often framed as being a result of disabilities themselves, effectively depoliticizing disability, I would argue that they are all evidence of systemic oppression within society, in which myths of independence, expectations of economic productivity, and abledness are glorified. This type of depoliticization obscures ableism as a root of these barriers to food access. Where connections to systemic oppression in the food system are commonly present in other analyses, they seem to be absent in regard to disability. Alison Kafer (2013, 10) asks questions I believe are useful to begin to deconstruct this: "How has disability been depoliticized, removed from the realm of the political? Which definitions of and assumptions about disability facilitate this removal? What are the effects of such depoliticization?"

The strategy of linking communities' material conditions to structural inequities, thereby politicizing marginalized communities' experiences, is of particular value in working toward a food justice movement informed by disability justice; this strategy was also fundamental to the food justice work of the Black Panthers.

I aim to illustrate that, much like inequities along the lines of other facets of identity, the barriers that people with disabilities face in the food system can also be read as a result of ableism in society. I consider the impact of ableism intersectionally, intertwined with those other facets of identity. Referring to women, people of color, and immigrants, Douglas Baynton (2001, 33) asserts, "The concept of disability has [also] been used to justify discrimination against other groups by attributing disability to them." This use of ableism as further justification of oppression against marginalized communities potentially provides a context for the absence of an analysis of ableism within the food justice movement. Delving into the origins of food justice elucidates why its activism is situated uniquely in its ability to affect transformation <u>beyond</u> food access.

Radical Black Origins of the Food Justice Movement

"The long black freedom struggle has repeatedly underscored the cultural and political significance of food, explicitly calling attention to structures of racism and social inequality" (Potorti 2014, 45). Carney (2013) illustrates this long black freedom struggle by characterizing enslaved African people's relationship to food in the context of the transatlantic slave trade and the ensuing realities of slavery. Indigenous African foods and related knowledge of food production sustained enslaved Black people and many others, but food was also strictly controlled and exploited by "plantation capitalism" (71–73). These, among others, are origins of unjust circumstances from which a Black politics around food in the United States, and throughout the African diaspora, sprung.

I believe it is fruitful to revisit and highlight the more radical Black legacy of food justice in order to illustrate how the politicization of food access was utilized to connect a range of issues and supported political actions from consciousness-raising to informing other types of political organizing. As early as the Great Depression the Alabama Sharecroppers Union organized against the race- and class-based oppression of Black sharecroppers within a radical communist framework (Potorti 2014, 45), but my focus here will be on the food justice programs of the Black Panther Party. The Party's Free Breakfast for Children Program, initially based in Oakland, California, synthesized their radical political analysis with the program's practical reach. It fed 250,000 children each day before school, nationwide, through forty-nine Party chapters, in partnership with other organizations (Holt-Gimenéz and Wang 2011, 89). This and their other food justice programs were a means to raise communities' consciousness by explicitly connecting "capitalism [and] social stratification [to] their own material deprivation and political marginalization" (Potorti 2014, 46, emphasis added). Of importance here, in addition to critiquing capitalism, the Party members demonstrated alternatives by sustaining this large-scale breakfast program solely with donations (45, 47).

The government sought to disrupt the food justice work of the Black Panther Party precisely because it was explicitly political rather than humanitarian (FBI as cited by Potorti 2014, 46); these disruptive tactics included shaming accusations of sexual deviance and sexually transmitted infections; harassment, questioning, and arrest; frivolous public health citations; and the destruction of food (46). The Black Panthers understood that concerns about obtaining the basic sustenance necessary for survival could divert Black communities' attention and energies away from linking a lack of sustenance to other "manifestations of egregious racism such as underemployment, economic exploitation, police brutality, and a skewed criminal justice system" (Holt-Gimenéz and Wang 2011, 89). Therefore they did not view food access as a goal in itself but as a necessary step on the way to Black liberation (Potorti 2014, 46).[5]

Observing this historical context can provide promising directions for food justice praxis, or the application of this knowledge, as it connects to realizing food justice for people with disabilities. First, however, it is important to take into account the influences of the environmental justice movement and the mainstream food movement on modern food justice (Alkon and Agyeman 2011, 7) in order to illustrate what further sets it apart from mainstream food and environmental movements.

Environmental justice breaks away from mainstream environmentalism, whose ideologies, discourses and practices have historically been aligned with colonialism and eugenics.[6] The environmental justice movement developed out of the civil rights tradition, with Black, Indigenous, and other women of color, particularly mothers, at the forefront of the fight to gain protection from and provide input about a number of their communities' environmental concerns, such as land and water rights, exposure to toxins, and unsafe living and working conditions (Alkon and Agyeman 2011, 7–8; Stein 2004, 2–3). While mainstream environmentalism asserts that nature is separate from (certain) humans and ranks nature above humans, "the environmental justice movement has instead defined the environment as 'where we live, work, play, and worship'" and firmly integrates humans with nature (Stein 2004, 1). The movement's strategy often employs data from community-based research to prove environmental and bodily harm and to advocate for legal protections and stewardship of their communities (Alkon and Agyeman 2011, 7). This framework is evident in the food justice movement's focus on the disproportionate food insecurity in poor communities of color, as well as in many activists' insistence that communities should determine how their food system operates (8). The centering of poor people and people of color in the food justice movement is also, in some ways, a rebuttal to the "predominantly white and middle-class" priorities of the mainstream food movement (2), which focuses "more on what people eat than how food is produced, works through the market, and for the most part punts on the question of inequality" (Guthman 2011, 141).

Although it is often referred to as the sustainable or alternative food movement, I will refer to it as the mainstream food movement to reduce confusion. (For instance, the food justice movement can also be considered a sustainable or alternative food movement.) Historically associated with the leftist counterculture of the 1960s, when initial concerns about increasing corporate consolidation and environmental exploitation in the food system began to appear, mainstream communal, organic, and local food operations came out of this framework (Guthman 2011, 142). While adopting similar operations but with less emphasis on organic, the food justice movement has drawn attention to the mainstream food movement's privilege since its strategy generally entails encouraging people to buy fresh, local, and organic food without consideration for the fact that the cost or availability may be prohibitive (Alkon and Agyeman 2011, 2–3). The food justice movement, however, has an opportunity to center the impact of ableism on food access for people with disabilities.

Politicizing Disability within Food Justice

In analyzing the mission statements of four Oakland-based food justice organizations, I became particularly interested in the discourses they contain regarding health, food access, and what constitutes food justice activism to ascertain the potential implications of these discourses in inhibiting or advancing food and disability justice.

The majority of the mission statements define health in ways that perpetuate the undesirability of disability, essentially defining disability as the antithesis of health. All four organizations explicitly posit restoring health, not ever explicitly defined, as one of the aims of their work; three of the four organizations position illness or disease as the opposite of health and, in doing so, employ the language of medicine and public health, specifically referring to "diet-related diseases," diabetes, hypertension, and heart disease alongside obesity and asthma. Categorizing people experiencing illness and other disabilities as unhealthy, and therefore abnormal, in need of fixing or curing, has been and continues to be a prominent ideology that fuels the oppression of disabled people.[7]

Scholars have finally joined disability rights, disability justice, and fat activists in drawing attention to the fact that this concept of health is not apolitical,[8] that it is "a term that speak[s] as much about power and privilege as about well-being. Health is a desired state, but it is also a prescribed state and an ideological position" (Metzl 2010, 1, emphasis added). Health as "a prescribed state and an ideological position" is an offshoot of ableism, and the depoliticization of this concept as such is in opposition to the vein of food justice that the Black Panther Party engaged in. If health is a defined goal of food justice activism, and health is the absence of illness or disease (which can include disability), then the root of food insecurity (ableism) of those who <u>cannot</u> attain health by this definition is obscured and normalized rather than recognized as a manifestation of ableist oppression. This depoliticization is a danger to disability justice much like the depoliticization of food justice was for the Black Panther Party.

Health, in this context, actually entails a normative state, and this can be directly traced to eugenics, and normalization impulses within medicine and public health. Although Guthman (2011, 41) set out to contribute a "political ecology of obesity," I am applying her insights regarding how "normal . . . became normative" in the context of disability. Guthman tracks this notion of "normal" bodies to the nineteenth-century application of statistical methods, particularly the bell curve, in public health and then medical practice; this led increasingly to the belief in the "average" within the population as the norm. Even further, the comparison of people based on "average" bodies made any outliers abnormal and pathological, the bodies against which normal was defined (41–42). Baynton (2001, 36) writes, "Although normality ostensibly denoted the average, the usual, and the ordinary, in actual usage it functioned as an ideal and excluded only those defined as <u>below</u> average." Medicine and public health are two factors in shaping bodily norms, often dominating society's views of what truly "healthy," "normal" bodies are, but bound with them is the legacy of eugenics.

Eugenics is "the social engineering project that sought to eradicate defective traits from a nation's hereditary pool" (Mitchell and Snyder 2010, 187). People primarily within marginalized communities have been targeted based on nonnormative traits of the bodymind, and eugenics programs have spanned and intersected with gender, race, and other identities—not just because of disability but also due to the <u>perception</u> of disability. Society's ableism has permitted science and medicine license to commit injustices in the name of health and normality, namely involuntary medical procedures and institutionalization, among other "cures" based in eugenics, against people with disabilities as well as others perceived to be defective (Wendell 2001; Gabel and Peters 2004; Mitchell and Snyder 2010). It is from these experiences that the social model arose, "the result of resistance to the medical model, to the oppression of disabled people, and to ableism" (Gabel and Peters 2004, 592). These ideologies are apparent in references to "diet-related" illness and disease, which imply that through appropriate diet one can—and, more importantly, should—"cure" oneself of diabetes, hypertension, and heart disease. This erases the agency of people who are sick and disabled, shames them, and does not take into account, for example, those for whom diet is not a primary cause of illness or disability, those who cannot be "cured" by adopting a produce-rich diet, or those who don't desire to be cured to an abled standard. Susan Wendell (1996, 94) refers to this as the myth of control, which also stems from and is perpetuated by medicine and public health, that "by means of human actions" we can control the near inevitability of illness and disability and the definite inevitability of death. This myth supports an increasingly common expectation that people "control" their bodyminds by whatever means necessary, which advances the notion that health is a matter of personal responsibility (Guthman 2011, 47). This idea of health as a matter of personal responsibility is abundantly clear in the case of antifat discourse within the food justice movement; Sonya Renee Taylor asserts, "We must ask who benefits from a war against people's bodies. Does it benefit communities to be at war with their bodies? If the benefit is not to the communities we serve then what makes the model a justice movement?" (qtd. in Duong 2013).

Because disability or perceptions of disability were, and often still are, used to justify continued oppression of multiply marginalized groups, it potentially clarifies why the food justice movement might hesitate to adopt a disability justice framework. Black experiences, as well as the experiences of other people of color, with medicine, public health, and eugenics (although by no means monolithic), have included medicalization and other ableist violences. This has often been characterized by simultaneous hypervisibility and invisibility or neglect, for example through forced medical experimentation as well as a lack of desired medical care (Nelson 2013, xiii).[9] For people who are already marginalized due to race, gender, sexuality, and more, distance from disability has been a method of gaining rights (Baynton 2001, 34)—but at what cost? This has translated into "a lot of people that are functionally disabled [but] who don't identify as disabled" (Patricia Berne as cited by Allen 2013) where there is a possibility for becoming "politically disabled" (Mingus 2010); this depoliticization and distancing from disability limits possibilities for mobilizing against ableism.

To illustrate just how far-reaching these normative ideas of the bodymind are, I interviewed four chronically ill women about their experiences with nonapparent disabilities. Because people make the determination of disability on the basis of "function and appearance" (Lennard Davis as quoted in Baynton 2001, 48), the impact of ableist ideals of the "normal," "healthy" bodymind feels intensely present for these women with nonapparent disabilities. There were three common threads among their experiences: people discount their disability or are skeptical of its existence or suspicious of the severity of their impairments; this denial of disability identity impacts whether their needs for access are taken seriously, let alone met; they must navigate others' expectations of the functioning of their bodymind based on social norms of abledness, exaggerated because, to others, they do not "look" like they have impairments; and they experienced difficulty claiming their agency because doctors encouraged them to use medical treatment to make them as "normal" as possible so they could pass as abled. Clearly ableism has a broad reach; however, by working toward politicizing disability and toward disability justice within the food justice movement, we may begin to resist disability as a basis of justification for oppression. Idealizing "healthy," "normal" bodyminds clearly stems from ableism and contributes to the oppression of people with disabilities.

Conclusion

As is now clear, the discourse of these select food justice organizations stem from particular ideologies advanced by medicine, public health, eugenics, and capitalism, even alongside the organizations' race and class analysis. It is important to contend with the material impacts of these ideologies in order to work toward disability justice as well as food justice. By engaging with a disability justice framework, I believe, the food justice movement can be a site for transforming oppressive beliefs about health and bodyminds. But what exactly does this look like?

The food justice movement's lineage from environmental justice often means that inequities in food access are articulated particularly through their impacts on the body, as previously illustrated. Kafer (2013, 158, emphasis added) aptly concludes, "What is needed, then, are analyses that recognize and refuse the intertwined exploitation of bodies and environments without demonizing the illnesses and disabilities, and especially the ill and disabled bodies, that result from such exploitation." This is an essential foundation to further analyses in regard to disability.

All of the food justice organizations I've included here have programs for community and political education; learning from those engaged in disability justice as part of their established political education efforts is one important aspect. Should the food justice movement deepen its analysis, and broaden the accessibility of its organizing, this could facilitate connections across movements and further the meeting of food and disability justice.

Also important to bringing food justice and disability justice together is a broader conception and practice of access. Food access is often defined in terms of proximity, cost, and education, but this is not enough when thinking about disability. I hope that this essay has illustrated that the scope of these barriers is wider than is usually articulated. Disability justice within this movement means there should be alternatives to solely labor-intensive methods of engaging with food production and organizing.[10] It means forms of transportation that are comfortable and reliable for a multitude of bodies and accessible options for people who are homebound or otherwise have difficulty getting to and/or preparing food. It entails incorporating more accessibility once people do get there, such as rest areas, Braille, and more affordable organic foods for those who experience injury from pesticides and other chemicals; it entails organizing against ableism throughout the food system, from production to reuse with a firm understanding of how ableism colludes with other forms of oppression, and how capitalism further impacts accessibility in this context.

This inherently also expands to relationships with other people, and interdependence is critical: what about those who are fed by others, or those with feeding tubes (Wilkerson 2011)? What about those whose pain or fatigue limits the cooking they can do, or who can consume only limited produce because fiber makes them ill (Sarah 2014)? These are all contexts that food justice can address if informed by disability justice, and my hope is that this increasingly will be the case.

NOTES

1. Food insecurity is defined by the USDA as "a household-level economic and social condition of limited or uncertain access to food." Low food security entails reduced quality, variety, or desirability of diet, with little to no indication of reduced food intake; very low food security indicates disrupted eating patterns and reduced food intake (U.S. Department of Agriculture, Economic Research Service. 2015). I diverge from this definition to claim that food insecurity is structural, affected on the household and even individual levels by systems of oppression.

2. See Berne (2015) of Sins Invalid, a disability justice organization cofounded with Leroy Moore, for the ten principles of disability justice.

3. Ableism creates hierarchical distinctions between abled and disabled as well as false distinctions between apparent and nonapparent disability. I do not seek to employ these types of neat distinctions. Rather I attempt to illustrate how these distinctions function to deny access to all people with disabilities, which can create fissures in relations across disability, as well as how they function to coerce chronically ill and nonapparently disabled people into what is in some ways a liminal space between abled and disabled should they not comply with performing ableness.

4. This could mean that food insecurity is actually much higher among disabled people, as those who, for myriad reasons, are not utilizing these programs are not represented. USDA Economic Research Service data from 2009–10 found that 33 percent of households that included an adult with a disability who was unable to work, and 25 percent of households with an adult with a disability that did not prevent him or her from working were food insecure, compared to 12 percent of households without an adult with a disability. The data also showed a whopping 38 percent of households including an adult with a disability had very low food security, as defined in note 1 (Coleman-Jensen and Nord 2013).

5. I define food access as the ability to easily produce or obtain, prepare, and consume food that nourishes on the physical, mental, emotional, cultural, and spiritual levels.

6. For more on the influences of colonialism and eugenics on mainstream environmentalism, see Ray 2013.

7. Like many others, I assert that being fat is not in and of itself an illness or disability; medicalization is, however, common among both people who are fat as well as those who are disabled, and fatness is also a basis of oppression.

8. The desire of disabled people to utilize agency as a way to care for our bodyminds, whether through medicine, food, or other means, does not invalidate this or automatically imply internalized ableism.

9. Washington (2008) provides a thorough history of forced medical examinations. The Black Panthers also organized to address the medical mistreatment of Black Americans (see Nelson 2013).

10. Credit to Toi Scott (http://www.afrogenderqueer.com) for being essential to initiating this conversation for me.

REFERENCES

Alkon, Alison Hope, and Julian Agyeman. 2011. "Introduction: The Food Movement as Polyculture." In Cultivating Food Justice: Race, Class and Sustainability, edited by Alison Hope Alkon and Julian Agyeman, 1–20. Cambridge MA: MIT Press.

Allen, D. 2013. "Liberating Beauty: A Conversation with Sins Invalid's Patty Berne." Feministing. http://feministing.com/2013/10/09/liberating -beauty-a-conversation-with-sins-invalids-patty-berne/.

Baynton, Douglas. 2001. "Disability and the Justification of Inequality in American History." In The New Disability History: American Perspectives, edited by Paul K. Longmore and Lauri Umansky, 33–57. New York: New York University Press.

Berne, Patricia. 2015. "Disability Justice—A Working Draft by Patty Berne." Sins Invalid, June 10. http://sinsinvalid.org/blog/disability -justice-a-working-draft-by-patty-berne.Carney, Judith. 2013. "Fields of Survival, Foods of Memory." In Geographies of Race and Food: Fields, Bodies, Markets, edited by Rachel Slocum and Arun Saldanha. 62–78. Burlington VT: Ashgate.

Coleman-Jensen, Alisha, and Mark Nord. 2013. "Disability Is an Important Risk Factor for Food Insecurity." U.S. Department of Agriculture, Economic Service Research, May 6. http://www.ers.usda.gov/amber

-waves/2013-may/disability-is-an-important-risk-factor-for-food
-insecurity.aspx#.vn-Zb8yhr8e.

Duong, Truong Chinh. 2013. "Reframing Food Justice with Body Love."
Oakland Local, October 12. http://oaklandlocal.com/2013/10/food
justicebodylove/.

Gabel, S., and S. Peters. 2004. "Presage of a Paradigm Shift? Beyond the
Social Model of Disability toward Resistance Theories of Disability."
Disability & Society 19, no. 6: 585–600.

Guthman, Julie. 2011. Weighing In: Obesity, Food Justice, and the Limits
of Capitalism. Berkeley: University of California Press.

Holt-Gimenéz, Eric, and Yi Wang. 2011. "Reform or Transformation?
The Pivotal Role of Food Justice in the Movement." Race/Ethnicity:
Multidisciplinary Global Contexts 5, no. 1: 83–102.

Kafer, Alison. 2013. Feminist, Queer, Crip. Bloomington: Indiana University Press.

Lamm, Nomi, Patty Berne, and Kiyaan Abadani. 2015. "This Is Disability
Justice." The Body Is Not an Apology, September 2. http://thebodyis
notanapology.com/magazine/this-is-disability-justice/.

Metzl, Jonathan M. 2010. "Introduction: Why 'Against Health'?" In
Against Health: How Health Became the New Morality, edited by
Jonathan M. Metzl and Anna Kirkland, 1–14. New York: New York
University Press.

Mingus, Mia. 2010. "Reflecting on Frida Kahlo's Birthday and the Importance of Recognizing Ourselves for (in) Each Other." Leaving Evidence,
July 6. https://leavingevidence.wordpress.com/2010/07/06/reflecting
-on-frida-kahlo's-birthday-and-the-importance-of-recognizing
-ourselves-for-in-each-other/.

Mitchell, David T., and Sharon L. Snyder. 2010. "Disability as a Multitude:
Re-Working Non-Productive Labor Power." Journal of Literary & Cultural Disability Studies 4, no. 2: 179–93.

Nelson, Alondra. 2013. Preface to Body and Soul: The Black Panther Party
and the Fight against Medical Discrimination. Minneapolis: University
of Minnesota Press.

Oakland Food Policy Council. N.d. "Food Access." http://oaklandfood
.org/our-work/policy-initiatives/food-access/.

Potorti, Mary. 2014. "Feeding Revolution: The Black Panther Party and the Politics of Food." Radical Teacher: A Socialist, Feminist, and Anti-Racist Journal on the Theory and Practice of Teaching 98: 43–51.

Rauscher, Laura, and Mary McClintock. 1997. "Ableism Curriculum Design." In Teaching for Diversity and Social Justice, edited by Maurianne Adams, Lee Anne Bell, and Pat Griffin, 335–358. New York: Routledge.

Ray, Sarah Jaquette. 2013. The Ecological Other: Environmental Exclusion in American Culture. Tucson: University of Arizona Press.

Sarah. 2014. "Food Is NOT Medicine." Skeptability, August 2. http://skeptability.com/2014/08/02/food-is-not-medicine/.

Slocum, Rachel, and Arun Saldanha. 2013. "Geographies of Race and Food: An Introduction." In Geographies of Race and Food: Fields, Bodies, Markets, edited by Rachel Slocum and Arun Saldanha, 1–24. Burlington VT: Ashgate.

Stein, Rachel. 2004. Introduction to New Perspectives on Environmental Justice: Gender, Sexuality, and Activism, edited by Rachel Stein, 1–20. New Brunswick NJ: Rutgers University Press.

U.S. Department of Agriculture, Economic Research Service. 2015. "Definitions of Food Security." September 8. http://www.ers.usda.gov/topics/food-nutrition-assistance/food-security-in-the-us/definitions-of-food-security.aspx#ranges.

Washington, Harriet A. 2008. Medical Apartheid: The Dark History of Medical Experimentation on Black Americans from Colonial Times to the Present. New York: Anchor.

Webber, Caroline B., Jeffrey Sobal, and Jamie S. Dollahite. 2007. "Physical Disabilities and Food Access among Limited Resource Households." Disability Studies Quarterly 27, no. 3. http://dsq-sds.org/article/view/20/20.

Wendell, Susan. 1996. The Rejected Body. New York: Routledge.

———. 2001. "Unhealthy Disabled: Treating Chronic Illnesses as Disabilities." Hypatia 16, no. 4: 17–33.

Wilkerson, Abby. 2011. "Food and Disability Studies: Vulnerable Bodies, Eating or 'Not Eating.'" Food, Culture, and Society 14, no. 1: 17–28.

15

Cripping Sustainability, Realizing Food Justice

Kim Q. Hall

> The shared meal is no small thing. It is a foundation of family life, and the place where our children learn the art of conversation and acquire the habits of civilization: sharing, listening, taking turns, navigating differences, arguing without offending.
>
> — Michael Pollan, <u>Cooked: A Natural History of Transformation</u>

> The table in its very function as a kinship object might enable forms of gathering that direct us in specific ways or that make some things possible and not others. Gatherings, in other words, are not neutral but directive.
>
> — Sara Ahmed, <u>Queer Phenomenology: Orientations, Objects, Others</u>

While many are familiar with the Brundtland Commission's 1987 definition of sustainability—meeting the needs of the present generation without compromising the ability of future generations to meet their needs—the conception of disability that informs the Commission's now mainstream conception of disability is less well known and certainly has not been a topic of conversation in mainstream U.S. environmentalism. In <u>Our Common Future</u>, the Brundtland Commission urges, "Sustainability must work to remove disabilities from disadvantaged groups in forests, desert nomads, groups in remote hill areas, and indigenous people of the Americas and Australasia" (World Commission on Environment and Development 1987, 53). Here the Commission associates disability with the vulnerability of indigenous populations,[1] an association that establishes the economic North as able-bodied and secure. The Commission's definition of sustainability presumes the perspective of the economic North that establishes disability and vulnerability as elsewhere. One wonders, does sustainability have anything to say about disabilities among the global elite? What does it mean to conceive of sustainability as incompatible with the presence of disability?

While it is crucial to address the connections between ecological devastation and disability, it is also important to question the understanding of vulnerability and security that informs assumptions about disability in the prevailing discourse of sustainability. After all, if sustainability involves economic, environmental, and social justice (and I believe it should), it is imperative to question the extent to which assumptions about sustainability that inform the U.S. alternative food movement are compatible with disability justice. As I use the term, disability justice involves both justice for disabled people and conceptions of sustainability and a sustainable world that include disabled people. As Alison Kafer (2013, 3) stresses, "In imagining more accessible futures, I am yearning for an elsewhere—and perhaps an 'elsewhen'–in which disability is understood otherwise: as political, as valuable, as integral." In other words, a sustainable world is an accessible world.

In this paper I build on Kafer's important connection between sustainability and accessibility and focus in particular on the meaning and possibility of sustainable foodscapes. I argue that the sustainable foodscapes that populate much contemporary food writing in the United States are heteronormative and able-bodied and, consequently, inaccessible and unsustainable. Moving toward sustainable foodscapes requires, I contend, cripping sustainability—a reorientation of foodscapes that resists heteronormativity and ableism, enabling the emergence of an alternative conception of sustainability that is accountable to different ways of being in the world and is, as a result, more conducive to food justice.

A foodscape, like food itself, is not a site through which one simply moves or an object that one consumes. Rather foodscapes emerge in the complex interactions of culture, economics, and politics that shape relations between food, processes and sites of food production, distribution and consumption, and eaters.[2] Thinking about how one might move toward sustainable foodscapes requires thinking about how one might be oriented within foodscapes in ways that either open or foreclose new modes of being and relationship in the world.

Building on Sara Ahmed's (2006) queer phenomenology, I analyze the paths constituted by prevailing understandings of sustainability and sustainable foodscapes, with particular attention to their accessibility. To what extent do these understandings of sustainability and sustainable foodscapes remain critically attuned to those whose lives are deemed not worth living or without a future in ways that facilitate the cultivation of a resistant imagination that opens the possibility of being and living otherwise?[3] As environmentalist literature about climate change reminds us, addressing climate change is not merely a matter of consulting scientific, technological, or economic experts. Rather addressing climate change means that global elites must learn to live otherwise, a change that requires a transformed orientation toward the world, oneself, and others (Jamieson 2008; Cuomo 2011; Gardiner 2011). According to José Medina (2013, 299), resistant imagination is the critical capacity necessary for knowing and realizing alternatives, "an imagination that is ready to confront relational possibilities that have been lost, ignored, or that remain to be discovered or invented." Resistant imaginations are pluralist and involve multiple perspectives and a turning toward that which has been cast outside social norms.

In order to orient my consideration of the place of disability and queerness in the imagined sustainable foodscapes that populate contemporary food writing, I turn to the central place of the table in the farm-to-table imaginary of the contemporary U.S. food movement. In Queer Phenomenology Ahmed (2006) offers a phenomenology of orientation in relation to writing and dining tables. Given that the table and the family meal are ubiquitous, taken-for-granted fixtures in the sustainable foodscapes of much contemporary writing about food, how does the table play an orienting role in contemporary food writing?

My consideration of these issues also draws on crip theory, which shares with queer theory a critical understanding of the fraught, contested, incomplete, and contingent nature of identity, as well as a persistent critique of forces of normalization. Crip theory values the "epistemic friction" (Medina 2013) in which what disability is or what it means to be disabled is a site of important political contestation and negotiation (Kafer 2013, 10). Both crip and queer theory share a political commitment to thinking and imagining otherwise (Sandahl 2003; McRuer 2006; Kafer 2013). In cripping sustainability I take up Stacy Alaimo's (2012, 562) question and ask: Who and what is sustained in sustainability discourse, and for what end? To answer these questions in relation to the meaning of sustainable foodscapes involves considering what is taken for granted as commonsensical about sustainability and whether the meaning of sustainability itself can be reconceived.

"An accessible society," writes Robert McRuer (2006, 94), "is not simply one with ramps and Braille signs on public buildings, but one in which our ways of relating to, and depending on, each other have been reconfigured." Rephrasing McRuer, an accessible foodscape is not simply one with raised garden beds that can be tended from a wheelchair in nursing home greenhouses. Accessible foodscapes are those that crip the meaning of sustainability itself by bringing to the foreground that which has been ignored in heteronormative and ableist idealizations of the family farm and table. In her discussion of nature as a built environment that reflects a heterosexist and able-bodied imaginary, Kafer (2013) considers how paths built for experiencing nature are often inaccessible for many disabled people. She points out that this built barrier that restricts nature experiences for many disabled people reflects and reinforces the assumption that disability is abnormal and unnatural and that disabled people do not belong in nature (131–32). My investigation of the heteronormative and able-bodied farm-to-table imaginary in contemporary food writing will proceed along the following paths: the path toward a common future that informs the Brundtland Commission's definition of sustainability, the path from the farm to the table that is so frequently celebrated in the U.S. alternative food movement, and the path toward cripping sustainability and realizing food justice.

Common Future, Common World

The Brundtland Commission's 1987 definition of sustainability has become, as Emma Foster (2011) puts it, part of the "common sense" within U.S. environmentalism and political and corporate appropriations of the discourse of sustainability. Today, in fact, it seems everything can become green, including capitalism, the military, and prisons (Parr 2009; Ridgeway 2011). Sustainability has become, in a word, institutionalized (Alaimo 2012). According to Foster (2011, 137), sustainability discourse's status as common sense enables it to circulate uncritically as a mode of environmental governmentality.

With its emphasis on the responsibilities of the present to future generations, institutionalized sustainability discourse tends to adopt a reproductive logic that assumes a seamless, untroubled line of inheritance that unites past, present, and future.[4] This line is seamless in the sense that it assumes a stable inheritance that can be retrieved, preserved, and passed on to future generations, provided we act now to adopt a more sustainable way of living or return to a simpler way of life. Jeremy Caradonna (2014, 17) asserts that the theme of return in sustainability tends to reject "industrialized society as weak and vulnerable to collapse, while the reorientation toward the local is offered as a strategy for societal resilience." In its orientation toward resilience, sustainability turns away from and denies loss. Industrialization and its resulting climate change have led to a loss of ecological and social integrity, and sustainability proposes to remedy loss by restoring balance and stability (20).

Aldo Leopold's (1966, 262) land ethic defines good action as that which "preserves the stability, integrity, and beauty of the biotic community." His philosophy continues to shape understanding about sustainability in mainstream U.S. environmentalism. But while Leopold offers an important critique of thinking about the value of the biotic community in exclusively economic terms, the concepts of stability and integrity (both of which he considers part of beauty) reinforce, even if unintentionally, ableist, heteronormative, and classist values. For example, in the United States stability is associated with home and property ownership,[5] heterosexuality, and nuclear families. Leopold himself emphasizes ethical actions of landowners (251), claiming that one can be ethical only toward that which one "can see, feel, understand, love, or otherwise have faith in" (251). While he admits the existence of (and critiques) unethical landowners, he also presents landownership as a potential opening for the development of familiarity that can lead to a more ethical relationship with the land.

To value stability is to value that which remains fixed and unaffected by change, a stance that devalues changing bodies and places. Similarly to value integrity is to value wholeness and to devalue incompleteness and brokenness. The devaluation of impurity and changing bodies and places that is associated with stability and integrity has informed heteronormativity, classism, racism, ableism, and sexism. The values of integrity and stability lead to a characterization of sustainability as resilience in the face of that which threatens to undo the present.

Within mainstream sustainability discourse the individual is responsible for working to restore balance and stability through acts that reestablish forgotten connections to land. By living within the confines of nature, humans can, this literature suggests, restore balance and leave a world that is as good for future generations. This theme is reflected in both Leopold's and Wendell Berry's (2009) discussion of the problem of the broken relationship between humans and land (or nature). Interestingly both emphasize the importance of farm ownership and farm labor as central to sustainability. Leopold (1966, 6–7) writes, "There are two spiritual dangers in not owning a farm. One is the danger of supposing that breakfast comes from the grocery, and the other that heat comes from the furnace. To avoid the first danger, one should plant a garden, preferably where there is no grocer to confuse the issue. To avoid the second, he should lay a split of good oak on the andirons, preferably where there is no furnace, and let it warm his shins while a February blizzard tosses the trees outside." As this passage makes clear, for Leopold restoring forgotten connections to the land community requires an ability to own and to labor on the land. It requires planting a garden, splitting one's own wood, and living far from grocery stores and furnaces. Disability is absent from, and in many ways incompatible with, this scene of reconnection. Leopold's discussion of the importance of farm ownership also ignores the histories of racism and classism that have resulted in the fact that most U.S. farms are owned by white people (Green et al. 2011; Getz 2011).

For his part Berry (2009) expresses concern about the emptying out of rural communities that he associates with the disappearing family farm in the age of agribusiness. Berry defines family farms as those farms that have been tended by the same family for at least three generations (32). He suggests that farms (and thus farm families) thrive when they operate according to the principle of "nature as measure" (7). Using nature as a guide, according to Berry, is crucial for the survival of rural agricultural communities, the family farms that are central to those communities, nature itself, and all humans because we must eat and cannot eat well in the absence of thriving family farms. Berry writes, "As the old have died, they have not been replaced; as the young come of age, they leave farming or leave the community. And as the land and the people deteriorate, so necessarily must the support system. None of the small rural towns is thriving as it did forty years ago" (4). For Berry the disruption of the line of inheritance, the line in which the old leave their way of life to the young who take their place, is at the heart of the disintegration of rural communities and the entire food system.

In their important efforts to name the cause of and connections between environmental and social devastation, both Leopold and Berry romanticize the family farm and rural life, a romanticization that denies the messiness and violence of the family and the past in favor of visions of a lost coherence that can be recovered through a right relationship to the land. Their nostalgia for the family farm and rural existence positions land as the stable ground of sustainability, as that which must orient conceptions of sustainability. But, as Steve Mentz (2012, 586, 590) points out, the centrality of land to mainstream conceptions of sustainability is odd given the fact that oceans constitute the majority of the Earth. While concerns about "the land" promise to ground sustainability and give it a connection to "reality," it also turns away from the arguable point that the ocean has a greater claim to being our world. Nonetheless the discourse of sustainability privileges land in its farm-to-table imaginary. The centrality of land to ideas about sustainability, according to Mentz, has produced an environmentalism oriented toward stability rather than change and disruption, which are part of the world (587–88). Following the path from farm to table in sustainability literature, I contend, makes visible the centrality of heteronormativity and able-bodiedness to conceptions of sustainability oriented toward the family farm and stability.

From Farm to Table

The family meal is a ubiquitous presence in the foodscape of mainstream sustainability discourse. Presented as both the end of agricultural production and the beginning of repairing damaged health and communities, the family meal is both the romanticized past and the desired future of sustainability. In many ways the family meal is one of the things sustainability wants to preserve and sustain. In the farm-to-table imaginary that informs mainstream ideas about sustainability in the United States, the table is often the point of arrival, the final destination in the sequence of events and interactions that ultimately produce the meal and promise to keep the family together. The table is the class-privileged, heteronormative, and able-bodied site where that meal is consumed by the family. In addition, as Elaine Gerber (2007) and Denise Lance (2007) note, the ritual of the family meal is governed by values of control and self-sufficiency that constitute the table as a site for the production and exclusion of disability. For example, eating at the table involves embodying a whole repertoire of culturally specific rules of appropriate eating. There are rules about what should and should not be eaten, when, and by whom. And there are rules about how one should comport oneself at the table. The scenes of family meals that pepper prevailing ideas about a sustainable foodscape do not include adults who require assistance eating or holding utensils with one's feet. In fact disability is erased from the scene of the sustainable family meal to the extent that it is posited as that which is prevented by sustainable eating practices. Disability, disruption, and vulnerability are conceived as the inevitable, undesirable results of being unsustainable, while able-bodiedness, stability, and integrity are conceived as the results of fidelity to the sustainable path from farm to table.

Class also informs the idealization of the family meal at the table in farm-to-table discourse. Within this discourse the shared family meal at the table is a line of defense against eating practices and lifestyles deemed unhealthy and unproductive. While much emphasis is place on distinguishing between bad and good food, it is assumed that meals at home are shared at the table. Eating on couches, on the floor, or in bed is a scene of shameful rather than healthy eating.[6] As Ahmed (2006) notes, the family table is a site of surveillance and disciplining. Families keep an eye out for that which is out of line, and the scene is defined by expectations that one will stay in one's place within the family. Similarly the dining table in farm-to-table discourse is a site of surveillance of what and how much is eaten; it is presented as crucial to socialization and as a defense against unhealthy and unproductive bodies and relationships.

Consider Michael Pollan's (2013) description of the family meal, quoted in one of this paper's epigraphs, where the purpose of the shared meal at the table is to civilize human beings. While Leopold (1966, 240) understood eating as that which demonstrates human and nonhuman similarity as living beings who are "plain members and citizens," not conquerors, of the land community, Pollan emphasizes human uniqueness in the preparation and consumption of food. Moreover in <u>Cooked: A Natural History of Transformation</u>, Pollan (2013, 1–2) contends that cooking is important because it enables self-sufficiency and freedom from the corporations that have dictated our diets and made us dependent upon them.

In his emphasis on self-sufficiency and independence, Pollan (2013) enacts a heteronormative and able-bodied imaginary of the family meal. The family meal shared at the table is valued for its potential to restore balance through self-sufficient use of nature's resources—a role that defines what it means to be human, for Pollan, and sustains and reproduces the family. The romanticized notion of the shared meal at the family table privatizes and naturalizes the family meal and the family itself.

Consider Pollan's (2013) discussion of gender politics and cooking. While he assures readers that he is not arguing for women's return to the traditional role of cook in the family kitchen and stresses that the kitchen needs to be a place for men and children too (10), his paean to home cooking and the shared family meal is nonetheless informed by an overall obfuscation of power within the home. His consideration of race and southern barbeque notwithstanding, his idealized home kitchens are white and class-privileged. He writes:

It is generally thought that the entrance of women into the workforce is responsible for the collapse of home cooking, but the story turns out to be a little more complicated, and fraught. Yes, women with jobs outside the home spend less time cooking—but so do women <u>without</u> jobs. . . . There is irony in the fact that many of the women who have traded time in the kitchen for time in the workplace are working in the food-service industry, helping to produce meals for other families who no longer have time to cook for themselves. These women are being paid for this cooking, true, yet a substantial part of <u>their</u> pay is going to other corporations to cook <u>their</u> families' meals. (182–83)

Pollan's account of U.S. women's move out of the home and into the food service industry ignores how class and race inform the gender politics of cooking. He falsely universalizes the experiences of white and class-privileged women in the United States and ignores the extent to which the food service industry relies on poor immigrants. As Saru Jayaraman (2013, 2) points out, seven of the ten lowest paying jobs in the United States are in the restaurant industry, in which racism creates a wage gap between white workers and workers of color (18). While Pollan proclaims that women working in food service are paid for their work, he ignores the exploitative conditions of this labor. Furthermore he assumes that women leave home to cook for others in restaurants, but, as Jayaraman reveals, many restaurant workers do not make enough to cover rent. Whether meals at home are prepared by men or women, Pollan's discussion of the importance of home cooking tends to portray it as a key element in sustaining heteronormative and class-privileged family connection.

Pollan (2013) presents the table as the scene where a proper relation to nature can be restored by eliminating one's dependence on processed ingredients. In so doing he relies on a distinction between natural and unnatural ingredients. While cooking certainly modifies foods, as Pollan admits, it is a mode of modification he perceives as most aligned with human species being. As such the proper line from the farm to the family table is through harvesting, hunting, fishing, foraging, or, when those activities are not possible, purchasing foods from people who have harvested, hunted, fished, or foraged for them. Who is able to gather at this scene of good eating, this table? To the extent that the family table is also a line of defense against impure foods and the health problems they cause, it is imagined as a scene where disability is absent and defended against through responsible food choices. This is an idealized scene of family eating that relies upon and perpetuates the stigmatization of disability. Disability thereby appears in this literature as incompatible with sustainability.

Further, in emphasizing local, homemade, and unprocessed ingredients, Pollan (2013) shapes a farm-to-table imaginary that homogenizes a past that was in fact quite diverse in its response to industrialization, so much so that the line between the authentic and the processed, the natural and the unnatural, is more porous than many in the alternative food movement seem to assume. After all, far from being mere objects for consumption, foods are embedded in social, political, cultural, and economic relationships. Those relationships materialize foods and establish their value for eaters. Elizabeth Engelhardt (2011, 8, 9) explains that "the story" of southern food and gender "does not follow a straight line." What is romanticized as the southern meal tends to focus on the homemade and the local, while ignoring the presence of processed ingredients that were also part of what we have come to associate with southern food, for instance, the Duke's mayonnaise on sandwiches and the highly processed white flour used to make the iconic southern biscuit. Some southern foods are natural and local; some are industrial and transnational. Engelhardt writes, "What looked like a quintessential southern drink, iced tea, was a distant remainder on the table of British colonial trade routes to India and China and the Atlantic slave trade triangle of Caribbean sugar, African labor, and European and U.S. capital" (11). Similarly nostalgia for the family meal tends to erase the hierarchies that structure the family, community, and the meal itself.

Idealization of the local ignores the persistence of racism, homophobia, ableism, classism, and sexism within local communities. As Sarah Jaquette Ray (2013, 3) puts it, the locavore movement is informed by a desire for "pure connections to land," by distinctions between "pure" and "impure" foods, people, and practices. Such a movement, she contends, stigmatizes certain foods and the people who eat those foods, creating "ecological others" against which mainstream U.S. environmentalism defines its aims (3). Pollan's (2013, 22) proposed solution is to devote more of "our leisure" time to cooking at home, a solution that assumes class privilege, whiteness, and able-bodiedness.

Pollan's idealization of the family meal echoes Berry's heteronormative farm imaginary. For Berry sustainable agricultural practices rely on, support, and mirror both nature and the division of labor in the patriarchal, heteronormative family unit. In "Nature as Measure," Berry (2009) critiques the destructive impact of industrial agriculture on families, communities, and farms. Farms must be small, and farmers must be able to know and love them as they know and love their neighbors and families (9). The inability to achieve this intimacy in farming "is a condition predisposing to abuse, and abuse has been the result. Rape, indeed, has been the result, and we have seen that we are not exempt from the damage we have inflicted. Now we must think of marriage" (9–10). In other words, small farms, small communities, and patriarchal heteronormative families mirror nature, and sustainable relationships with farms and nature are most appropriately conceptualized as marriage.

So far I have discussed how the table has appeared in prevailing conceptions of sustainable foodscapes as nostalgic, romanticized scenes of a right relationship to nature and as the scene of the family meal that ensures the security of farms and farm communities. What are we to make of these tables? How do these tables orient us in relation to sustainability and food justice? In her discussion of queer phenomenology, Ahmed (2006) reflects on the orienting function of the table in the discipline of philosophy and life. Tables, like other objects, are, for Ahmed, "orientation devices"; they orient us in space, providing direction and perspective. Orientations take a point of view as given (14). When one is oriented in space, one is pointed in a certain direction, enabling one to find one's way. Tables, like other objects in our world, are able to function as orientation devices in large part because of the ideas that constitute them as recognizable objects in our world. Because we are able to recognize those objects, we are able to reach out to them and find our way. It is, in other words, their familiarity, their relationship to our past, that orients us in relation to the familiar object and makes it possible for the object to direct us toward a horizon of possible experience. By contrast, Ahmed explains, when surrounded by unfamiliar objects, we become disoriented and thus unable to find our way.

Like other objects, the table becomes what it is as we turn toward it, and our turning is shaped by assumptions, values, and interactions that direct us in our relationship to it. Orientation, according to Ahmed (2006, 8), establishes the relation between here and there, between the present and the future. Becoming oriented directs one in certain ways that brings some things to our attention and turns us away from other things, relegating them to the background (17).

Following Ahmed (2006, 169), queer moments disrupt familiarity in their presentation of that which seems strange or out of place in a space. To queerly negotiate space is to turn toward more distant, less obvious objects—to take what is in the background and bring it to the foreground (167). Queer orientations move out of line and off the path that points in the direction of that which is deemed good, natural, and normal. Queer orientations enable the emergence of new meanings and new possibilities (169, 171). As Ahmed puts it, "Orientations shape not only how we inhabit space, but how we apprehend the world of shared inheritance, as well as 'who' or 'what' we direct our energy toward. A queer phenomenology . . . might start by redirecting our attention toward different objects, those that are 'less proximate' or even those that deviate or are deviant" (3). A queer table, according to Ahmed, is not so much a matter of who has a seat at the table as how they are oriented toward it and the paths that orientation makes possible.

Ahmed's discussion of queer phenomenology is useful for understanding the heteronormative and able-bodied orientation of much of contemporary food writing, an orientation in which the farm-to-table narrative treads the well-worn path of idealizing the heteronormative family and erasing and pathologizing disability. Rather than understanding disability and queerness as alternative resources for reconceptualizing sustainability, the line from farm to table relegates both to the background. The family meal and the family farm are presented as vital to individual and community well-being. Queers and crips have no place in this family portrait of sustainability. Put another way, idealizations of the happy family meal are made possible by turning away from and relegating to the background queer crip lives and experiences.

Cripping Sustainability

How might our understanding of and orientation in foodscapes shift if we crip sustainability, drawing attention to what is ignored, kept out of reach and in the background in the line from farm to table? To crip sustainability means valuing disability as a source of insight about how the border between the natural and the unnatural is maintained and for whose benefit. It means understanding a sustainable world as a world that has disability in it, a perspective that recognizes the instabilities, vulnerabilities, and dynamism that are part of naturecultures. Cripping sustainability resists understandings of sustainability that are oriented toward a preservation of the same in the future. It means, as Kafer (2013, 142) puts it, "approaching nature through the lens of loss and ambivalence." It means not turning away from the wounds of the world that disrupt ideals of stability, integrity, and beauty. Cripping sustainability attends to those who are left out of the picture of the perfect, happy family meal. In its orientation toward stability and security that seeks a straight line of inheritance connecting past, present, and future, heteronormative and able-bodied farm-to-table imaginaries fail to attend to alternatives that could move closer to realizing food justice. Queer, for Ahmed (2006, 178), names that which refuses to follow a straight "line of inheritance," opting instead for other possibilities of inhabiting the world (178).

So what are examples of an alternative way of dwelling in the world occasioned by cripping sustainability? One is ways of living in the world that trouble straight lines by striving to attend to that which is kept in the background and, thus, resist the forces that work to keep it out of view. To think about this, I turn to two paintings of tables: Normal Rockwell's iconic Freedom from Want (1943; figure 15.1) and Frank Moore's Freedom to Share (1994; figure 15.2). Rockwell's painting depicts an all-white family seated at the table, enjoying each other's company, while the grandfather and grandmother stand and present a huge roasted turkey. The grandmother wears an apron and is setting down the turkey platter at its assigned place at the head of the table, indicating that she has prepared the feast. The grandfather stands behind her, waiting to carve the bird and take his place at the head of the table. Rockwell's painting has come to represent the ideal of the American family. It is also a good illustration of how the table is an orienting device in the heteronormative and able-bodied ideal of the family meal. Each person gathered at the table has an assigned place in the family line and within the context of white supremacy. The family's racial homogeneity is a sign that it has stayed in line and thus reproduced both whiteness and heteronormativity. Any visible marker of disability is hidden from view. The family is also free from want; everything family members need is around and on the table.

Compare Rockwell's painting to Moore's. Moore was a gay AIDS activist who died of HIV/AIDS in 2002. He was also the designer of the red ribbon for AIDS activism and awareness. In Freedom to Share the viewer is presented with a defamiliarization of Rockwell's scene of American family togetherness. In inviting the viewer to "look and look again" (Smith 2012), Moore brings to the foreground some of what remains hidden in Rockwell's painting, and indeed, as the painting hints, all family stories. Moore's painting brilliantly critiques the myriad disabling effects of the industrial food system, pharmaceutical industry, and heteronormative family and simultaneously foregrounds (without pathologizing) that which remains hidden, erased, ignored, and rendered impossible and unthinkable in Rockwell's painting.

First, Moore's family disrupts the whiteness of Rockwell's American family ideal and portrays the family meal as an interracial gathering. In doing so Moore makes explicit the myth of purity

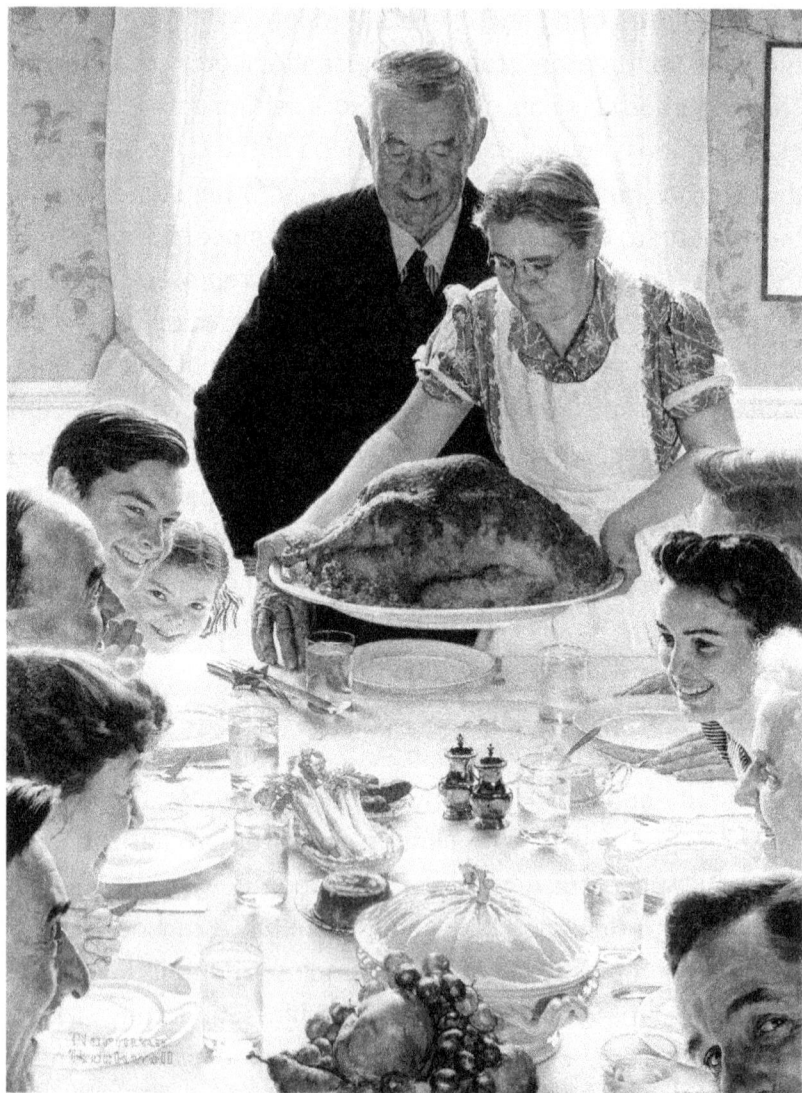

Fig. 15.1. Norman Rockwell, <u>Freedom from Want</u>, 1943. Reprinted by permission of the Norman Rockwell Family Agency. Copyright © 1943 the Norman Rockwell Family Entities.

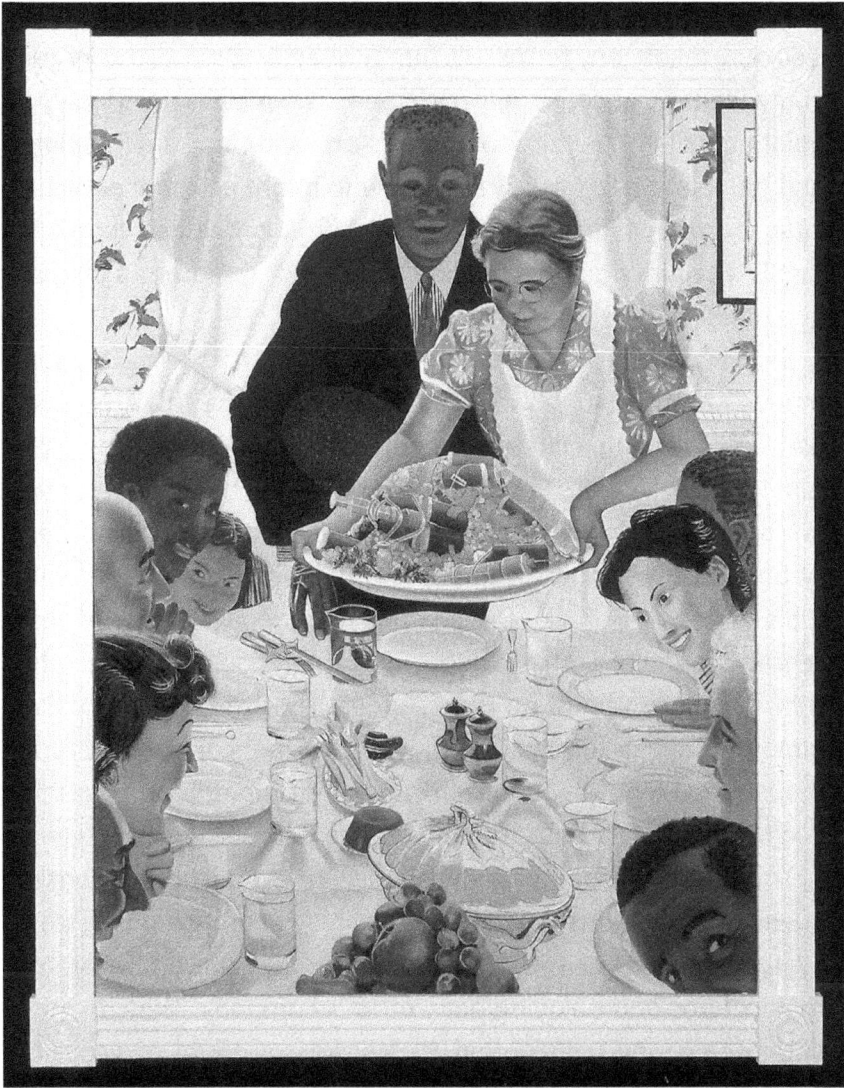

Fig. 15.2. Frank Moore, <u>Freedom to Share</u>, 1994, oil and glass beads on canvas on wood with frame, 60 × 46 in. © Gesso Foundation/Frank Moore Estate. Courtesy of Sperone Westwater, New York.

that defines assumptions about whiteness and implies that families may take many forms. His family queerly disrupts the image of the ideal American family portrayed in Rockwell's painting. The painting's title, Freedom to Share, is an invitation to participate and an opening to possible others who might be there or arrive later. By contrast Rockwell's Freedom from Want underscores the family's security against outside forces that threaten to disrupt and undo it.

Second, Moore draws attention to the fact that the heteronormative American family ideal itself, as well as the "all-American diet," is making us, and the animals consumed at the American family table, sick. Instead of serving a turkey the grandmother in Moore's painting presents a platter filled with pills, pill bottles, IV bags, and syringes. A queer crip perspective on the family table portrayed in Rockwell's painting might notice that everyone seated around the table is happy and laughing and wonder why that is. Moore's painting may suggest that the illusion of the happy American family (and the happy American family meal) is sustained by many pharmaceuticals that numb participants against the dysfunctions that threaten to disrupt the happy scene.

Third, Moore's painting makes visible the disabling consequences of the industrial food system in a nonpathologizing way. Everyone seated at the table is eagerly anticipating his or her medications and enjoying each other's company. They are disabled and happy, a disruption of ableist associations of disability with tragedy and unhappiness. At the same time the presence of pharmaceuticals critiques the food industry and nostalgic scenes of happy family gatherings. Happiness, pain, and woundedness are entangled in this scene and create a productive tension for opening more critical, resistant thinking about the shared meal, families, and disability than those found in the mainstream U.S. food movement.

Fourth, Moore's painting does what the United States does not do with HIV/AIDS or any other disease: it makes treatment freely available to all who need it. While Rockwell's painting depicts a family giving thanks for the fact that their private needs have been met (they are free from want), Moore's painting emphasizes community responsibility and sharing with others (freedom to share). Rockwell's table is closed and inaccessible to others, who can look and want but not share. Moore's table, by contrast, remains open to those who aren't there but who are invited to share.

Moore presents a view of disability that is not romanticized or pathologized. All seated at the table need their medications and want to share them with others who also need them. Disability is depicted as part of a desired community. While Moore's painting points to the industrial food system as harmful to health, he leaves room for multiple possible disability identifications. Disability in Moore's painting is a point of departure for political critique and a site of community, family, and coalition. Its political orientation toward disability characterizes the painting's queer crip perspective. While Freedom from Want reflects the white, heteronormative, and able-bodied family seated around the table that is idealized as the desired goal in much contemporary food writing, Freedom to Share presents an example of how cripping sustainability and sustainable foodscapes opens the possibility of realizing a more coalitional conception of food justice that attends to, rather than ignores, other modes of injustice and the connections between them.

NOTES

1. See Cuomo 2011 for a discussion of how emphasizing the vulnerability of indigenous populations devalues their epistemic agency.
2. My critique of the flattening and homogenizing of foodscapes is indebted to Sarah Jaquette Ray's (2013) critique of how the landscape appears in environmentalist literature. Despite its commitment to place and the local, environmentalism tends to ignore the complex histories and social hierarchies that shape place and various degrees of agency in place (25–30).
3. See Medina 2013 for more about the resistant imagination.
4. Lee Edelman (2004) also critiques the concept of the future as reproductive and heteronormative. For a queer crip feminist engagement with Edelman's discussion that shares Edelman's critique of heteronormative futures while rejecting the notion that the future is necessarily heteronormative, see Kafer 2013; Hall 2014.
5. Many thanks to Sarah Jaquette Ray and Jay Sibara for pointing out the connections between stability and property ownership in the United States.
6. Thanks to Ray and Sibara for suggesting this example of eating on couches.

REFERENCES

Ahmed, Sara. 2006. Queer Phenomenology: Orientations, Objects, Others. Durham NC: Duke University Press.

Alaimo, Stacy. 2010. Bodily Natures: Science, Environment, and the Material Self. Bloomington: Indiana University Press.

———. 2012. "Sustainable This, Sustainable That: New Materialisms, Posthumanism, and Unknown Futures." PMLA 127, no. 3: 558–64.

Berry, Wendell. 2009. Bringing It to the Table: On Farming and Food. Berkeley: Counterpoint.

Caradonna, Jeremy L. 2014. Sustainability: A History. New York: Oxford University Press.

Cuomo, Chris J. 2011. "Climate Change, Vulnerability and Responsibility." Hypatia: Journal of Feminist Philosophy 26, no. 4: 690–714.

Edelman, Lee. 2004. No Future: Queer Theory and the Death Drive. Durham NC: Duke University Press.

Engelhardt, Elizabeth D. 2011. A Mess of Greens: Southern Gender and Southern Food. Athens: University of Georgia Press.

Foster, Emma A. 2011. "Sustainable Development: Problematizing Normative Constructions of Gender within Global Environmental Governmentality." Globalizations 8, no. 2: 135–49.

Gardiner, Stephen M. 2011. A Perfect Moral Storm: The Ethical Tragedy of Climate Change. Oxford: Oxford University Press.

Gerber, Elaine. 2007. "Food Studies and Disability Studies: Introducing a Happy Marriage." Disability Studies Quarterly 27, no. 3. http://dsq-sds.org/article/view/19/19.

Getz, Christy. 2011. "Race and Regulation: Asian Immigrants in California Agriculture." In Cultivating Food Justice: Race, Class, and Sustainability, edited by Alison Hope Alkon and Julian Agyeman, 65–85. Cambridge MA: MIT Press.

Green, John J., Eleanor M. Green, and Anna M. Kleiner. 2011. "From the Past to the Present: Agricultural Development and Black Farmers in the American South." In Cultivating Food Justice: Race, Class, and Sustainability, edited by Alison Hope Alkon and Julian Agyeman, 47–64. Cambridge MA: MIT Press.

Hall, Kim Q. 2014. "No Failure: Climate Change, Radical Hope, and Queer Crip Feminist Eco Futures." Radical Philosophy Review 17, no. 1: 203–25.

Jamieson, Dale. 2008. Ethics and the Environment: An Introduction. Cambridge, UK: Cambridge University Press.

Jayaraman, Saru. 2013. Behind the Kitchen Door. Ithaca NY: Cornell University Press.

Kafer, Alison. 2013. Feminist Queer Crip. Bloomington: Indiana University Press.

Lance, G. Denise. 2007. "Do the Hands That Feed Us Also Hold Us Back? Implications of Assisted Eating." Disability Studies Quarterly 27, no. 3. http://dsq-sds.org/article/view/23.

Leopold, Aldo. 1966. A Sand County Almanac. New York: Ballantine Books.

McRuer, Robert. 2006. Crip Theory: Cultural Signs of Queerness and Disability. New York: New York University Press.

Medina, José. 2013. The Epistemology of Resistance: Gender and Racial Oppression, Epistemic Injustice, and Resistant Imaginations. New York: Oxford University Press.

Mentz, Steve. 2012. "After Sustainability." <u>PMLA</u> 127, no. 3: 586–92.

Parr, Adrian. 2009. <u>Hijacking Sustainability</u>. Cambridge MA: MIT Press.

Pollan, Michael. 2013. <u>Cooked: A Natural History of Transformation</u>. New York: Penguin.

Ray, Sarah Jaquette. 2013. <u>The Ecological Other: Environmental Exclusion in American Culture</u>. Tucson: University of Arizona Press.

Ridgeway, James. 2011. "The Overseer." <u>Mother Jones</u> 46, no. 4: 44–51.

Sandahl, Carrie. 2003. "Queering the Crip or Cripping the Queer? Intersections of Queer and Crip Identities in Solo Autobiographical Performance." <u>GLQ: A Journal of Gay and Lesbian Studies</u> 9, nos. 1–2: 25–56.

Smith, Roberta. 2012. "Where Anxieties Roam: 'Toxic Beauty: The Art of Frank Moore' at N.Y.U." <u>New York Times</u>, September 6. http://www.nytimes.com/2012/09/07/arts/design/toxic-beauty-the-art-of-frank-moore-at-nyu.html?_r=0.

World Commission on Environment and Development. 1987. <u>Our Common Future</u>. New York: Oxford University Press.

Section 4   CURING CRIPS?
NARRATIVES OF
HEALTH AND SPACE

16

The Invalid Sea

Disability Studies and Environmental Justice History

Traci Brynne Voyles

Invalidism and Invalidity in the Desert

The Salton Sea is a body of water of almost five hundred square miles east of San Diego and southeast of Los Angeles in southern California's Riverside and Imperial counties. It sits in a deep basin sunk hundreds of feet below sea level, in the mountain-ringed Colorado Desert, named for the Colorado River, which borders it on the east. If you have heard of the Salton Sea, you probably know it for its notorious environmental problems, possibly for the number of spectacularly large fish and bird die-offs that have occurred there in the past three decades. The Salton Sea has been called an environmental disaster, a dying sea, a sewer, "nature's magnificent mistake," and "a death trap for wildlife."[1] Almost in the same breath, however, the sea is known as one of the most important water resources for migrating birds in the Southwest and a major stopover on the Pacific Flyway. As such the Salton Sea hosts more diverse bird populations than even the Florida Everglades—by one count as many as 3.5 million birds on any given day.[2] Because of the near wholesale destruction of most other southern California wetlands, the Salton Sea is a crucial resource for these birds, many species of which are threatened or endangered.

Since the 1920s the Salton Sea's water level has been sustained almost entirely by drainage from the farms of the Imperial and Coachella valleys and inflow from the Alamo and New rivers, which originate in Mexico and are both considered among the most polluted waterways in the United States.[3] As the sea's water evaporates under the fierce desert sun, heavy metals and carcinogens—to say nothing of salt—become increasingly concentrated, making the salinity levels 50 percent higher than the Pacific Ocean's (and climbing).[4] The sea is clearly a study in contradictions, so much so that it reveals the limitations of the vocabulary we use to describe environments: it can be described neither as entirely natural nor entirely human-made; it is both an astoundingly rich environmental resource and an astoundingly polluted hazardscape; it is a wetland in a desert. It is most frequently described in the news media as a "dying sea," to the annoyance of scientists who tout its biodiversity and ability to support a wide range of wildlife despite its environmental challenges.[5]

This state of contradictions leaves writers of all kinds—scholars, journalists, bloggers—at loose ends when it comes to describing the Salton Sea; is it "a natural wonder, a national embarrassment, paradise, [or] the ecological equivalent of the Chernobyl disaster"?[6] In a series of articles over the course of more than a decade, the Los Angeles Times has taken to describing the Salton Sea as "California's environmental invalid" and a "sickly sea," descriptors that put a fine point on general understandings of the sea as diseased, moribund, and deeply in need of recuperation.[7] These intimations about the state of the sea, caught up as they are in socially constructed ideas about health and ill health, are damning in a discursive context in which "Americans, the celebrants of robust heartiness and self-sufficiency, are suspicious of illness" as being the fault of those marked as "ill."[8]

The Salton Sea as an "environmental invalid," a "sickly" or "dying" sea, thus provides an appropriate node from which to explore the resonances between environments and ability (and disability) and between ideas about "valid" and "invalid" human bodies as well as bodies in nature. "Invalidity," or sickliness, has long been used to mark people as Other; in Margaret Atwood's prose an invalid is simply "one who has been invalidated."[9] Invalidism, in short, is a social construction that changes over time, space, and culture to mark bodies seen as nonnormative or sickly and also to relationally construct healthy as a normative bodily state. The cultural figure or trope of the invalid has very particular resonances with regard to gender, race, and social and environmental location, which I explore more closely below. Like invalidity (being invalidated), disability "takes much of its meaning from the coordinate concept of able bodied," according to Bonnie Smith; in this sense viewing the Salton Sea as an environmental invalid—in other words viewing it principally through culturally and historically specific notions of disease, disability, and, crucially, dependence—requires an implicit agreement about what constitutes a valid or able environment.[10] Moreover illness, whether for human bodies or sickly seas, "is experienced by both sick and robust bodies," making ill health not so much an objective, unchanging state as "a jumble of ideas that shifts among groups over time" and "a cultural artifact configured in . . . bodies."[11]

In this essay I explore the multiple social constructions of invalidism and invalidity in the history of the Salton Sea and the desert surrounding it, both "invalid" as in constructed notions of infirmity, convalescence, weakness, and disease, and, relatedly, "invalidation," as in viewing something or someone as unacceptable, unsound, or illogical. To imagine the Salton Sea as an environmental invalid is to implicate it as both invalid and invalidated and, perhaps more urgently, to mark it with social signifiers of invalidity, ill health, and disability that have historically been used to shore up what the disability studies scholar Alison Kafer and others call "compulsory able-bodiedness."[12] Moreover to see the Salton Sea as an environmental invalid is to envision it as itself a pollutant to the Colorado Desert, something unnatural, impure, diseased or disease-causing, and intimately bound to <u>human</u> rather than natural history (as though those histories can be divorced). After all, what is pollution but that which invalidates an environment, rendering it impure or in need of remedy and recuperation? The fact that the Salton Sea's creation can be seen as perhaps the ultimate hybrid between nature and culture, between the organic and the technological, makes its twentieth-century relegation to the deeply human realm of pollution that much more ripe for analysis.

The Salton Sea, as it turns out, is not the first occupant of this part of California to be marked as invalid, sickly, or diseased. From the late 1880s to the early 1910s this part of California was perhaps best known for its reputation in hosting sanitariums and health resorts for "health seekers": people with ailments or perceived ailments ranging from tuberculosis and rheumatism to asthma and insomnia, hysteria and neurasthenia.[13] Many of these health seekers arrived in the desert having been multiply dislocated: first from eastern cities, traveling to southern California as part of a transformative "health rush" that populated cities like Los Angeles with tens of thousands of what one historian described as "rich, idle, aging, and sickly [white] Americans" and plenty of people of ill health who were neither rich nor white.[14] Their second dislocation from the city to the desert occurred once tuberculosis, by far the most common health complaint among these new denizens of Los Angeles (who Stanford University's David Starr Jordan referred to as the "one-lunged people" of southern California), was confirmed to be highly contagious, at which point "visibly diseased guests were no longer welcome" in Los

Angeles hotels, and rampant disdain for sickliness pushed people out of cities to "isolated desert quarantine stations."[15] A group of Los Angeles doctors, in fact, requested that the State Board of Health deport people infected with tuberculosis, evidence of the way compulsory able-bodiedness functions through institutionalized practices of physical force and coercion.[16]

I read these two histories of invalidism and invalidation in the desert (first, the push to move people of ill health out of the city and, second, the push to view the Salton Sea itself as a sickly environmental invalid) as deeply connected components of the region's larger environmental history. The link between them is not causal; one did not lead to or precipitate the other in any strict sense (although I argue that making the desert a settlement for people marked as invalids and shunted east into the desert was causally related to Americans' larger attitude toward deserts as Othered ecologies and invalids as Othered bodies). But neither is the link merely metaphorical; it is rather a conceptual tool, a way of looking at the environmental history of this region that can help us more fully understand how to think about and act on environmental problems that defy standard categories of culture and nature, human and nonhuman. I look to the ways late nineteenth-century invalids were marked as diseased or sickly bodies through related understandings of environment, race, and gender, and I look to the Salton Sea through the lens of social constructions of human (discursive) disablement, invalidity, and invalidation. As the environmental historian Linda Nash points out, when we "focus on the human body" in environmental history, "the boundary between the human and nonhuman world, the actors and their objects, becomes much more fuzzy and the distinction much more tenuous." I propose to take up this project and add a kind of productive inversion: to focus on the Salton Sea as a body and itself an agent of change. Human and environmental bodies alike can be seen as both "agents of environmental change but also objects of that change."[17] These shifting roles of human bodies and bodies of water become increasingly important to how we imagine, describe, and react to conundrums in the socionatural world around us.

What does it mean for a sea to be an invalid? What would constitute a valid sea? What implications does this projection of human notions of sickness and disability (and, by extension, ability) onto landscapes have for how we imagine and engage with nonhuman nature? What promises does invalid nature hold for a postenvironmental future? I explore these questions, arguing that the meaning projected onto the Salton Sea, the surrounding desert, and various of its human denizens has long been caught up in ideas of validity, invalidity, gender, race, and ability—in other words, notions of <u>human</u> and social difference projected onto the nonhuman world.

Invalidation and the Desert

Invalidism in the United States in the late nineteenth and early twentieth century was to a large extent imagined to be an effect of one's environment and social location.[18] Middle- and upper-class easterners in increasingly crowded cities with increasingly sedentary lifestyles were seen to take sick because of the weakened state of their bodies and being forced to constantly breathe in the "foul air" of a "sheltered life." Throughout the West the draw of arching skies and low population density was often imbricated in the promotion of good health. In western states and territories sanitariums cropped up designed specifically to attract easterners of ill health, particularly those suffering from respiratory diseases. Southern California stood out as one of the most attractive of these "healthy" western regions, and southern California boosters touted the glories of the area's fresh air for "debilitated mankind."[19] Railroad companies were a powerful institution in promoting the region "to catch the early influx of invalids" from the East.[20] The vigorous outdoor lifestyle that characterized southern California was a powerful counterpoint to the closed-in, crowded lifestyle of eastern cities, with their foul and polluted air. Southern California's Colorado Desert in particular was seen as having "no equal in America," with a "warm, dry climate" that was "an elixir for the invalid, especially those afflicted with throat and lung trouble and rheumatism."[21]

People who were deemed invalids, this subset of "debilitated mankind" who were told they could be cured by fresh air, dry climate, and open vistas, were environmental invalids in the sense that it was their environment—closed in, overcrowded, cold, and befouled—that, so the thinking went, had made them sick in the first place. A different environment could be their salvation, an "elixir" for their ailments. Concerns over the "health rush" to California, however, made people who were perceived as invalids in another sense environmentally invalidated: as they arrived in increasing numbers in southern California cities, anxieties arose that the chronically ill were themselves a threat to the perceived healthiness of the state. One journalist compared their diseased bodies directly to environmental pollution, arguing, "Like the oil derricks in the city . . . we shall probably have to consider this branch of immigration as a necessary evil." (Luckily there was an upside: "in both cases" of the "health rush" and oil derricks "there is a considerable revenue derived.")[22] Also of concern, Europeans too "select[ed] California as the burial ground for their sick rather than the Riviera and the hills of Algeria."[23] At a time when immigration from Europe, particularly from the racially maligned southern and eastern European countries, was a (rather hyperbolic) concern across the United States, the convergence of immigration and disease was particularly troubling.[24]

The "tubercular" or "consumptive" was a notorious cultural trope, a signifier of the (often highly racialized) threat of contagion and an inverse corollary of the imagined healthy subject. The consumptive was "a physical wreck—pale, haggard, and debilitated" in the popular imagination.[25] This powerful trope justified quarantine, segregation, and institutionalization of people suspected of having tuberculosis, just as related tropes have long shored up such policies to coerce and control people deemed disabled, diseased, or infectious.[26] During this time tuberculosis was compared to leprosy, and more than one public health official suggested that "marriage between the infected should be looked upon as a crime," gesturing not only to the stigma attached to ill health but also to the use of biopolitical social policy about marriage and reproduction to shape population outcomes.[27]

Increasingly the solution to hosting California's health seekers, particularly those suffering from tuberculosis, was to construct sanitariums far from coastal cities and towns. The Colorado Desert, just east of San Diego and southeast of Los Angeles, provided an ideal location for this kind of segregation and institutionalization. Sending consumptives to the desert served two ends: it removed the risk of infection from the more densely populated coastal cities and increased the possibility of their being cured by the preferable environmental conditions of the desert climate. By the mid-1890s the Colorado Desert was "conceded to be the ideal location for the planting of tuberculosis," which was an "imperative" move, "when we come to consider the formidable numbers that come to this Coast every year from all parts of the world—come here in all likelihood to die."[28] In time, some suggested, "the high mountain regions of Southern California and out on the desert" would contain whole "settlements" for invalids "where diseases of the lungs will be made a specialty."[29] Palm Springs, for example, was touted as having mineral springs with "waters

[that] are most efficacious for the cure of rheumatism."[30] At Indio a large hotel catered to "such invalids whose presence by reason of their infirmities would be irksome to the general public."[31] It is worth noting that, while moving these contagious individuals from the coastal cities would certainly protect those cities from the risk of infectious diseases, moving them to settlements in the deserts exposed an entirely different population to the threat of tuberculosis: the Natives who still outnumbered non-Natives in the Colorado Desert by a significant margin and who often provided the labor that built, maintained, and served the desert's sanitariums, hot springs hotels, and other infrastructure.[32]

Culturally the figure of the invalid has taken on specifically gendered and classed meanings. As the historian Diane Price Herndl points out, regardless of actual rates of diagnosis of maladies, "invalidism" has been closely aligned with the nineteenth-century, middle- or upper-class "sickly woman" trapped in the ideological and embodied effects of the "cult of female frailty."[33] The "urbanization of the United States and the shift to industrial capitalism," as Herndl puts it, produced a "dynamic struggle among competing ideologies to define gender roles (for both sexes) and to gain control of people's bodies. Increasingly, this conflict became a struggle to define women's bodies as sickly."[34] Conditions of "nervous prostration"—neurasthenia, hysteria, anxiety, insomnia—were largely seen as the effect of the emasculating tendencies of late nineteenth-century modern middle- and upper-class lifestyles, particularly in cities. Cures for these ailments, famously taken by none other than Theodore Roosevelt, who claimed his childhood asthma was cured by his living "the strenuous life," were often located in the ruggedly masculine open air of the West, where the effete environment of eastern city life was countered by wide western skies, rough climbs up rocky mountain passes, and the manly thrills of big game hunting.

Invalidism, in short, was feminized in distinct ways: as weakness rather than strength, dependence rather than independence, sickliness, frailty, urban rather than rural. Women and men of poor health were thus similarly feminized within their bodily and environmental contexts. The influx of health seekers to the Colorado Desert, dislocated from eastern and then from California cities, was likewise predicated on the (imagined) benefits of the rugged outdoor life on the (imagined) physically weak, effete, or feminized body. As these feminized invalids sought to gain strength from the clear air and warm climate, the desert itself took on feminine characteristics: it was the nurturer, the home, the all-sacrificing source of endless comfort, the private space of recovery—characteristics central to the notion of white femininity as enshrined in the Cult of True Womanhood. Invalids, according to the logic of the time, were understandably drawn "from the hyperborean East to the sensuous West."[35]

This feminization of the desert, however, was a slippery thing. While providing good motherly nurturance, the desert could not entirely escape the American environmental imagination that regarded deserts generally with anxiety and apprehension. The result: a feminized desert that tended to fluctuate from a glorified to a threatening femininity, from sensuous and nurturing to scary and inconstant. The Palm Springs mineral bath, for example, though "remarkable" in its curative abilities, was "as variable in its moods as a woman. Now a quiet pool of water, then again a bubbling, fretful lake, and then again a seething, howling, hissing, mud-spouting volcano."[36] These inconstant slippages between glorified and threatening femininity reflected larger racializations and class characterizations of women, particularly mothers, at the time. While middle- and upper-class white women were revered as the site of True Womanhood, mothers of color and working-class mothers were generally regarded with apprehension as the literal and figurative sites of the reproduction of unwanted bodies.[37] The historian Lorna Duffin points out that "middle-class women in the home were pure" even when afflicted with illness, but "working-class women outside the home were able-bodied but contaminated and sickening," threats to both racial purity and environmental health.[38] This slippage between glorified and "sickening" femininity was highly local: the Native tribes of California were alternately seen as an unredeemably savage menace or a submissive and romantic bunch. The contradiction in these two racializations is exemplified in two highly influential nineteenth-century literary treatments: Mark Twain's 1872 travel book <u>Roughing It</u>, wherein he famously dubs California Natives "the despised" "Digger Indians," and Helen Hunt Jackson's 1884 novella <u>Ramona</u>, in which southern California tribes are humanized and romanticized (and the violent racism of white California settlers taken considerably to task).[39] This is a familiar racial binary in which representations of people of color jolt "from subhuman to superhuman," but they "are rarely perceived as being [simply] human."[40]

The ideological and material uses of the Colorado Desert during this time thus came to revolve around two related recuperations of the feminized: the recuperation of the (monstrous and diseased) feminized invalid body and the recuperation of the (nurturing yet unpredictable) feminized desert environment. Through hosting settlements of the sickly and thus providing a regional barrier "protecting the well from the sick,"[41] the desert took on meaning and purpose that distinguished it from its previous identity as unredeemable wasteland.

The Salton Sea, Environmental Invalid

Even as desert towns like Indio were busily building sanitariums for the sick, plans were under way that would again transform the environmental and sociopolitical history of the Colorado Desert in dramatic ways. The desert, which featured a basin that dipped two hundred feet below sea level, known as the Salton sink, had long been the setting of various irrigation schemes that envisioned rich farmlands nourished by water diverted from the Colorado River. The fact that this sink had once been a great sea, which geologists called Lake Cahuilla, told would-be developers that it had potentially rich soil, but it didn't seem to indicate to them that it might once again be filled with a great inland body of water. The feminized desert that "sooth[ed]" invalids required only "water to convert it into a productive [read: masculine] region."⁴²

By the fall of 1904 this transition from a desert that nurtured those seen as convalescent and infirm to a desert deeply imbricated in the masculine project of productive yeoman agriculturalism seemed to be off to a successful start. The fact that the burgeoning Imperial Valley farms were seen as a wholesale (and, again, successful) manipulation of nature only bolstered the triumphant glee of developers; as one writer put it, the success of the valley came from "the systematic and thorough operations that will ultimately hold the [Colorado River] in perpetual bondage," and in turn allow "fecund Mother Earth [to] continue to pour forth her abundant riches."⁴³ The Imperial settlers, the desert, and the river, in short, were linked in a kind of patriarchal matrimony, she in "perpetual bondage" and limited to a "fecund" reproductive capacity, he in a productive role of using her resources to remake the world.

This "perpetual bondage" of the West's most powerful river was famously short-lived: in the winter of 1905 the Colorado River began to flood the Salton sink, as it had many times before, inundating small towns, drowning settlers' new fields of melon, asparagus, and alfalfa, chasing the railroad out of the desert basin, and cutting enormous new courses—some more than one hundred feet deep—through the dry desert soil as it rushed downhill to the Salton sink.[44] It took nearly two years, thousands of laborers (many of them Native workers culled from the local tribes, many others Mexican and Mexican American), and hundreds of thousands of pounds of dirt and rock to stop the flooding. During these months of flooding the Colorado River re-created a smaller version of Lake Cahuilla, the Salton Sea, inundating almost five hundred miles of the sink by the time the floods were controlled in the winter of 1907. The floods had quickly remade the ecology of the desert, wiping out stands of mesquite trees and dispersing their seeds, bringing "vast numbers of aquatic birds—ducks, geese and pelicans," as well as freshwater fish swimming "above the desert floor where men had died of thirst."[45]

At first settlers and outside observers looked on the new Salton Sea with a kind of startled wonder. For Imperial Valley settlers the floods had been a violent undoing of the heady triumph of desert reclamation, and the role of nature in westward expansion in general. For the larger American public who read newspaper accounts of the floods the "extraordinary picture of a great railroad," the Southern Pacific, "being chased over a bone-dry desert by a flood" was an unsettling image of nature displacing the very technology that symbolized and served westward expansion.[46] (Certainly the flood "chasing" out the railroad served as a dramatic counterpoint to the image of the railroad barreling through great herds of bison as it cut through the Great Plains half a century earlier.)

Very quickly, however, the sea took on new meaning and a new relationship to settler agriculturalism: as a much-needed repository for the fields' wastewater, a kind of sacrifice zone necessary for the survival of Colorado Desert farms. Within two decades of agriculture on the sea's northern and southern shores, irrigation water seeping into the desert threatened to bring ruin to farmers whose own fields were raising the desert's groundwater levels. This problem only increased with the rapid development of new acreage: in just five years, from 1915 to 1920, Imperial Valley increased its irrigation by nearly 100,000 acres. Nearby, Mexicali—just on the Mexican side of the U.S.-Mexico border—stepped up its irrigation by 150,000 acres.[47] Problems of rising groundwater and surface accumulation of alkaline salts caused this newly reclaimed desert land to "revert to worse than its native state," requiring massive drainage infrastructure to draw water out of the fields and away from the Imperial Valley farms. The Salton Sea, it seemed, finally had a purpose: it "blessed" the farmers by providing a "natural dumping basin for the entire valley."[48] In 1923 the problem of building a drainage infrastructure to properly utilize that "natural dumping basin" was taken on by the new Imperial Irrigation District (IID), which quickly became the largest irrigation district in the country, controlling 600,000 acres of farmland.[49] In time the IID would oversee a complex system of drainage canals that would draw wastewater away from Imperial Valley farms and down into the Salton Sea.

The Salton Sea, in the meantime, was in the process of rapidly evaporating under the sweltering desert sun. As it had so many times in the past, the sea would vanish entirely within a relatively short number of years; because it has no natural inflows except for the desert's anemic annual rainfall and more or less negligible drainage from the New and Alamo rivers, most observers predicted that, without efforts to artificially sustain it, the sea would evaporate entirely by the early 1930s. A 1924 study by the Interior Department confirmed the rapid decline of the sea, finding that in one year alone the shoreline had dropped a full foot. It now sat 248 feet below sea level, newly exposing over thirteen thousand acres of shoreline.[50] Such evaporation, observers fretted, would mean losing the farmers' "natural dumping basin" and would also bring to a close "another episode in the history of the most genuine desert region in the United States": the 1905 floods that brought a "sudden inrush of the most vital factor in desert life"—water.[51] The sea's fortunes were clearly imbricated in the settler narrative of the valley, in which "hardy, courageous men and women . . . wrung a livelihood from Mother Nature in her fiercest phase, and made a spot of beauty on her breast." The wastewater from the IID thus seemed to serve the multiple purposes of artificially sustaining the sea's water level, saving Imperial Valley farmers from alkaline-clogged fields, and sustaining a narrative of settlers "wresting victory from the desert wastes."[52]

The Salton Sea, in the end, did not evaporate as it had in the past. A 1924 Executive Order by the Coolidge administration made the Salton Sea a permanent drainage basin for local farmers, a move justified in large part by the widespread notion that the "Salton Sea furnishes a natural outlet" for drainage.[53] In this context notions of nature and pollution were inverted: rising water tables in the desert were deemed pollutants by virtue of the threat they posed to farmers raising crops in a desert, and sustaining the Salton Sea with wastewater runoff was understood as a natural solution to the drainage problem. In the 1920s, it seems, the Salton Sea was far from an environmental invalid. Quite the opposite: its role in Colorado Desert agriculture was seen as both natural and, counterintuitively, worth artificially sustaining. In fact when Imperial Valley farmers began to find ways to conserve water in the mid-1920s, which resulted in less wastewater and less runoff into the Salton Sea, farmers were chided that their conservation had single-handedly caused the sea's shoreline to drop even more rapidly than had been anticipated.[54]

Throughout subsequent decades the sea was sustained almost entirely by multiple, increasingly polluted inflows. The rapid development of chemical pesticides in the wake of World Wars I and II meant that Imperial Valley farms were dousing their crops (and, lest we forget, their workers) with chemical pesticides ranging from DDT to organophosphates. The water draining out of these farms correspondingly brought with it industrial pesticides to the ever-more saline sea.[55] In addition to the drainage of wastewater from Imperial and Coachella valleys, inflow came from the Alamo and New rivers, both of which pass through the cities of Mexicali, on the Mexican side of the US-Mexico border, and Calexico, on the California side. As these border cities became industrialized in the latter decades of the twentieth century, the area transitioned from agricultural to industrial economies. Mexicali came to host a significant number of maquiladoras, factories that notoriously produce dangerous amounts of unregulated industrial waste, much of it liquid. The liquid waste of the Mexicali maquiladora corridor runs directly into the New River, and thence into the Salton Sea.[56]

Less literal kinds of pollution have likewise shaped the sea's environment and history. In the 1960s, when developers sought to make the Salton Sea "California's Riviera," complete with beachfront resorts and a lush golf course, one hundred million tilapia were introduced as a means of controlling the weeds and mosquitoes that collected near agricultural drains.[57] The presence of tilapia contributed to the decline of the sea's only native fish species, the endangered desert pupfish, which, because of its ability to survive in extremes of temperature, pH, and salinity, once thrived in the lower Colorado basin and the Gulf of California.[58] Other species of nonnative fish, such as sargo, orange mouth corvina, and croaker, were all introduced for the benefit of tourists as other, less hardy fish populations died out in the sea's increasingly salty waters.[59]

The sea has thus become a kind of sacrifice zone for multiple types of pollution. Through the sacrifice of its environmental health, and the associated sacrifice of fish and bird life, the sea has allowed farms to bloom in "the most genuine desert region in the United States," providing "the source of early fruits and vegetables of the famous Imperial Valley."[60] Artificially sustained by agricultural runoff, the sea transitioned from being a temporary nature-culture border-crosser in the desert to a confounding environmental problem—an "environmental invalid," an infirm and convalescent body of water. In the process it has come to be imagined as more than just a polluted landscape; it is a diseased and dying one, a "sickly" one, imperiled by a systemic, debilitating condition that may in fact be incurable. Through this disease the sea is rendered invalid in what disability studies scholars call the medical model of disability, which sees disability as an objective medical state, unlike the social model, which sees disability as contextual, contingent, and socially constructed.[61]

This projection of invalidism, however, is deeply relational. Just as late nineteenth-century health seekers were constructed as a diseased social class in relation to the rest of "healthful" California, the Salton Sea is diseased only in relation to an imagined self-sufficiently healthy environment. The relationality of health and disease—or of validity and invalidity, purity and pollution—is built on a constitutive, binary opposition that is perceived (as are all hegemonic binaries) as exclusive, universal, and hierarchical. As Nash points out in reference to modern conceptions of health in human bodies, "health" has come to "connote primarily the absence of disease; it implies both purity and the ability to fend off harmful organisms and substances"; at bottom, cultural understandings of health have become "a quality possessed (or not) by an individual body rather than a dynamic relationship between a body and its environment."[62] Like human bodies, environments that are perceived as pure (healthy) or polluted (diseased) are held in contrast to one another, despite the fact that, materially speaking, those contrasts are thin at best. Take the Sierra Nevada mountains, the California range that was the subject of John Muir's most poetic environmental prose and thus arguably the landscape where contemporary environmentalism was born (namely in the form of Muir's Sierra Club). This mountain range is a place that, in our environmental imaginary, simply "is nature—it must be."[63] Such landscapes present a seemingly stark opposition to places like the Salton Sea. While the former seems to be pure nature, eminently protectable, the latter seems to be no more than a "toxic catastrophe" and "a fetid swamp not worth saving."[64] And yet there are myriad ways in which the Sierras are indeed polluted, from the nonnative livestock that use the mountain ranges to the mercury that still lingers in streams and streambeds as a legacy of the gold rush.[65] Lamentations of the Salton Sea as a sewer and an environmental disaster deny and occlude its history as a powerfully natural-cultural environmental body, just as celebrations of the Sierras as pure nature deny and occlude the same kinds of natural-cultural co-constitution.

Conclusion: Belonging and Pollution

Through the lens of invalidism and invalidity, of what does and does not belong, these histories of desert sanitariums and a desert sea become inextricably bound. Practices of making social and cultural meaning of the desert—itself a specter and a conundrum in the American environmental imagination—here are shaped as much (and perhaps more) by the arrival of health seekers the disease-phobic and ableist public of coastal cities regarded as "polluted" outsiders as by the desert itself. For people of ill health arriving from eastern and coastal cities, the desert came to embody a kind of feminine nurturance, a motherly home for the weak, the convalescent, and the infirm, or, worse, the contagious. The Salton Sea itself has functioned as a kind of feminized sacrifice zone for the increasingly polluted wastewater of adjacent farmlands, sustained entirely by agricultural drainage. The sea is, in very real ways, limited to a marriage of "perpetual bondage" to large-scale Imperial Valley agriculture.

The conundrum of the Salton Sea, and of "saving" it, is in part a conundrum of whether or not it belongs in the desert. Its belonging has been contested, rejected, or affirmed for a range of reasons: it belongs as a natural repository of polluted water but does not belong as a body of water that needs to be managed and maintained through human action. Thinking of the sea as an infirm body, as invalid and invalidated, negotiates this conflict between belonging and not belonging, the sea's border crossing between natural and unnatural. Like the health seekers who made their home in the desert, the sea's presence made the Colorado Desert a useful and productive place. It gave the desert meaning outside of its reputation as a savage and deadly wasteland.

The Salton Sea has historically been feminized in its enabling role to the Imperial and Coachella valleys. To borrow Adrienne Rich's concept of compulsory heterosexuality, the sea's role, like that of femininity and womanhood, has been as a default economic and symbolic resource for masculinity.[66] But, as I've argued throughout, it has also been inconsistently imagined as either able-bodied (a valid and natural feature of the landscape) or disabled (invalid and invalidated, itself a pollutant of the surrounding desert). There is no question that in recent decades the sea has come to occupy the latter side of the able/disabled binary, at least in popular and journalistic accounts of its current status.

As an environmental problem, one that has no solution that seems to satisfactorily be understood as pure or natural, the Salton Sea and its surrounding environment provide an intriguing test case for other environmental problems that have no readily apparent solutions: climate change, persistent organic pollutants, invasive species, mass extinctions, and the complex natural-cultural nexus of our own bodies.[67] These problems, like the sea itself, will require us to think differently about human relationships to what is not-human. It might, in fact, require us to decolonize the epistemologies that so emphatically insist that the somatic, material world live up to our constructed artifices of it as at once self-sustaining, independent, and strong (qualities inherent in pure environments and bodies that are littered with social—and gendered—meaning). This is a kind of Western, settler colonial, and deeply ableist environmental epistemology that is of a piece with the notion that all human bodies are able and normative; those bodies, both human and more-than-human, that exist outside or at the margins of this social construction of pure health are invalid, invalidated, and deemed unworthy of inclusion. To uphold this normative dichotomization of health and disease, purity and pollution, validity and invalidity is to accept the logic that different bodies—human or water, infected or polluted—occupy opposite banks of a wide and impassable sea.

NOTES

1. Lupi Saldana, "Salton Sea Booming: Recreation Mecca Created by Mistake," Los Angeles Times, April 16, 1965; Kaiser, "Bringing the Salton Sea Back to Life," 565.
2. Cohn, "Saving the Salton Sea."
3. Crepeau et al., Dissolved Pesticides in the Alamo River and the Salton Sea.

4. Setmire et al., <u>Detailed Study of Water Quality, Bottom Sediment, and Biota Associated with Irrigation Drainage in the Salton Sea Area</u>; Glenn et al., "Science and Policy Dilemmas in the Management of Agricultural Waste Waters," 413.
5. Diana Marcum, "7.6 Million Fish Die in a Day," <u>Los Angeles Times</u>, August 12, 1999; Kaiser "Bringing the Salton Sea Back to Life," 565; Matt Simon, "The Salton Sea: Death and Politics in the Great American Water Wars," <u>Wired</u>, September 14, 2012, online.
6. Simon, "The Salton Sea."
7. Tony Perry, "Salton Sea Study Findings Are Encouraging," <u>Los Angeles Times</u>, May 23, 1999; Tony Perry, "Salton Sea Sticking Point in Water Deal," <u>Los Angeles Times</u>, April 14, 2002; Tony Perry, "A Fresh Battle between Southern California Water Adversaries," <u>Los Angeles Times</u>, October 18, 2010.
8. Herndl, <u>Invalid Women</u>, xiii.
9. Margaret Atwood, <u>The Handmaid's Tale</u>, quoted in Herndl, <u>Invalid Women</u>, xvii.
10. Smith, introduction, 2.
11. Ott, <u>Fevered Lives</u>, 2.
12. Kafer, "Compulsory Heterosexuality, Compulsory Able-Bodiedness," 77–89.
13. "The Desert Area: Animal Life, Soil and Climate. The Desert for Invalids," <u>Los Angeles Times</u>, January 1, 1897.
14. Gendzel, "Not Just a Golden State," 351; Abel, <u>Tuberculosis and the Politics of Exclusion</u>, 1–2.
15. Gendzel, "Not Just a Golden State," 354.
16. Gendzel, "Not Just a Golden State," 355; Kafer, "Compulsory Heterosexuality, Compulsory Able-Bodiedness," 79.
17. Nash, <u>Inescapable Ecologies</u>, 8.
18. Frawley, <u>Invalidism and Identity in Nineteenth-Century Britain</u>.
19. Norman Bridge, "The Sun-and-Air Cure: Out-Door Life in California, and Its Value," <u>Los Angeles Times</u>, January 1, 1898.
20. Baur, "The Health Seekers and Early Southern California Agriculture," 347.
21. "A Voice from the Desert: Christmas Day at Springs—The Climate and the People," <u>Los Angeles Times</u>, December 29, 1892.

22. "Care of the Body: Valuable Suggestions for Acquiring and Preserving Health," Los Angeles Times, August 27, 1899.

23. John Hamilton Gilmour, "A Danger Signal: Another Warning against the Deadly Health Resort," Los Angeles Times, June 5, 1894.

24. Ngai, Impossible Subjects.

25. Abel, Tuberculosis and the Politics of Exclusion, 1.

26. Ott, Fevered Lives, 112–13. Kafer designates this kind of bodily violence and control one of the primary functions of compulsory able-bodiedness ("Compulsory Heterosexuality, Compulsory Able-Bodiedness," 79).

27. Letter from Dr. Francis L. Haynes to John Hamilton Gilmour, reprinted in Gilmour, "A Danger Signal"; Foucault, History of Sexuality.

28. Gilmour, "A Danger Signal," emphasis added.

29. "Care of the Body."

30. "The Desert Area."

31. "Progress of the Coast," San Francisco Chronicle, December 7, 1897.

32. In 1892 Palm Springs reportedly was home to "thirty white people and one hundred Indians" ("A Voice from the Desert"). .

33. Herndl notes that, despite the fact that men's health was probably as bad as or worse than women's, "the public perception . . . was that women were truly at risk" (Invalid Women, 21, 24, 25). Perhaps the most famous literary depiction of the lived reality of these inter-secting ideological and embodied forms of invalidation is Charlotte Perkins Gilman's The Yellow Wallpaper (1892).

34. Herndl, Invalid Women, 22–23.

35. Gilmour, "A Danger Signal," emphasis added.

36. "The Desert Area."

37. Irving, Immigrant Mothers; Davis, "Racism, Birth Control, and Repro-ductive Rights." It is important to note here that in this historical context "nonwhite" referred to different categories of raciality than it does today; women excluded from the privileged category of "white" in the 1890s included Chinese, Japanese, and Indian women, African Americans and Native Americans, but also Germans, Armenians, Italians, Irish, Romanians, and a range of other categories we would, in time, include under the rubric of "white" (Jacobson, Whiteness of a Different Color).

38. Duffin, "The Conspicuous Consumptive."
39. Gendzel, "Pioneers and Padres," points out that Twain's disdain for California tribes was shared among most Americans, while Jackson's romanticization of the tribes was exceptional. Gendzel also notes that this deeply antagonistic portrayal of California Natives was, at least in part, a settler attempt to rationalize and explain the Spanish failure to fully "'civilize' the Indians after decades of effort" (74).
40. Dower, War without Mercy, 99. It is worth noting the resonance between racial "subhumans" and "superhumans" and work done in disability studies on "supercripdom," a trope of disability in which a disabled person is lauded for achievements in overcoming disability—in short, relying "upon the perception that disability and achievement contradict one another" Clare, Exile and Pride, 8).
41. Gilmour, "A Danger Signal."
42. "The Desert Area."
43. "The Clouds over Imperial," Los Angeles Times, December 21, 1905.
44. DeBuys, Salt Dreams, 99–121.
45. Roger Birdseye, "America's Dead Sea Is Curbed Forever," New York Times, March 29, 1925.
46. Birdseye, "America's Dead Sea Is Curbed Forever."
47. U.S. Senate, "Problems of Imperial Valley and Vicinity."
48. Robert Benson, "How the Imperial Valley Is Solving Its Drainage Problem," Los Angeles Times, January 27, 1924.
49. "Bill Proposes Salton Sea as Drainage Basin," Los Angeles Times, December 8, 1925.
50. "Salton Sea Is at Low Level: Surface Nearly Foot under Last Year's Mark," Los Angeles Times, June 25, 1924; Birdseye, "America's Dead Sea Is Curbed Forever."
51. Birdseye, "America's Dead Sea Is Curbed Forever."
52. "Wresting Victory from the Desert Wastes," Los Angeles Times, May 17, 1925.
53. "Bill Proposes Salton Sea as Drainage Basin," emphasis added.
54. "Salton Sea Is at Low Level."
55. Orlando et al., Pesticides in Water and Suspended Sediment of the Alamo and New Rivers, Imperial Valley/Salton Sea Basin, 365; May et al., Total Selenium in Irrigation Drain Inflows to the Salton Sea.
56. Neville, "Who's Singing the Mexicali Blues"; Cass, "Toxic Tragedy."

57. Cohn, "Saving the Salton Sea."
58. The pupfish was listed by the federal government as endangered in 1986.
59. Cohn, "Saving the Salton Sea."
60. Birdseye, "America's Dead Sea Is Curbed Forever."
61. Wolbring, Advances in Medical Sociology, 94.
62. Nash, Inescapable Ecologies, 12.
63. Warren, "Paths toward Home," 3, emphasis added.
64. Simon, "The Salton Sea."
65. Warren, "Paths toward Home."
66. Rich, "Compulsory Heterosexuality and Lesbian Existence."
67. Nash, Inescapable Ecologies.

BIBLIOGRAPHY

Abel, Emily K. Tuberculosis and the Politics of Exclusion: A History of Public Health and Migration to Los Angeles. New Brunswick, NJ: Rutgers University Press, 2008.

Baur, John E. "The Health Seekers and Early Southern California Agriculture." Pacific Historical Review 20, no. 4 (1951): 347–63.

———. "Los Angeles County in the Health Rush, 1870–1900." California Historical Society Quarterly 31 (1952): 13–31.

Cass, Valerie. "Toxic Tragedy: Illegal Hazardous Waste Dumping in Mexico." In Environmental Crime and Criminality: Theoretical and Practical Issues, edited by Sally Mitchell Edwards, Terry D. Edwards, and Charles B. Fields, 99–119. New York: Garland, 1999.

Clare, Eli. Exile and Pride: Disability, Queerness and Liberation. 1999; Cambridge MA: South End Press, 2009.

Cohn, Jeffrey. "Saving the Salton Sea." BioScience 50, no. 4 (2000): 295–301.

Crepeau, Kathryn L., Kathryn M. Kuilila, and Brian Bergamaschi. Dissolved Pesticides in the Alamo River and the Salton Sea, California, 1996–97. U.S. Geological Survey Open-File Report 02–232. Sacramento, 2002.

Davis, Angela. "Racism, Birth Control, and Reproductive Rights." In Women, Race, and Class, 202–71. New York: Vintage Books, 1981.

deBuys, William. Salt Dreams: Land and Water in Low-Down California. Albuquerque: University of New Mexico Press, 1999.

Dower, John. War without Mercy: Race and Power in the Pacific War. New York: Pantheon Books, 1986.

Duffin, Lorna. "The Conspicuous Consumptive: Woman as an Invalid." In The Nineteenth-Century Woman: Her Cultural and Physical World, edited by Sara Delamont and Lorna Duffin, 26–56. New York: Routledge, 1978.

Foucault, Michel. History of Sexuality, Volume 1: An Introduction. New York: Vintage Books, 1990.

Frawley, Maria H. Invalidism and Identity in Nineteenth-Century Britain. Chicago: University of Chicago Press, 2010.

Gendzel, Glen. "Not Just a Golden State: Three Anglo 'Rushes' in the Making of Southern California, 1880–1920." Southern California Quarterly 90, no. 4 (2008–9): 349–78.

———. "Pioneers and Padres: Competing Mythologies in Northern and Southern California, 1850–1930." Western Historical Quarterly 32, no. 1 (2001): 55–79.

Glenn, Edward P., Michael J. Cohen, Jason I. Morrison, Carlos Valdés-Casillas, and Kevin Fitzsimmons. "Science and Policy Dilemmas in the Management of Agricultural Waste Waters: The Case of the Salton Sea, CA, USA." Environmental Science & Policy 2, nos. 4–5 (1999): 413–23.

Herndl, Diane Price. Invalid Women: Figuring Feminine Illness in American Fiction and Culture, 1840–1940. Chapel Hill: University of North Carolina Press, 1993.

Irving, Katrina. Immigrant Mothers: Narratives of Race and Maternity, 1890–1925. Urbana: University of Illinois Press, 2000.

Jacobson, Matthew Frye. Whiteness of a Different Color: European Immigrants and the Alchemy of Race. Cambridge MA: Harvard University Press, 1999.

Kafer, Allison. "Compulsory Heterosexuality, Compulsory Able-Bodiedness." Journal of Women's History 15, no. 3 (2003): 77–89.

Kaiser, Jocelyn. "Bringing the Salton Sea Back to Life." Science 287, no. 5453 (2000): 565.

May, T. W., M. J. Walther, M. K. Saiki, and W. G. Brumbaugh. Total Selenium in Irrigation Drain Inflows to the Salton Sea, California, April 2009. U.S. Geological Survey Open-File Report 2009–1230. Reston VA, 2009.

Nash, Linda. Inescapable Ecologies: A History of Environment, Disease, and Knowledge. Berkeley: University of California Press, 2006.

Ngai, Mai. Impossible Subjects: Illegal Aliens and the Making of Modern America. Princeton NJ: Princeton University Press, 2004.

Neville, Martha. "Who's Singing the Mexicali Blues: How Far Can the EPA Travel under the Toxic Substances Act?" Washington Journal of Urban and Contemporary Law 265 (Fall 1999): 265.

Orlando, James L., Kelly L. Smalling, and Kathryn M. Kuivila. Pesticides in Water and Suspended Sediment of the Alamo and New Rivers, Imperial Valley/Salton Sea Basin, California, 2006–2007. U.S. Geological Survey Data Series 365. Reston VA, 2008.

Ott, Katherine. Fevered Lives: Tuberculosis in American Culture since 1870. Cambridge MA: Harvard University Press, 1996.

Rich, Adrienne, "Compulsory Heterosexuality and Lesbian Existence." Signs 5, no 4 (1980): 631–60.

Setmire, J., R. Schroeder, J. Densmore, S. Goodbred, D. Audet, and W. Radtke. Detailed Study of Water Quality, Bottom Sediment, and Biota Associated with Irrigation Drainage in the Salton Sea Area, ca, 1988–1990. U.S. Geological Survey, Sacramento, 1993.

Smith, Bonnie G. Introduction to Gendering Disability, edited by Bonnie G. Smith and Beth Hutchison, 1–8. New Brunswick NJ: Rutgers University Press, 2004.

U.S. Senate. "Problems of Imperial Valley and Vicinity." In Senate Documents, volume 2. 67th Congress, 2nd Session. Congressional Serial Set. Washington DC: Government Printing Office, 1922.

Warren, Louis S. "Paths toward Home." In A Companion to American Environmental History, edited by Douglas Cazaux Sackman, 3–32. New York: John Wiley & Sons, 2010.

Wolbring, Gregor. Advances in Medical Sociology. Vol. 15: Ecological Health: Society, Ecology, and Health. London: Emerald Group, 2013.

17

La Tierra Pica/The Soil Bites

Hazardous Environments and the Degeneration
of Bracero Health, 1942–1964

Mary E. Mendoza

On a frigid evening in Ysleta, Texas, during the winter of 1958, Adolfo Ramírez Bañuelos was rushed to the hospital from the farm where he worked as an agricultural laborer; he could not breathe. In the midst of a two-day cold snap a few of Bañuelos's coworkers had turned on the heat in their bunkhouse and gone to sleep. The next morning, according to Bañuelos, "they woke up dead."[1] The pipes in their room were leaking gas, and carbon monoxide—a colorless, odorless killer—suffocated the men while they slept. Without having repaired the leak and without opening any windows to air out the building, the rancher in charge ordered Bañuelos to remove his dead companions and clean the room. By evening Bañuelos too nearly fell victim to the poisonous gas.

Bañuelos and his coworkers had traveled from Mexico to participate in the Bracero Program. Under the auspices of this program, which lasted from 1942 until 1964, the United States and Mexico collaborated to bring Mexicans as guest-workers to the United States. Originally intended to fill labor shortages after the U.S. entry into World War II, the program proved so beneficial to southwestern agribusiness that growers lobbied to extend it well after the war had ended.[2]

When Bañuelos arrived at a hospital near El Paso, he learned that the noxious air he had spent the day inhaling had caused severe damage to one of his lungs and half of the other. Once

U.S. Department of Labor officials learned the extent of the damage and realized that Bañuelos would no longer be able to fulfill his work duties, they deported the newly disabled man to Juárez. Mexican doctors operated, and although he lived for several decades following the surgery, Bañuelos was never able to work again. For the remainder of his life he struggled to catch his breath. And because he could not provide for his family, his children had to quit school and work so they could support themselves and their disabled father.

When Bañuelos crossed the border into the United States to begin work, he—like all Mexicans participating in the Bracero Program—underwent a mandatory health examination. This examination, during which U.S. Public Health Service (USPHS) officials stripped, washed, and deloused Mexicans, was part of a concerted and coordinated effort on the part of the USPHS to create a "medical border" along the international boundary.[3] During the Bracero era USPHS and other U.S. government officials had serious concerns about Mexicans and their health. But they did not worry that Mexicans would fall ill while working in the United States; instead they worried that Mexicans would carry disease into the country when they crossed the border.

These medical examinations at the border had roots in the early twentieth century, when smallpox and typhus outbreaks near the border compelled public health officials to examine and vaccinate Mexicans crossing into the United States in search of seasonal work or day labor. But the examination process was discriminatory on several levels. First, USPHS officials conflated Mexicanness, bad hygiene, and bad health, and the institutionalized cleaning process was part of an effort to transform presumably filthy bodies into what authorities considered clean ones. This process, though, rendered Mexican people "dirty" and "diseased" and marked them as racially inferior.[4] Second, officials also subjected migrants to a screening process to weed out those they considered disabled. The treatment Mexicans received at the border was both a direct result of and directly contributed to both racist and ableist practices. John McKiernan-González has noted that the medicalization and racialization of the border solidified racialized notions of Mexicans as inferior, since white Americans crossing the border were not subject to health examinations meant to decipher both personal hygiene and physical ability.[5] This essay builds on this notion of medicalized racialization, revealing the combined forces of racism and ableism over the course of the Bracero Program through the lens of environmental history.

Public health–based perceptions of race at the border developed in the midst of the first wave of immigration reform, when the U.S. Congress outlined who could be excluded from entering the country. These immigration laws reflected Progressive Era fears of epidemics and contagion. As Douglas Baynton explains, immigration laws reflected a growing desire to exclude <u>any</u> inferior person, including people officials found "mentally or physically defective."[6] As such, medicalization of the border not only fueled racialization in a world where dirt represented germs and disease, marking people as "others." It also increased scrutiny of bodies with regard to their ability to physically perform labor, which reflected and encouraged an ableist view of the immigrant body. These Progressive Era exclusionary practices based on physical health and ability continued well into the twentieth century and later dictated who could and could not participate in the Bracero Program.

But Bañuelos's story, like the stories of many other Mexicans who crossed the border to work in the United States, demonstrates the cruel irony behind health officials' concerns during the Bracero era: rather than Mexicans bringing sickness to the United States, working in the United States often made Mexicans sick or disabled. While inside U.S. borders, braceros were exposed on a daily basis to environments that carried the risk of disease, malnutrition, exhaustion, injury, poison, even death. And while public health officials sought to control the spread of communicable diseases, workplace injuries and illnesses leading to hospitalization or deportation only fueled racialized notions of Mexicans as filthy, diseased, and inferior. Beyond the exposure to disease and the risk of disablement, Bañuelos's story reveals how ableism and racism—two separate systems of power—were deeply entangled during the Bracero era.

As health officials decided who was fit to be laborers, Mexican nationals entered the United States only to find themselves placed in debilitating or hazardous conditions that undermined those very conceptions of fitness. Long-standing notions of Mexicans as dirty and racially inferior justified the placement of their bodies in toxic, hazardous environments that posed the risk of bodily harm, disablement, or even death. In the case of Bañuelos, once he became disabled, officials saw him as useless and then used ableist justifications to deport him. This progression from racially inferior to both racially inferior and disabled created conditions in which Mexican guest workers found themselves double-othered. That is, health examinations at the border marked Mexicans as racial others, but once these migrants crossed the border they faced dangerous environments that caused many of them to become disabled others as well. Put succinctly, the racialized perception of bodily difference produced bodily difference in the form of disease and disability.

Mexican Bodies as Racial Others

In the early 1940s collaborative initiatives like the Bracero Program ostensibly laid the groundwork for a changing view of the Mexican body. In 1941, when the United States entered the war, farmers across the country lacked laborers "because of the necessity for increasing armed forces and the movement of farm workers into industry."[7] Farmers wrote letters to bureaucrats in the Departments of Labor and Agriculture requesting that the agencies find and import laborers. In response the U.S. Employment Service and Farm Security Administration worked with the departments on a plan to "import labor from Puerto Rico, Cuba, and other areas to the south."[8] On July 23, 1942, the U.S. government entered into a bilateral agreement with Mexico to send Mexican nationals as laborers for the shortage. The USDA oversaw the program through the Farm Security Administration, and the first braceros arrived in Stockton, California, in September 1942.[9]

Shortly after the Bracero Program began, newspapers, magazines, and the U.S. Office of War Information created posters and covered stories about Mexican nationals and their laudable efforts to help the United States. The Office of War Information commissioned the artist Leon Helguera in 1943 to create a poster that represented the new bilateral agreement. On the poster Helguera printed, "Americanos todos luchamos por la victoria / Americans all, let's fight for victory."[10] The bilingual posters sought to sway both U.S. Americans and Mexicans to achieve solidarity. The design includes an image of two arms reaching out in unison, one belonging to a Mexican and holding a sombrero, the other belonging to Uncle Sam, who holds his top hat (see figure 17.1). News articles portrayed Mexican Braceros as "good neighbors . . . helping to harvest victory in [the] western farmland."[11] This propaganda effort implied that Mexicans aided the United States in the war effort and should see themselves and be seen as "American" and "neighborly."

Beyond propaganda purporting that Mexicans and Americans were "all [equal and] Americans," the agreement itself stipulated that braceros "shall not suffer discriminatory acts of any kind,"

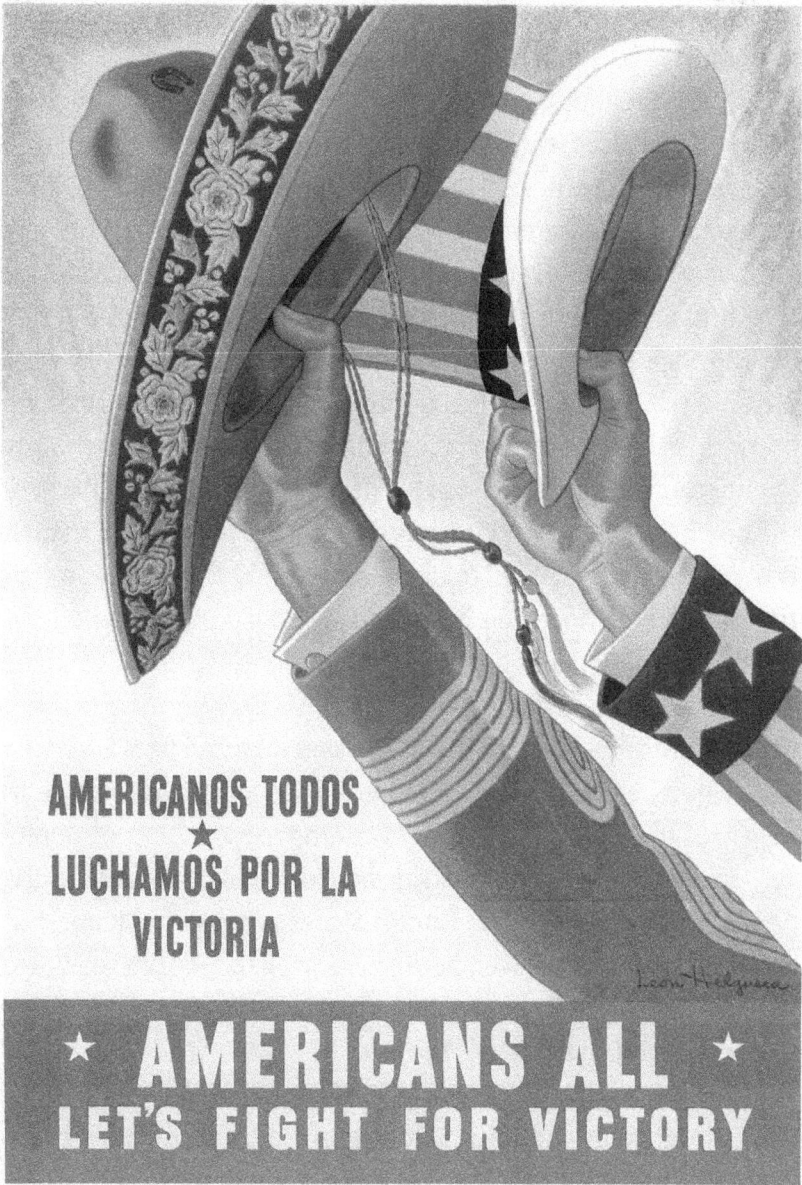

Fig. 17.1. "Americans All," 1943, a poster from the World War II era designed to attract Mexican laborers to the United States to work. Image provided by the Eagle Commons Library, University of North Texas, Denton, Texas.

that "housing conditions, sanitary, and medical services . . . shall be identical to those enjoyed by other agricultural workers in the same localities," and that workers should "enjoy as regards occupational disease and accidents the same guarantees enjoyed by other agricultural workers under United States legislation."[12] In this mutual agreement it seemed as though Mexican laborers might have some leverage to lobby against the bodily scrutiny they had endured since the early twentieth century.

But in spite of the inter-American cooperation and images praising and encouraging the efforts of Braceros, the Mexican body remained threatening in the eyes of Americans. Early twentieth-century ideas about Mexicans carrying disease north of the border persisted, and the guest-worker agreement stipulated that all Mexicans needed to undergo detailed physical examinations before leaving their home state.[13] Once they reached the border they underwent additional inspections, including stripping and delousing; so instead of one health examination, as earlier migrants faced, these guest workers endured two. Even at a time when the U.S. government petitioned Mexicans to come to help with the war effort as part of a larger American community U.S. government officials still viewed Mexicans as a threat to the health of the country. The United States wanted the labor, but not the human beings who performed it.[14] Reluctant to see these Mexicans as sanitarily equal, the inspection policies reduced them to carriers of disease.

Medical practitioners in Mexico performed the workers' preliminary health examinations. Sometimes these exams took place in the migrants' hometown, but most often applicants traveled to recruitment centers across Mexico, where they underwent a series of examinations.[15] At the centers doctors sometimes examined many men all at once. One aspiring bracero noted that there were so many contenders for the program that "the recruitment sites were converted to a Bracerópolis"[16] In his study of the program the sociologist Henry P. Anderson reported, "In peak seasons, when as many as 2,500 men may be processed in a single day, 4 or 5 physicians are employed. Each concentrates on a particular area: one auscultates the chest; one examines for gross evidence of venereal disease or hernia; one examines eyes, ears, nose, and throat; one conducts an anal examination; and one conducts a simple neurological and musculoskeletal examination."[17] Doctors also looked for signs that braceros had the wherewithal and physical ability that agricultural work required. In his memoir of life as a bracero, Jesús Topete remembered seeing applicants trying to "make callouses on their hands" so they would appear to be well seasoned and physically able to withstand tough working conditions harvesting crops.[18]

After the initial examination in Mexico, braceros who met all of the requirements for the program traveled by train or bus to the border, where they experienced a second, more thorough examination. Officials like Julius Lowenberg of the U.S. Public Health Service led the Mexicans from cattle trains or buses, where they had spent hours and sometimes days, to processing centers. In an oral history interview about his experience Lowenberg said hundreds, sometimes thousands of men would arrive for processing. He remembered one group in particular that "smelled bad."[19] This was an early instance in which an <u>assumption</u> of filth actually produced the reality of it. This group had arrived in cattle cars that had traveled all the way from Yucatán—the southeastern-most region of Mexico—and had likely been forced to stay in the cars for days, with only a few short stops en route. Lowenberg suspected that the trip to the border was the worst part of their enlistment process.

Marcelo Zepeda, a bracero who enlisted in the program in 1945, described the screening process: "First they will look at our hands, looking for callouses. For them, this was an indication of a hard-working man, used to tough work. After this we had a physical exam. They didn't want us to bring disease to the United States."[20] The physical screening took place in bathhouses where USPHS bureaucrats like Lowenberg stripped, bathed, and then dowsed the men with polvo, or powder. Then USPHS employees would wash the migrants' clothes and American doctors would examine the laborers thoroughly, looking for signs of illness or weakness. Lowenberg took chest x-rays and doctors or nurses took blood (see figure 17.2).[21]

The trip north required youth and health, and the two health examinations nearly guaranteed that the braceros were healthy when they left home and remained healthy after the arduous journey. The screening process, though it probably did not catch everything, likely yielded a particularly healthy population of laborers.

Producing Disease, Disability, and Death

Braceros' health began to decline almost as soon as they crossed into the United States. When the braceros left the processing centers at the border, they carried the stigma of filth, disease, and racial inferiority to the fields. As their U.S. employers welcomed them to their orchards and farms, they did not see these Mexicans as "equal Americans." The same racialized notions that provoked public health officials to examine and delouse Mexicans crossing the border also justified the provision of poor housing and abysmal working conditions once they arrived at their destination.

Work contracts stipulated that employers provide "hygienic lodgings adequate to the climatic conditions of the area of employment."[22] But employers repeatedly placed migrants in subpar housing, creating an environment optimal for the contraction of disease and the endangerment of bodies. Most Mex-

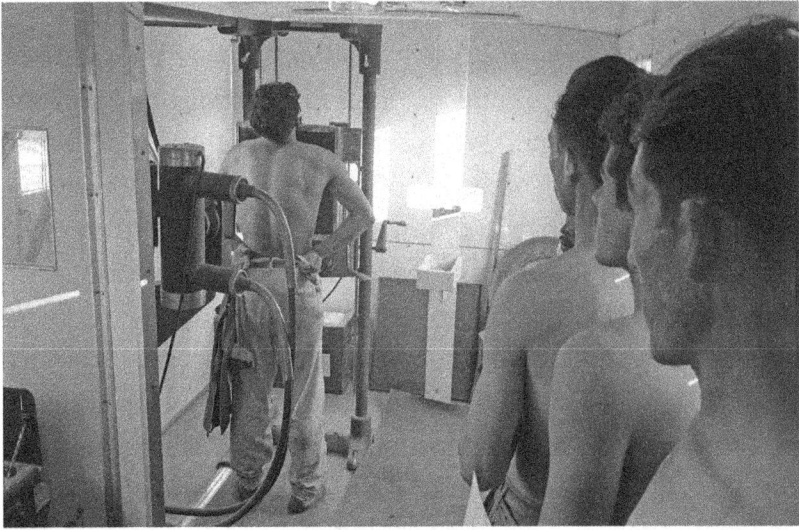

Fig. 17.2. "A Bracero Receives a Chest X-Ray," 1956, Leonard Nadel Photographs, provided by the Archives Center, National Museum of American History, Smithsonian Institution.

ican nationals lived in migratory labor camps where employers expected them to cook, eat, and sleep. The housing ranged from old shacks and barns to dorm-like buildings with beds. Food rotted due to improper storage or was otherwise unsuitable for human consumption. In a Department of Labor memorandum a field inspector described the labor camp conditions as "a scene of a filthy over crowded barracks, with double bunks stacked side by side, without allowance for walking space between beds, forcing workers to crawl over each other to get to their resting places. . . . [On] the inside of a long crumpled down barrack, . . . one side [was] lined with broken beds, and on the other stoves, food, and garbage; here the workers were forced to live, cook, eat, and sleep."[23] Such conditions created "an outstanding health hazard" to those forced to live in them and could exacerbate epidemics of communicable diseases such as typhoid fever and tuberculosis.[24]

Many camps crammed large numbers of people into small rooms and lacked working toilets. Mexicans in one camp in Arlington Valley, California, endured "improper garbage disposal and lack of toilet sanitation." When camps such as these experienced typhoid outbreaks, some U.S. officials claimed that Mexicans brought the disease with them. But even if some Mexicans did slip through the screening at the border, the conditions in which they lived caused their illness to flare up or spread (see figure 17.3). As one physician pointed out, "Tuberculosis may flare up if a person with the disease does not eat properly, sleep properly, or if he works too hard. Almost all of these conditions exist [for the Mexican workers]."[25] Even if the Mexican workers enjoyed adequate time to sleep, they could hardly do so soundly when forced to crawl over one another to get to and from their tightly packed barracks.

For many Mexican workers the food situation aggravated an emergent health crisis in the camps. According to the Anderson study, there were three causes of food poisoning. First, because the camps provided only small cooking facilities for large numbers of workers, they could rarely prepare and serve food at the same rate it was acquired. Consequently uncooked food often sat in inadequate storage facilities until consumed. Second, the men who prepared the food often did not have adequate sanitation facilities. Third, men who worked far from camp would often consume meals hours after preparation. On February 7, 1955, for instance, thirty-seven men in the San Fernando Valley fell ill four hours after eating. Their symptoms included vomiting, diarrhea, cramps, chills, fever, and dizziness. Upon investigation the Los Angeles Health Department found that the lunch they consumed at noon had been prepared at 1:00 a.m.[26]

Anderson's study also found that in some labor camps employers spent very little money on the food they fed the Mexican

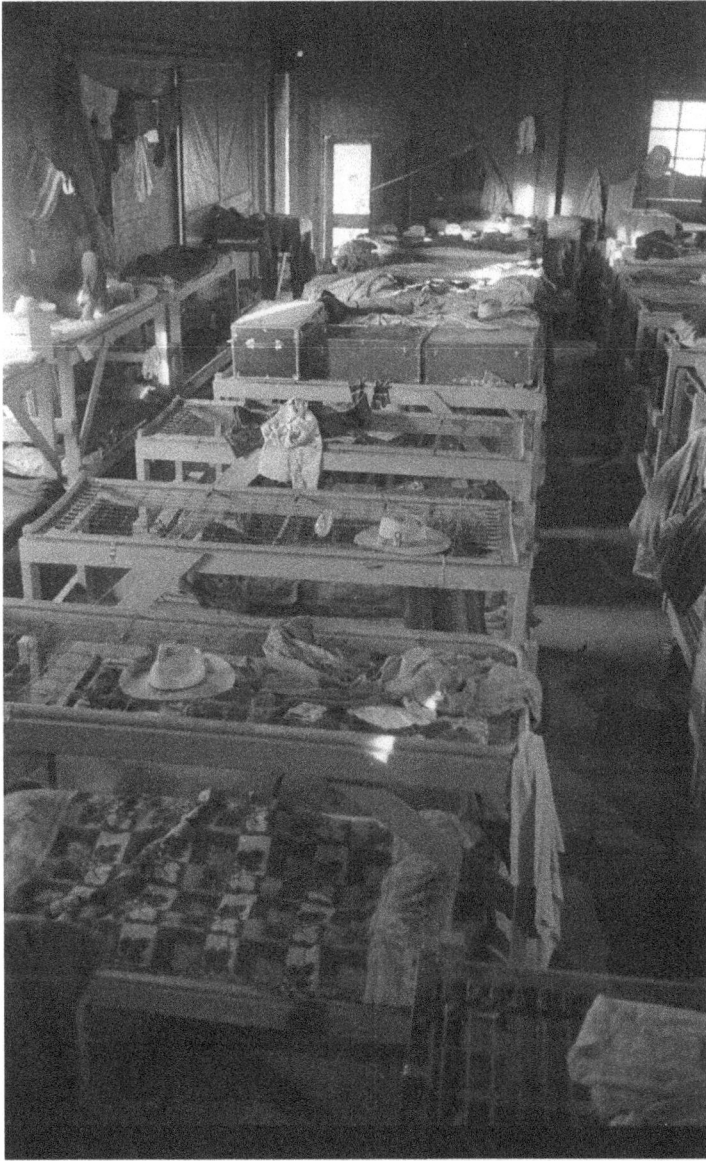

Fig. 17.3. "A View into a Living Quarter," 1956, Leonard Nadel Photographs, provided by the Archives Center, National Museum of American History, Smithsonian Institution.

workers. One interviewee said, "A friend of mine up in —— runs a sick cow business. 'Canceroid cows,' he calls them. . . . They're the most revolting sight you ever saw. . . . The operators of Bracero camps in the three county area . . . come in to buy these things at auction." Farm owners fed their workers cheap, unhealthy food to maximize profits. As a result Mexicans acquired parasites and suffered from food poisoning and dietary deficiencies. Some died of starvation. An investigator of these incidents reported:

> [One] man had been in the United States six months, and during that time all he had to eat were tomatoes, which he got from the fields where he was working, and yeast, which apparently he had heard somewhere was good for him. . . . This was a young man, 26 years old; who was as far as we know was [sic] in perfect health before he came here. . . .
>
> I investigated another Mexican National death near San Jose. This was another case of a young man who died mysteriously. No signs of violence, no signs of illness. Well, it turned out that all he had been eating was a pail of pears a day. . . . He was working in pears at the time, you see, he didn't have to pay anything for them. . . . It appeared likely that this man had simply starved to death.[27]

Dietary deficiencies were a major problem for impoverished Mexican workers who depended on employers for food. A 1951 report to the President's Commission on Migratory Labor concluded that "the diet of migrant farm laborers is insufficient to maintain health, as is their shelter."[28]

In theory the USDA mitigated poor housing situations by assigning agents to inspect labor camps and ensure that employers provided adequate housing. Individual states, at the direction of the USDA, oversaw and performed inspections. In practice, however, poor housing persisted even when state agents performed inspections and mandated improvement. In a report generated by Ernesto Galarza, the research director for the National Agricultural Workers Union, one bracero described his California camp's lack of water:

> Our camp was without water for a week.... There was a small rusty pipe that brought enough water for washing hands and the face but we could not wash our clothes and we could not take a bath for a week. The day I did not work an inspector came.... He ordered the pump to be fixed right away. Now the water from the baths and from the washing is pumped out of a big hole and it flows through a ditch between the bunkhouse and the tents. When it makes warm weather [sic] it smells very bad.[29]

In this case, even after an inspector demanded that the employer repair the water pipe, the repair was questionable. This situation was not unique to California. States across the country placed Mexican workers in inadequate labor camps. The chairman of the Governor's Committee on Migrant Labor described a facility in Fort Collins, Colorado: "I have never been as shocked as when I entered the one-room shacks with old iron bedsteads and thin pads, with one shaded bulb, in which as many as eight to ten people sleep, and with an old cook stove, dirt just as thick as you could find it, no toilet facilities, no water facilities." At a labor camp in Florida a public health official found that "180 people liv[ed] in 60 rooms, with only one toilet stool that work[ed]."[30]

Numerous reports similarly reveal that the USDA did not enforce compliance with the standards outlined by the international agreement. In a response to Galarza's report, the Region X office of the Bureau of Employment Security lamented that

Galarza ignored places where housing conditions were not so dreadful, but then confessed, "We cannot pretend that our own field representatives inspect more than a small percentage of the thousands of housing units in California where Mexican workers are lodged."[31]

The work environment did not promote good health any more than the environment of the labor camps did. The original agreement between Mexico and the United States stipulated that all braceros in the program work in the agriculture industry, one of the most dangerous professions.[32] A handout on safety for recruited farm help printed by the National Safety Council in 1943 listed the range of work performed on different kinds of farms and the gamut of risk for injury and illness. The handout also encouraged those considering agricultural work to have a checkup, as "physical exertion may aggravate a hidden weakness."[33] Migratory Labor in American Agriculture: A Report of the President's Commission on Migratory Labor in 1951 confirmed, "Migratory workers are more subject to sickness and have a higher death rate than most other sections of the population."[34] Mexican workers in the Bracero Program often worked long hours in fields in extreme, unfamiliar weather, handled dangerous equipment, and came into close contact with pesticide-treated plants and dirt, all posing risks for illness, injury, or death.

Given the required health examinations, reports of death or injury often mystified families back home. On July 3, 1945, José Luis Fuentes of the Instituto Nacional de Migración (National Migration Institute) wrote to Sra. Mercedes García de Haro in Zacatecas to inform her that her husband, Jesús de Haro Camacho, had died while working as a bracero in Syracuse, New York. Fuentes told the señora that her husband had been hospitalized while working and had died from "acute aortitis," an acute inflammation of the aortic wall.[35] After learning of her husband's untimely death she wrote a letter to the secretary of labor stating that her husband had been healthy when he left Mexico: "Upon being contracted as a Bracero under the number 724-16-3241, [he] was examined by the doctors . . . and they did not find any cardiac condition or anything else that would have affected his ability to become a Bracero." According to Sra. García, her husband must have developed his condition after he left "for reasons that [she] did not understand." "Whatever the reason," she added, "it has left my children orphans and me without the resources to survive." She asked the secretary to request that the U.S. government or her husband's patrón pay her the indemnities that they saw fit.[36] Sra. García was baffled that her husband, who had been declared healthy by not one but two doctors, had suddenly died. But he was one of many whose hidden condition was aggravated by overexertion.

Anderson's study showed that in California from 1953 to 1961, while injury rates in other industries declined, the number of agricultural injuries continued to rise. In an interview with Anderson in 1956, one U.S. Department of Labor field representative said, "Most of the sickness that we get in this area comes from the fact that Braceros are not used to our weather. They usually come from either a place that has a very high altitude, and is very dry, or from the coast of Mexico where it is very hot and humid. Here in the central coast area of California, it is different. They have a hard time adjusting to it, many of them. You'll see them with colds all the time."[37]

As more braceros traveled north for work, many Mexicans became aware of the risk that came with the journey and the job. In Mexico labor unions fought to ensure better care for their compatriots, noting that the working conditions in the United States were deplorable. In 1944 members of the Confederación de Trabajadores de México (Confederation of Workers in Mexico) wrote a memo outlining the terrible conditions braceros faced and urging the union to put pressure on the Mexican government to act: "Our compatriots that work on the other side of the border return victims of dysentery, Tuberculosis, Dermatitis, venereal infections, and [are] either partially or totally disabled because of work accidents, negligent medical attention, bad food, etc." The union members noted that it was the responsibility of the Mexican government to ensure workers' safety while abroad and to care for those who returned injured.[38]

The lack of concern among government officials on both sides of the border provoked fear in some laborers. In 1945 Pedro Pérez Lara wrote to Mexican president Manuel Ávila Camacho begging for protection from deportation while he helped to care for his friend Pedro Calzada, who had recently suffered an accident while working and had to have his arm amputated. After seeing his friend lose a limb, Pérez Lara wanted to give up his contract to avoid suffering from a similar injury, but he also hoped to stay in the United States until he could escort his incapacitated friend back to Mexico.[39] Many others also opted to give up their contracts once they realized the dangers of the work. One Mexican bracero stated, "My friends and I had contracts with the Yuma Producers Cooperative Association. Our contracts have not expired, but we are leaving. Two men in our area died recently from heat exhaustion. Others have become sick. We want to get out of this country while we are still alive."[40]

Exposure to different climates, wind patterns, and temperatures rendered Mexicans susceptible to illness as they suffered dehydration, their skin burned, or they became chilled.[41] Roberto García Estrada described the heat as so intense that he and his coworkers had to take salt pills to replace what they lost in sweat while working under the hot sun.[42] The bracero Topete recorded that his friend became sick from the freezing rain and snow just three months after he arrived in the United States. Unable to work in the new, harsh climate, the man decided to return to Mexico.[43]

The massive undertaking of this agricultural work—in effect the transformation of the U.S. soil from an unkempt landscape to groomed fields of production—also required the use of hazardous tools and equipment, which often led to injury. One of the most common tools employed by the workers was the "cortito," or short-handled hoe (seen in figure 17.4). Mexican men using this tool were stooped over for hours in the heat. Their employers preferred the short-handled hoe to a hoe with a longer handle because it allowed for more precision; in theory a worker who was physically closer to the crop was more likely to accurately chop away at weeds and harvest the plants without damaging them.

But the short-handled hoe created significant problems and pain for the laborers. Rodolfo Jacobo Páramo described how he felt abused because his boss would not allow him to stand up to stretch his back. "They did not want to see anyone standing up," he recalled. "They said they wanted to see us bend like staples."[44] Bernabé Alvarez Díaz, who worked in beet fields, described working with the hoe in the heat as strenuous and painful.[45] Like Díaz, many Mexican workers complained of musculoskeletal distress in the lower back "as a consequence of prolonged hours of repetitive motions and postures for which the human anatomy is poorly adapted." While many Anglo-Americans viewed Mexican bodies as filthy and diseased, they contradictorily viewed them as immune to the effects of exhausting and abusive labor conditions. One farm placement representative stated, "I've seen Mexican nationals work stooping over for hours at a stretch, without straightening up. An Anglo simply couldn't take it. But it didn't seem to bother these boys a bit. Don't ask me what it is. Maybe it's because the Mexicans are a good deal shorter than Anglos—they're built closer to the ground."[46] Though Americans

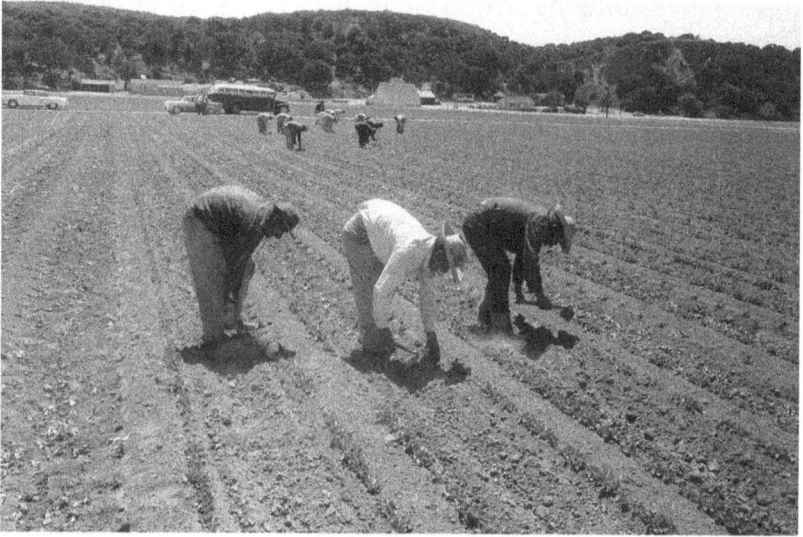

Fig. 17.4. "Braceros Perform Stoop Labor," 1956, Leonard Nadel Photographs, provided by the Archives Center, National Museum of American History, Smithsonian Institution.

viewed Mexicans as subhuman with regard to cleanliness, health, and hygiene, they viewed them as superhuman with regard to their capacity to perform otherwise back-breaking work. But even when describing the Mexicans' superhuman powers, the language Americans used reflected their racist attitudes.[47]

During the Bracero era occupational hazards increased with the mechanization of agricultural work. The 1951 report to the President's Commission noted, "The use of tractors and other machines, of knives and other cutting tools, of high ladders, and noxious gases in fumigation, as well as the truck transportation of workers . . . have all contributed to mak[ing] the accident rate in agriculture one of the highest."[48] In 1952 José Barajas Chávez, who was harvesting lettuce with a short-handled hoe, had to race a machine as he worked. As he picked the heads of lettuce, a machine followed right behind to pick them up and wrap them. "We couldn't stop even to stretch our backs," he said. "If we did, the machine would run right over us." One day, rushing to beat the machine, Chávez cut his own hand instead of the lettuce. Upon realizing that he could not stop the bleeding, he asked the white woman operating the machine for help, but she refused. Afraid of losing his job if he stopped, Chávez wrapped his hand and continued to work. When his foreman realized he had hemorrhaged all over the lettuce, he told Chávez that he was going to have to eat the lettuce that he had bled on. "No one asked if I was all right," Chávez recalled. "I hid my pain."[49]

Transportation to and from worksites in open grain trucks also caused injury and death. Galarza found repeated violations of transportation safety regulations on farms in California, including one incident that resulted in the injury of seven Mexican nationals, as well as the death of seven others and the contractor who was driving.[50] The archives reveal case after case of injury or death due to tractor or car accidents.[51]

The historian Linda Nash has explained how "noxious gases in fumigation" generated a health hazard new to the bracero era. The fairly recent development and use of pesticides such as DDT caused a series of reactions among braceros who had direct contact with the chemically treated plants. Many laborers worked on land that was treated with these chemicals to control pests, and ironically many of the braceros themselves had been sprayed with DDT upon entry to ensure they were healthy. By 1955, 7.1 million acres of land were treated with these chemicals in California alone. In addition to DDT, the most common chemical used, braceros also worked with DDE, endrin, aldrin, dieldrin, and toxaphene.[52]

While it is difficult to track the long-term effects of these chemicals on Mexican workers, the Anderson study provides some evidence of the short-term effects. One worker reported, "My fingernails became infected as a result of poison that was on the tomato plants." Others who worked with cotton contracted infections of the skin and fingernails as well. Some had allergic reactions around their mouth from eating the plants. In many places even organic soil irritated the skin. Anderson reported that in San Joaquin County's delta the peat dirt, which had high organic content, induced pain. One Mexican worker said, "La tierra pica [the soil bites]."[53] José Luis Gutierrez Navarro, who entered the program in 1959, noted that working in fumigated fields was "one of the hardest jobs" because "after working for three or four hours, our skin would break out in rashes of little red dots and we did not receive any medical attention."[54] These environmental conditions contributed to the poor and declining health of these Mexican workers. Unfamiliar climates, dangerous chemicals, and machines had endogenous and exogenous effects on the Mexican body, in spite of the American opinion about the Mexicans' ability to bear these hazards.

The relationship of the farm owner, or patrón, to the Mexican worker likely also exacerbated poor health. Relations were rarely friendly, and many Mexicans worried that complaining of pain or illness would result in unemployment and deportation.[55] One laborer explained, "These things have to be tolerated in silence because there is no one to defend our guarantees. In a strange country you feel timid—like a chicken in another rooster's yard."[56] Though some Mexicans did report their pain, the majority kept it to themselves until their contracts expired or their pain was so great they could no longer ignore it. As a result, when compared to Anglo-American agricultural workers, Mexican workers suffered a greater number of injuries—it was not only the material environment that led to bodily degeneration but the bureaucratic environment as well. Of those reported in California, Mexican injuries and health problems exceeded, in number and in gravity, those of their Anglo-American counterparts in every category from infectious diseases to injuries of the bones and organs.[57]

Hundreds of braceros like Adolfo Ramírez Bañuelos traveled from Mexico to the United States in search of an opportunity to improve their lives but returned to Mexico with some kind of sickness or injury. Thinking back on his time in the United States, Topete wrote that a number of his friends and colleagues suffered and that "a considerable percentage of Mexicans" experienced various hardships related to illness or poor treatment.[58]

Conclusion

In her study of disease and the environment Nash argues that the "history of health and disease is not fully divorced from place."[59] This relationship is particularly evident during the bracero era. From 1942 to 1964 many of the Mexican diseases and deficiencies that U.S. Public Health officials fought so fiercely at the border were actually born within the borders of the United States. As public health officials treated Mexicans as unhygienic and sought to transform their filth into cleanliness, they perpetuated ideas of the racialized Mexican, which justified placing Mexican workers in substandard housing and work environments. This treatment, in turn, actually transformed healthy people into diseased and disabled people and created a feedback loop that only fueled the racialization process. Beyond that, while agricultural work underlined Mexican bodies, it further enabled healthy American consumer bodies as Mexican workers harvested crops in American fields. Anglo-American perceptions of Mexican bodies as dirty, diseased, and sometimes disabled led to racist and ablest treatment of Mexican workers. This treatment then propagated a stigma against Mexicans as unfit and inferior beings, a stigma with a long and unbroken legacy. The environments in which braceros lived and worked ended up sickening or disabling many of them. But the perception that these conditions created extended beyond the braceros themselves to the Mexican population as a whole and lasted long after the guest-worker program ended.

NOTES

The author would like to thank Susan Burch, Gail Glover, Katherine Johnston, Ari Kelman, Kathy Morse, Sarah Jaquette Ray, Jay Sibara, and Traci Voyles for their help and vital feedback during the completion of this essay.

1. Selfa Chew, "Manuel Ramírez," item 236, Bracero History Archive, 2005, http://braceroarchive.org/items/show/236, my translation.
2. See Kelly Lytle Hernández, Migra! A History of the U.S. Border Patrol (Berkeley: University of California Press, 2010); Calavita, Inside the State; Deborah Cohen, Braceros: Migrant Citizens and Transnational Subjects in the Postwar United States and Mexico (Chapel Hill: University of North Carolina Press, 2011); Peter Andreas, Border Games: Policing the U.S.-Mexico Divide (Ithaca NY: Cornell University Press, 2009); Mae M. Ngai, Impossible Subjects: Illegal Aliens and the Making of Modern America (Princeton NJ: Princeton University Press, 2004); Nash, Inescapable Ecologies.
3. McKiernan-González, Fevered Measures, argues that health examinations at the border created a "medicalized" border in which well-being, as defined by American bureaucrats, determined whether or not an individual could enter the United States.
4. See Nayan Shah, Contagious Divides: Epidemics and Race in San Francisco's Chinatown (Berkeley: University of California Press, 2001); Alexandra Minna-Stern, "Buildings, Boundaries, and Blood: Medicalization and Nation-Building on the U.S.-Mexico Border, 1910–1930," Hispanic American Historical Review 79 (February 1999): 41–81; Natalia Molina, Fit to Be Citizens? Public Health and Race in Los Angeles, 1879–1939 (Berkeley: University of California Press, 2006); McKiernan-González, Fevered Measures.
5. McKiernan-González, Fevered Measures, 11.

6. Immigration Act of 1907, 34 Stat. 898, 59th Cong., 2nd sess., February 20, 1907; Baynton, "Defectives in the Land," 33.

7. Assistant to the secretary, letter to G. A. Blots, January 27, 1942, entry 17, Gen. Corresp. 1906–1975, Employment, 1942, box 636, Record Group 16: Records of the Office of the Secretary of Agriculture, National Archives and Records Administration, College Park MD.

8. Assistant to the secretary, letter to Powell W. Price, January 26, 1942, entry 17, Gen. Corresp. 1906–1975, Employment, 1942, box 636, Record Group 16: Records of the Office of the Secretary of Agriculture, National Archives and Records Administration, College Park MD.

9. Galarza, Strangers in Our Fields, 5; Subject Files of Sec. James P. Mitchell 1953–60, NC 58, entry 36, box 140, Record Group 174: General Records of the Department of Labor, National Archives and Records Administration, College Park MD. See also Mexican Commissioners Ernesto Hidalgo and Dr. Abraham J. Navas and American Commissioners Joseph F. McGurk, John O. Walker, and David Meeker, letter to the attorney general, August 29, 1942, entry 17, Gen. Corresp. 1906–1975, Employment, 1942, box 636, Record Group 16: Records of the Office of the Secretary of Agriculture, National Archives and Records Administration, College Park MD.

10. Americans All, Let's Fight for Victory: Americanos todos, luchamos por la victoria, UNT Digital Library, http://digital.library.unt.edu/ark:/67531/metadc426/.

11. Grace McGrady, "Manpower from Mexico," Herald Tribune, November 18, 1943, Office Files of the Rep in Mexico, binder 4, Mexicans, Record Group 211: Records of the War Manpower Commission, National Museum of American History Archives, Washington DC.

12. Quoted in Jacobo, Los Braceros, 25–27.

13. Annette Shreibati, "José García Díaz," item 356, Bracero History Archive, 2006, http://braceroarchive.org/items/show/356.

14. Calavita, Inside the State, 6.

15. Anderson, The Bracero Program in California, 17.

16. Topete, Aventuras de un Bracero, 11. All translations from this source are mine.

17. Anderson, The Bracero Program in California, 17.

18. Topete, <u>Aventuras de un Bracero</u>, 14.
19. Richard Baquera, "Julius Lowenberg," item 68, Bracero History Archive, 2003, http://braceroarchive.org/items/show/68.
20. Quoted in Jacobo, <u>Los Braceros</u>, 48.
21. Baquera, "Julius Lowenberg."
22. Qtd. in Galarza, <u>Strangers in Our Fields</u>, 25, citing Article 2 of "Work Contract Provisions." See also Mexican Commissioners et al., letter to the Attorney General.
23. "A Report on 'Strangers in Our Fields,' Region X, Regional Office, Bureau of Employment Security, Attachment Number 1: H. R. Zamora, memorandum to A. J. Norton, August 10, 1956, Subject Files of Sec. James P. Mitchell 1953–60, NC 58, entry 36, box 140, Record Group 174: General Records of the Department of Labor, National Archives and Records Administration, College Park MD.
24. U.S. House of Representatives, <u>Hearings before the Select Committee to Investigate the Interstate Migration of Destitute Citizens</u>, 76th Cong., 3rd session, H. RES. 63 and H. RES 491, Part 9: December 11, 1940, and February 26, 1941, Holt-Atherton Special Collections and University Archives, University of the Pacific, Stockton, California.
25. Anderson, <u>The Bracero Program in California</u>, 222.
26. Anderson, <u>The Bracero Program in California</u>, 101, 103.
27. Anderson, <u>The Bracero Program in California</u>, 103, 83.
28. <u>Migratory Labor in American Agriculture: A Report to the President's Commission on Migratory Labor, 1951</u>, HD 1525.U 518m c3, 154, History of the INS Historical Reference Library, Washington DC.
29. Galarza, <u>Strangers in Our Fields</u>, 23. Translation from Spanish to English in original source.
30. <u>Migratory Labor in American Agriculture</u>, 154, 155.
31. "A Report on 'Strangers in Our Fields.'"
32. Mexican Commissioners et al., letter to the attorney general.
33. National Safety Council, Inc., "Safety for Recruited Farm Help," April 10, 1943, entry 17, Gen. Corresp. 1906–1975, Employment, box 841, Record Group 16: Records of the Office of the Secretary of Agriculture, National Archives and Records Administration, College Park MD.
34. <u>Migratory Labor in American Agriculture</u>, 153.

35. José Luis Fuentes, letter to Sra. Mercedes García de Haro, July 3, 1945, file 4-357-1-1945-2844, El Archivo Histórico del Instituto Nacional de Migración, Mexico City, my translation.
36. Sra. Mercedes Garcia de Haro, letter to Jose Luis Fuentes, [?1945], file 4-357-1-1945-2844, El Archivo Histórico del Instituto Nacional de Migración, Mexico City, my translation.
37. Anderson, The Bracero Program in California, 213, 218.
38. Enrique A. Lorenzo, letter to C. Fidel Velázquez, Secretario General de la Confederación de Trabajadores de México, October 3, 1944, Camacho Presidential Files, file 546.6/120, Archivo General de la Nación, Mexico City, my translation.
39. Pedro Pérez Lara, letter to President Manuel Ávila Camacho regarding accident of bracero worker Pedro Calzada de Rodríguez, September 17, 1945, Camacho Presidential Files, file 546.6/120-32, Archivo General de la Nación, Mexico City.
40. Anderson, The Bracero Program in California, 218.
41. Similarly, in his work on New Orleans Ari Kelman writes, "Immigrants unfamiliar with an environmental area are prone to illness" (A River and Its City, 88).
42. Veronica Cortez, "Roberto García Estrada," item 396, Bracero History Archive, 2006, http://braceroarchive.org/items/show/396.
43. Topete, Aventuras de un Bracero, 118.
44. Quoted in Jacobo, Los Braceros, 98.
45. Alejandra Díaz, "Bernabé Alvarez Díaz," item 663, Bracero History Archive, 2008, http://braceroarchive.org/items/show/663.
46. Anderson, The Bracero Program in California, 217.
47. Migratory Labor in American Agriculture.
48. Migratory Labor in American Agriculture, 158.
49. Quoted in Jacobo, Los Braceros, 90.
50. Galarza, Strangers in Our Fields, 53.
51. For example, see the following folders in the Archivo Histórico del Insitituto Nacional de Migración, Mexico City: 4-357-1945-2086, 4-357-1-1945-2844, 4-357-1-1946-6306, 4-357-1-1944-1900, 4-357-1954-9101, 4-357-1-1945-2857, 4-357-1-1945-2866, 4-357-1-1945-2854.
52. Nash, Inescapable Ecologies, 133.

53. Anderson, <u>The Bracero Program in California</u>, 213, 216, 219.
54. Jacobo, <u>Los Braceros</u>, 84.
55. <u>Migratory Labor in American Agriculture</u>, 156.
56. Galarza, <u>Strangers in Our Fields</u>, 75.
57. Anderson, <u>The Bracero Program in California</u>, 207.
58. Topete, <u>Aventuras de un Bracero</u>, 118.
59. Nash, <u>Inescapable Ecologies</u>, 9.

BIBLIOGRAPHY

ARCHIVES

Archivo General de la Nación, Mexico City.
Archivo Histórico del Insitituto Nacional de Migración, Mexico City.
Bracero History Archive, Roy Rosenzweig Center for History and New Media, George Mason University, http://braceroarchive.org/.
History of the INS Historical Reference Library, Washington DC.
Holt-Atherton Special Collections and University Archives, University of the Pacific, Stockton, California.
National Archives and Records Administration, College Park MD.
National Museum of American History Archives, Washington DC.

PUBLISHED WORKS

Anderson, Henry P. <u>The Bracero Program in California: With Particular Reference to Health Status, Attitudes, and Practices</u>. New York: Arno Press, 1976.
Baynton, Douglas C. "Defectives in the Land: Disability and American Immigration Policy, 1882–1924." <u>Journal of American Ethnic History</u> 24, no. 3 (2005): 31–44.
Calavita, Kitty. <u>Inside the State: The Bracero Program, Immigration, and the I.N.S.</u> New York: Routledge, 1992.
Galarza, Ernesto. <u>Strangers in Our Fields</u>. Washington DC: Joint United States–Mexico Trade Union Committee, 1956.
Jacobo, José-Rodolfo. <u>Los Braceros: Memories of Bracero Workers 1942–1964</u>. San Diego: Southern Border Press, 2004.
Kelman, Ari. <u>A River and Its City: The Nature of Landscape in New Orleans</u>. Berkeley: University of California Press, 2003.

McKiernan-González, John. Fevered Measures: Public Health and Race at the Texas-Mexico Border, 1848–1942. Durham NC: Duke University Press, 2012.

Nash, Linda. Inescapable Ecologies: A History of Environment, Disease, and Knowledge. Berkeley: University of California Press, 2006.

Topete, Jesús. Aventuras de un Bracero. 2d ed. México DF: Editoria Grafica Moderna, 1961.

18

Cripping East Los Angeles

Enabling Environmental Justice in Helena María
Viramontes's Their Dogs Came with Them

Jina B. Kim

In Helena María Viramontes's East Los Angeles the construction
of the 710 and Pomona 60 produces a fractured, maligned, and
thoroughly disabled urban environment. Viramontes's novel Their
Dogs Came with Them (2008), a Chicana coming-of-age narrative set in the age of freeway expansion, employs images of
bodily mutilation to dramatize the effects of urban displacement.
Freeways "[amputate] the streets into stumped dead ends"; an
unfinished overpass "[resembles] a mangled limb"; and nearly
every character carries the somatic imprint of prolonged systemic
neglect (33, 169).[1] Yet while disability operates as shorthand
for communal and geographic rupture in this historic Chicana/o
enclave, it does not act as a mere "narrative prosthesis."[2] Rather
it grants key entry to the novel's formal and political concerns.
As I argue in this paper, these fractured landscapes generate
an infrastructural counterimaginary, one that offers alternative mappings of East Los Angeles via the support networks on
which it depends. As one might expect, this ecology of support
diverges from the dominant urban imaginaries offered by Los
Angeles metropolitan growth coalitions.[3] But it also diverges from
the narrative of self-ownership so central to ethnic American
literary studies.

As the literary scholar Rey Chow has observed, ethnic subjectivity has largely been conceptualized in terms of the teleologi-

cal protest narrative, in which the subject as "resistant captive" engages in a linear "struggle toward liberation," an endpoint imagined as "self-ownership and self-affirmation in both individual and collective senses."[4] This is, in many ways, the ur-narrative of ethnic studies: the recovery of a sovereign, self-determining subject through practices of resistance. In this essay I argue that Viramontes's novel posits a different relation between ethnic subjectivity and literary narrative, one that instead prioritizes the avenues afforded by bodily vulnerability and nonautonomous personhood. Far from a protest novel, Their Dogs Came with Them is an account of human enmeshment within and dependency upon systems of social support. In Viramontes's novel the conditions of environmental injustice invite critiques of self-sustaining personhood, as individual and social bodies become the sum of their disabling entanglements with the cityscape. Yet at the same time that the novel's disabled bodies offer their testimony to urban redevelopment's destructive force, they also become the foundation for a politics and aesthetics of interdependency.[5] Rather than mobilizing narrative toward claims of self-determination or community coherency, then, Their Dogs Came with Them derives narrative and political strategies from the fractured landscape of East Los Angeles, evoking a disability politics that highlights our shared need for assistance. Throughout this essay I demonstrate how the novel's infrastructural counterimaginary underpins an account of human-environmental interconnection as well as a material politics of care.

This essay proceeds in three parts. First, I situate Viramontes's novel in relation to the celebratory discourses of Chicana/o cultural nationalism and Los Angeles freeway expansion, both of which roughly coincide with the novel's 1960–70 timeline. I argue that both nationalism and freeway boosterism rely upon ableist rhetorics to champion, respectively, a unified Chicana/o community and a unified Los Angeles region. In contrast Their Dogs centers disability in its figuration of East LA, thereby offering a narrative of Chicana/o urban life incommensurate with the still resonant discourse of cultural nationalism. In the second section I demonstrate how Viramontes's novel presents an account of human-environmental interpenetration, an enmeshment of skin and smog that suggests the impossibility of self-ownership. Drawing together theories of new materialism and disability studies, I highlight the little explored links between urban redevelopment, environmental racism, and mass disablement, foregrounding disability as a generative site that capacitates alternative political projects and urban epistemologies. In the final section I shift from discussing disabling state infrastructures (the freeway) to informal infrastructures of care, developing further the novel's politics of interdependency. Here I examine how Their Dogs figures the communal networks of material support both paved over and necessitated by freeway construction. Rather than devaluing or disavowing racialized, impoverished, or disabled lives, I argue, the novel highlights the support systems that enable their endurance. In so doing it proffers a narrative of ethnic American subjectivity centered around disabled embodiment.

Freeway Boosterism, Cultural Nationalism, and the Discourse of Ability

Set between the years of 1960 and 1970, Their Dogs Came with Them documents the everyday lives of several young characters growing up in the midst of freeway expansion and Chicana/o cultural nationalism, two discourses central to the novel that I will briefly gloss. In particular I highlight how both redevelopment and Chicana/o nationalism idealize able-bodied subjects and communities, yoking the health of the region and nation to the health of the body. While freeway expansion devastated communities of color, and, in contrast, cultural nationalism vied for the survival of Chicana/o community, both discourses nonetheless mobilize ableist metaphors of bodily wholeness to advocate for their respective sites, the city of Los Angeles and the Chicana/o spiritual homeland of Aztlàn.

Traveling toward East Los Angeles and Boyle Heights, free-way users encounter the concrete jumble known colloquially as "the stack," a "four-freeway interchange," according to Mary Pat Brady,[6] that funnels "547,300 cars a day through the Eastside" (Their Dogs, 169). Together East LA and Boyle Heights, the his-toric Chicana/o enclaves that host Their Dogs, contain no fewer than six major freeway systems. Between 1953 and 1972 East Los Angeles became "home to more freeways than any place in the country," despite decades of complaints by local residents.[7] As the scholars Raúl Homero Villa, Eric Avila, and Rodolfo Acuña have noted, these networks upended Chicana/o community in the postwar period, disrupting families, businesses, and neigh-borhood life.[8]

To justify these intrusions into Chicana/o neighborhoods urban planners seized upon the medical language of blight. Conflating racial difference with physical disability, the rhetoric of blight envisions racialized and low-income neighborhoods as diseased sites waiting for excision. Indeed the predominant urban-planning discourses of 1940s Los Angeles, which advocated both slum clearance and highway construction, cast professional plan-ners as "surgeon generals" vying for the "physical, economic, and moral health of the metropolitan body."[9] Their Dogs makes reference to such medically inflected policing by way of the Quarantine Authority, a fictional state entity that imposes on Eastsiders a mandatory neighborhood-wide curfew, ostensibly to contain a rabies outbreak. The casting of racialized neighbor-hoods as public health hazards, as the Quarantine Authority aptly demonstrates, subtends the regulation of these communities as well as their elimination.

Described by the editors of Westways magazine as the "sinews of a supercity," the burgeoning freeway network was cast in terms of physical hyperability.[10] Espousing a similar rhetoric, the architecture critic Reyner Banham, in Los Angeles: The Architecture of Four Ecologies—the "academic codex of the freeway faithful"[11]—celebrates the heightened sense of physical mobility the freeway imparts. He argues for mobility as itself a type of language, stating, "The city will never be fully understood by those who cannot move fluently through its diverse urban texture."[12] Far from claiming an exceptional viewpoint, Banham and the Westways editors mirrored the sentiments of other well-circulated and contemporaneous cultural narratives. From Disneyland's Autopia ride to Thomas Pynchon's 1966 novella, The Crying of Lot 49, the open road in the postwar LA imaginary functioned as a narrative site of self-determination. And in accordance with this ableist rhetoric the freeway was further imagined as a mechanism of regional cohesion. Expansionist boosters touted the freeway system as the unifying thread of the Los Angeles metropole, one that solidified a disjunctive collection of neighborhoods and towns into a cohesive whole. "Before an inch of concrete could be laid down," writes Brady, the region's "scalar imaginary" underwent a dramatic renovation, in which neighborhoods like Boyle Heights, Long Beach, and Pasadena became "mere nodules on a vertical and greatly expanded scaffold imaginary where the region claimed larger and overriding significance."[13] The freeway, then, was envisioned as vital to Los Angeles, as it maintained the health and physical integrity of the city and region.

Arising at the tail end of freeway expansion, Chicana/o cultural nationalism similarly traded on metaphors of physical ability to articulate communal cohesion. A call for ethnic liberation grounded in decolonization, the Chicana/o movement (el movimiento) promoted ethnic and spiritual unity, identifying "the pre-Columbian Mexica (Aztec) homeland of Aztlàn as the basis for Chicana/o claims to cultural and political self determination."[14] El Plan Espiritual de Aztlàn, a manifesto penned in 1969 by the poets Alurista and Rodolfo "Corky" Gonzales, articulated the ideas that would come to define Chicana/o nationalism. And akin to freeway boosterism, Chicana/o nationalist rhetoric also idealizes an able-bodied subject and community. The literary scholar María Josefina Saldaña-Portillo identifies the ideological overlap between between postwar revolutionary projects and neocolonial development projects, both of which retrench an independent "agent of transformation . . . one who is highly ethical, mobile, risk-taking, and masculinist."[15] El Plan Espiritual explicitly celebrates such an agent. The document's privileged subject was not only "male, working-class, heterosexual and racially marked as Indian/ mestizo" but, as Julie Avril Minich observes, also endowed with the "capacity for physical labor."[16] "Aztlàn," El Plan states, "belongs to those who plant the seeds, water the fields, and gather the crops."[17] Evoking images of laboring bodies, Chicana/o nationalism envisioned a unified homeland peopled by hale, able-bodied subjects.

Their Dogs Came with Them suggests alternatively that a just social order cannot lay claim to bodily integrity—that integrity is, in fact, a fiction. Foregrounding the toxicity generated by freeway expansion, Viramontes's novel instead charts the possibilities of political projects and narrative forms grounded in human-environmental interpenetration. As Stacy Alaimo has argued, the "recognition that human bodies, human health, and human rights are interconnected with the material, often toxic flows of particular places" profoundly affects the ideologies of movements such as cultural nationalism, civil rights, and identity politics, which take for granted that individuals are "bounded, coherent entities."[18] Following this, Their Dogs intervenes into the imaginaries of urban redevelopment and cultural nationalism by centering the disabled figures and environments excised from idealized visions of Los Angeles.

The novel presents a set of characters—mainly young women—irrevocably shaped by the "material, often toxic flows" of environmental racism. Ermila is an orphaned teenager who finds solace in her women's social circle, the "F-Troop"; Ana, a mixed-race, low-paid administrative worker, looks after her troubled brother, Ben; Turtle is a transmasculine gang member of the McBride Boys and recently homeless drifter; and Tranquilina, a Christ-like religious worker, runs a charitable ministry with her parents on the Eastside. As some of the Eastside's most vulnerable and impoverished residents, these characters cannot find affirmation in the movement's idealization of an abstract and cohesive community. These are the inhabitants of what the Chicana feminist Gloria Anzaldúa once termed "El Mundo Zurdo," or "the left-handed world": "the colored, the queer, the poor, the female, the physically challenged."[19]

Given Viramontes's documented dedication to Chicana and women-of-color feminisms, one might expect skepticism toward an undeniably masculinist movement, which often sidelined feminist concerns to promote "la familia de la raza."[20] Indeed much in Their Dogs critiques nationalist discourse. The novel features characters who are notably bad political subjects and who dismiss the project of protest central to the Chicana/o movement. After her initial introduction, Turtle comes across as a "Che Guevara wannabe" with a "brown beret flopped on his head," a figure we later identify as Ben (17).[21] This encounter broadcasts contempt for nationalist devotees, writing off the iconic brown beret with a simple declaration: "What a loser" (17). Later we learn that

Ben dons the beret only after meeting an attractive USC student at the MEChA table, who hands it to him as a gift (118). "Confused and terrified by the antiwar salvo of chanting and pro–civil rights demonstrations," the mixed-race Ben refuses "to be clearly defined as a Chicano" (118). And though Ermila and her teenage friends attend Garfield High, a key site of the burgeoning student movement, they pointedly do not identify as "politically active" (49). They attend a single meeting of the Young Citizens for Community Action, for "the fun of it," "ditching school, rabble-rousing, everyone else thinking they held up banners or raised fists to demand a better education, declare Chicano Power" (49–50). In contrast to the ethnic subject constituted through protest, Viramontes's characters gesture toward the limitations of protest as a mechanism of cultural solidarity; they explicitly seek out other modes of inhabiting the world.

Rather than the independent "agent of transformation," then, Their Dogs traffics in ethnic subjects, communities, and landscapes constituted by their disabling encounters with environmental racism. Through the novel's temporal and spatial formal aspects, as well as its content, Viramontes generates an infrastructural imaginary that evokes the destructive process of freeway construction. In an interview she describes the stories that make up the novel as "[multiplying] like freeway interchanges."[22] Their Dogs toggles unpredictably between 1960 and 1970, featuring an inconsistent, stuttering temporality that parallels the fractures and fissures divvying up the urban landscape. It unfolds in a process of recursion, with each character arc resting loosely on the scaffolding of another. And though the storylines stack one upon the other, much like the Eastside's four-freeway "stack," they "touch and intersect but never precisely connect."[23] Through these nodal points Their Dogs records the subplots and sites of its characters' respective lives, which become increasingly intertwined as the story progresses. Characters traverse the same streets, pass the same landmarks, and share memories of the same geographic touchstones: the unevenly demolished block on First Street; Whittier Boulevard, the "main cruising drag of the Eastside"; and the freshly built intersection connecting the 710 and the Pomona 60 (50).

While the novel's first section documents a series of passing daytime encounters, by its final section the characters are collectively linked through a dual murder: one gang-related, one state-sanctioned. On the eve of his return to Reynosa, Ermila's love-struck cousin, Nacho, locks Ermila's boyfriend, the gangbanger Alfonso, in a lifeguard booth. Enraged, Alfonso commands his gang, the McBride Boys, to "waste" Nacho and encourages Turtle to deliver the final blow. While combing the Eastside streets for Ben, who has gone missing, Ana and Tranquilina come across Nacho's slain body, recently murdered by Turtle. They then witness Turtle's untimely death by Quarantine Authority officers, who have been ordered to aerially observe and shoot all "undomesticated mammals" (54).

In the novel's somber ending we mourn the material and social costs of environmental racism, which rend apart body, landscape, and community. Rather than narrating a "resistant captive" grasping toward self-ownership, the novel registers the dispersal of the ethnic subject across a toxic environment and the vulnerability of brown bodies within a predatory landscape.[24] By decentering community, individual, and territorial unity as the foundation for a progressive Chicana/o politic, Viramontes's novel diverges from the dominant rhetorics of cultural nationalism and brings disability into the orbit of ethnic cultural production and critique.

A Disabled Somatics of Place

Envisioned in postwar LA iconography as an instrument of hyperability and hypermobility, in Their Dogs the freeway instead initiates a cycle of debilitating exchange between the local environment and its inhabitants. Freeway construction and its aftermath generate what I term "a disabled somatics of place," wherein the violated, ruptured bodies of people and landscape invite a heightened transference of matter, and human and environment begin to mirror one another. Laden with leaky imagery Their Dogs traffics in partial pieces, fragmented figures, and open forms as a means of illustrating the porous interface linking human and environmental elements.[25] This interface assumes the form of "tar feet," "tar-smudged" faces, "tobacco-stained" hands, human indentations on chairs and books, landscapes with "cesarean scars," and rotting houses featuring curling "tongues of paint" (4, 5, 325, 14). Through the disabled somatics of place, an aesthetic mode in which disability operates as environmental ambience rather than personal attribute, Their Dogs proffers a narrative world centrally defined by disabled embodiment. Yet the novel's disabled bodies do not function as signs of "political failure and decline," as the protest narrative might suggest,[26] but as sites of knowledge production in their own right. While the disabled somatics of place may recall the oft-critiqued characterization of disability as pathology, impairment, or lack, the social politics that Viramontes puts forth situates disability as a generative site, one that (1) intervenes in a Chicana/o nationalism predicated on false bodily integrity, (2) gives narrative form and urgency to the slow violence of environmental racism, and (3) complicates the dominant theoretical models governing our understanding of disabled subjectivity.

Akin to the eco-materialist focus on the significance of nonhuman agents—what the new materialist critic Jane Bennett terms the "force of things"[27]—Viramontes's novel redraws the lines of relation between people and their surroundings, indicating a mutual and debilitating exchange. That is, the fragments, leaks, and disappearances that constitute the disabled somatics of place signal the interpenetration of human and landscape and, further, emblematize the violence enacted through ostensibly neutral urban policy. This porous transit evokes what Alaimo terms "trans-corporeality," an ontological model in which "the human is always enmeshed with the more-than-human world." Recognition of our porous condition, Alaimo contends, will foster an "environmental ethos" that cultivates a "tangible sense of connection to the material world."[28] And in acknowledging human contingency on the "more-than-human world" this ethos implicitly dispels the fantasy of self-ownership and suggests that a more just social order must begin by acknowledging the body's permeability.

In Their Dogs human-environmental interconnection is envisioned through and intensified by the phenomenon of environmental racism, a disabling transit between body and landscape. While eco-materialist critics insist upon recognizing our enmeshment with the environment and, similarly, disability studies scholars "remind us that all bodies are shaped by their environments at the moment of conception," Viramontes's novel suggests that such reminders of human-environmental interdependency prove unnecessary and unexceptional for her Eastside characters.[29] Presenting a city steeped in pollutant byproducts, she employs dirty and invasive imagery to highlight the racially uneven consequences of urban redevelopment and the disproportionate toxic load borne by racialized communities. Indeed communities of color, according to environmental justice scholars such as Robert D. Bullard, "are subjected to a disproportionately large number of health and environmental risks in their neighborhoods . . . and on their jobs."[30] Race further impacts "accessibility to health care" and the proximity of "freeways, sewage treatment plants . . . and other noxious facilities" to neighborhoods.[31] And for those subject to these pernicious effects, the porous transit between human and landscape, which fosters a "tangible sense of connection to the material world," is all too often incapacitating.

Yet while studies of environmental racism invariably reference disability to denote environmental harm, few if any address the phenomenon from a critical disability perspective. In these primarily sociological studies, which seek to "quantify, measure, and 'prove' that environmental racism exists," disability is a constitutive feature of environmental racism but is treated simply as a transparent measure of inequity.[32] In contrast Viramontes's novel enables a consideration of disability vis-à-vis environmental racism that goes beyond quantifiable evidence. In Their Dogs disability operates as a mechanism of knowledge production and cultural critique. It posits modes of narrating and "knowing" the Eastside barrio grounded in disabled experience and of narrating and knowing disability via the Eastside barrio. In this way the novel demonstrates one of the political labors specific to literary fiction: the excavation of occluded systems of knowledge and the imaginative recuperation of fragmentary, peripheral, or ephemeral information absent from the historical record.

Across a range of physiological and psychological states disability is a definitive characteristic of Viramontes's Eastside community. The landscape and residents alike bear the stigma of poverty-induced environmental stress: years of manual labor, inadequate health infrastructures, forced displacement, and freeway construction. Subject to an erratic upbringing and a traumatic truck accident, the once promising student Ben Brady grapples with waves of an undisclosed mental illness. He struggles to secure adequate care from the public hospital system, which can only offer him seventy-two hours' worth of medical attention, thereby signaling the inadequacy of public infrastructure aimed at supporting Eastsiders (90). Lollie, one of Ermila's high school girlfriends, endures "degrees of deafness" due to the "bombarding pinions of earsplitting stitching" at her mother's garment factory (188). And though we never learn the occupation of Ermila's Grandfather Zumaya, references to his "hunchback stuffed with endless scolding" and "steel-tip leather boots" suggest a lifetime's worth of stiffening labor (10).

With its leaky cache of images <u>Their Dogs</u> gives form, momentum, and story to the quiet, quotidian theater of environmental racism. The novel's disabled somatics of place, which offer an alternative conceptual map of East Los Angeles, operate as a form of testimony: a living archive in which the body itself operates as documentation. This aesthetic mode materializes the often imperceptible and slow-moving intrusions of toxic exposure, which, in Viramontes' novel, are quite literally written on the body. It renders material the microscopic, slow-paced, and everyday intrusions not easily captured in narrative representation, the toxic everyday theorized by the literary critic Rob Nixon as "slow violence."[33] These miasmatic phenomena become concrete through the novel's disabled landscapes and bodies and their constant transit. The toxic byproducts of freeway construction circulate throughout the novel and the bodies of Eastside residents, narrativizing the freeway's often invisible, slow-paced effects on community health. Clouds of dirt, exhaust, and noise permeate both domestic interiors and public spaces, subjecting Eastsiders to a constant and inevitably lethal onslaught of contaminants. The residents of First Street, for example, must endure the "black fumes of the bulldozer exhaust hovering over the new pavements," the "jackhammering blasts and cacophony of earthmovers," and "floodlights [jetting] through the drawn blinds, drone of engines in and out of the hours" (8, 27, 75). Schoolchildren enjoy recess under the haze of a smog alert, and Ermila's grandmother breathes air "too thick to filter through her lungs," indicating future ill health (129). Fractured, overwhelming, and often threatening, the environment presses upon the reader's consciousness, and the background matter of East LA accelerates to the fore, "[becoming] available for progressive acts of reading and perhaps even for change."[34] That is, while sociological studies of environmental racism cast disability as a mere metric of injustice, in Their Dogs disability functions as a platform for epistemological and social transformation.

The disabled somatics of place too solicit a revision of the dominant paradigms that have come to govern the field of disability studies. For many scholars of disability, disability theorizing has frequently "[worked] from the assumption that disability is a minority subject position" and thus conceives of disability as "any departure from an unstated physical and functional norm."[35] That is, disability studies, and first-wave disability scholarship in particular, posit disability as a category of minority identity to which civil rights can adhere. In Their Dogs, however, disability is the norm and mass disablement a symptom of prolonged physical duress and insufficient infrastructural support. Conceptions of disabled embodiment grounded in minority identity are thus contested by Viramontes's Eastside, in which the confluence of racism, sexism, and poverty render disability nearly ubiquitous. In turn the ubiquity of disability foregrounds the relation between systemic racism and the creation of disability, positing disability as a standard feature of low-income and racialized communities. To borrow a formulation from the disability scholar Nirmala Erevelles, disability in Viramontes's novel functions as not a "condition of being but of becoming," a dynamic rewriting of the flesh. Rather than a static category of minority identity, disability operates here as a "historical event," embedded in processes of neocolonialism, structural racism, and urban displacement.[36] The "eventness" of disability in Their Dogs is inextricably linked to postwar urban redevelopment, a form of neocolonial displacement that fractured landscape and community alike. Diverging from the theories of minority identity that have come to define the category of disability,[37] disability functions here as atmosphere, as ambience, as an event that unfolds through the interpenetration of human and environment. The disabled somatics of place, then, demonstrate once more how "transcorporeality" provokes a reconceptualization of identity categories. And through the disabled somatics of place Their Dogs compels us to reconsider the theoretical parameters of disability as category and demonstrates how environmental racism solicits new theories of disabled embodiment.

Shaped by a public infrastructure system more invested in the flow of capital than the well-being of the least powerful, the disabled bodies and landscapes of Their Dogs offer a "space for reading the way that bios is determined by history,"[38] as well as the disabling transit between body and landscape amplified by processes of environmental racism. Though East Los Angeles is rent and covered up by freeway construction, these bodies testify to the intrusions of a metropolitan order governed by white supremacy. And in offering an epistemology of somatic witness Their Dogs reconfigures the way we think about ethnic American subjectivity vis-à-vis literary production. The disabling traffic between human and "more-than-human nature" narrates a Chicana/o subject and community that is not self-contained and self-affirming but violated and transformed by the toxic flows of city life.[39]

Infrastructures of Care as Environmental Justice
Given the concentration of disabled figures in Viramontes's East Los Angeles, how does the novel portray the process of healing, or even simply managing the onslaught of environmental

duress? Notably this is not a rehabilitative narrative in which one "overcomes" disability, an ableist storyline thoroughly critiqued by disability scholars. Viramontes refuses to organize the anarchic material of environmental crisis into a linear narrative of healing, one that papers over the ongoing toxicity generated by systemic racism.

To begin, Their Dogs suggests that the debilitating processes of environmental racism necessitate alternative forms of social, political, and cultural expression—narratives that, in short, go beyond the teleological narrative of self-ownership. To be clear, while I do not wish to dismiss the project of Chicana/o self-determination, and in fact insist upon its continuing relevance, I nonetheless contend that social justice models—and "progressive" models of literary interpretation, for that matter—cannot be wholly conditioned by the binaries of resistance or complicity, protest or acquiescence. And so rather than mapping the barrio exclusively in terms of "blight" or political resistance, Their Dogs charts the relations of care that underpin neighborhood life. It exhumes the sites and figures that salve environmental racism while critiquing the conditions that necessitate these informal support networks. The novel figures ostensibly public infrastructures, such as the freeway and the General Hospital, as contributing to the community's ill health and constructs an alternative infrastructural imaginary by underscoring informal systems of support. In short, it envisions environmental and social justice in terms of interdependency; here environmental justice entails enabling the survival of vulnerable life.[40]

To articulate a politics of interdependence, Their Dogs foregrounds the marginal figures and sites that simply make life more possible: Ermila's social circle, an elderly woman's nurturing blue house, Turtle's sibling bond with Luis Lil Lizard, and Tranquilina's charitable ministry. These informal safety nets, which I term "infrastructures of care," have received scant attention in the novel's critical reception despite underpinning what I identify as its primary vision of social recuperation. However, even these safety nets do not escape critique and raise a battery of questions: Does the lack of adequate public infrastructure force Eastsiders to construct informal support structures, thereby generating an extra burden of labor? Do these informal infrastructures allow the city to shirk its responsibilities, thereby coercing its residents to make do with fewer and fewer resources? The novel's ambivalence toward some of these informal networks, such as Tranquilina's ministry, provokes reflection on the dilemma of state care in an era wrought by infrastructural abandonment. On the one hand, state infrastructures and safety nets work to discipline the racialized poor and thus will always operate as mechanisms of violence, yet, on the other hand, informal infrastructures and privatized models of care erode state accountability to the public. Through its ambivalent figuration of informal infrastructure Their Dogs complicates the roles that nurturing elders and local charities serve in impoverished urban communities, thus disallowing any easy romanticization of "community."

Though the novel offers no easy remedies, it nonetheless elicits reflection on the supporting operations of East Los Angeles and the ways subjects and communities simply cannot make do without safety nets. Indeed, as Mitchum Huehls argues, the Eastsiders in the novel have "immediate material [needs]" that must be addressed one way or another.[41] Most significantly it hinges survival upon an acknowledgment of the self and community as multiply determined and embedded in wider webs of support. The only "independent" subject in the novel, Turtle Gamboa, inevitably perishes. Stripped of home, resources, family, and friends, she simply cannot survive.

Their Dogs foregrounds care as, above all, a social project to be shouldered by all rather than a private endeavor relegated to the domestic sphere. Resonant with feminist disability scholarship's "ethic of care," the novel's figuration of disability suggests that "human interdependence and the universal need for assistance" fundamentally affect narrative forms—like the protest narrative— that shore up a self-governing ideal of subjectivity. And in contrast to the widespread devaluation of care work, which leads in part to the "asymmetries of care relations," Their Dogs pays proper homage to the sites and figures that provide support.[42] The novel foregrounds Freudian "anaclitic love," or what Judith Butler describes as "the type of love that is characterized by the need for support or by the love of those who support."[43] And certainly anaclitic love on a "wider social scale" guides much of the affective force behind the novel's intimate descriptions of Chicana/o urban life.[44] Viramontes offers a paean, a "kind of praise-song for laboring Chicana/os," for the nannies, house-keepers, nursing aides, and garment workers that sustain the city's everyday operations.[45] While such laboring figures often occupy the margins of consideration, here they emerge made of "gut and grist and a gleam of determination as blinding as a California sun" (176).

In parallel Their Dogs begins with an elegy for the elder Chavela's house, which provides a much needed refuge for the neighborhood's children. It is also one of the first houses destroyed by the freeway expansion. At this initial scene of displacement we observe Chavela organizing her belongings into boxes and inventorying her life: "Cobijas, one note said; Cosa del baño, said another. No good dresses. Josie's typewriter. Fotos" (5). Her exhaustive list lends detail and texture to a house marked for removal, a seemingly marginal site that gives sanctuary to the neighborhood's children. Ermila, then identified as the "Zumaya child," visits with Chavela to escape the disciplinary atmosphere of her grandparents' house, luxuriating in the old woman's company (5). Following Chavela's removal, Ermila feels a "slow swelling lump of desire for Chavela and the blue house on First Street with its damp scent of tobacco and burnt out matchsticks" (144). Associated throughout the novel with ferns and hibiscus, Chavela tends a small yard with a "lemon tree that yielded lemons every other year," "potted ferns" that "[hang] from the shanty arbor built by a married man she had once loved," and "shrubs of bursting red hibiscus bushes that bloomed lush and rich as only ancient deep-rooted hibiscus shrubs can do" (7). Her yard anchors intimate histories; indeed the earthmovers not only displace people; they also uproot "vast networks of affiliations and place-linked memories."[46] Though she, and later Ermila, attempt to commit the details of her beloved house to memory, Chavela warns Ermila to always "pay attention" because "displacement will always come down to two things: earthquakes or earthmovers" (8). With this piece of counsel she suggests that land and property can never serve as the foundation for a communal politics, implicitly challenging the mythological ideal of Aztlàn, the nationalist spiritual homeland. Instead of lobbying for "solid tierra," Chavela offers restorative gestures that reinforce the value of racialized, impoverished, and disabled life, demonstrating a practice and politics of interdependency.

While the novel makes social and environmental support vital to Viramontes's Eastside, it also problematizes the systematic privatization of care that has transformed East LA's landscape. Much in Their Dogs meditates on the problem of offering love and shelter in a place where protective acts are anathema. The absence of truly supportive public infrastructures for Eastsiders yields informal infrastructures, represented in part by Chavela's house and Tranquilina's charitable ministry. Peopled on its peripheries by "congealed squatters like scabs on a wound" (276), East LA's unsupported populace gives rise to what Michael Dear and Jennifer Wolch term "zones of dependence," urban sites "dominated by service clients and their professional helpers."[47] Accelerated by welfare state restructuring in the 1970s, community care has undergone a "programmatic deinstitutionalization of social support," and the labor of care "is increasingly provided by a diverse, non-government human service sector, made up of a panoply of voluntary and for-profit agencies." This transition exemplifies the shifting of public responsibility to the private sphere; "any 'contracting out' of human services by the state is a form of privatization, irrespective of whether the supplier is motivated by profit or by altruism."[48] And as Eva Feder Kittay, Evelyn Nakano Glenn, and other feminist scholars have noted, these workers are given little to no financial compensation, devaluing further the labors of care.[49] Viramontes's East LA teems with the latest incarnation of community care. In addition to the Little Brothers of the Poor Rest Home, where Turtle gulps "lukewarm broth," and the Sacred Heart Church, where migratory laborers gather in search of employment, Tranquilina, Mama, and Papa Tomás run a ministry that doles out spiritual and physical sustenance to the Eastside's most impoverished, dependent, and disabled residents (18). They index the apparatus of charity that emerges in the absence of public support.

Grappling with the conundrum of public care in the midst of welfare erosion, Viramontes's figuration of their charitable ministry expresses both hesitation toward and recognition of their work's necessity. Tranquilina, the primary person in their trinity of caretaking, has reservations about the ministry despite laboring tirelessly to provide "simmering beef cocido," comfort, and attention to parishioners (84). "The constant flow of pitiless doubters and forever larger supply of ravished believers" strains her vigilance, her dedication now "buried in layers of decaying convictions" (31) Her efforts to shift the ministry sermon to topics of immediate material concern—the "quarantine and the roadblocks"—are met with Mama's refusal, as their church "had no room for a discussion regarding government rules" (86). Though Mama and Papa Tomás cling to the idea of spiritual uplift for Eastsiders, Tranquilina recognizes that the ministry operates best as an instrument of bodily rejuvenation. She knows that, for the down-and-out parishioners, "their ministry was no better than another bottle of Thunderbird wine, a quick fix of heroin, another prescription drug for temporal relief" (97).

Regardless, Tranquilina remains dedicated to meeting the yawning material needs of the Eastside: "Even with assassinations, assaults, and the slaughter of planet and people, [her] love for this world remained a conflicted, loyal love . . . because everything happened here on these sidewalks or muddy swamps of vacant lots or in deep back alleys, not up in the heavens of God" (34). At thirty-three she is explicitly associated with Christ and commits herself to the earthly concerns of the Eastside. Yoking herself to the ministry's needy in an interdependent, trans-corporeal relation, Tranquilina believes that "boundaries didn't exist between her life and their lives" and desires to be "their nourishment, their milk and muscle" (97, 37). Like Chavela, she practices a politics of care for the dependent body, administering to some of its most basic, sensuous needs. And yet in expressing frustration at the sheer volume of parishioners, she also implicitly critiques the injustices of environmental racism and the systemic production of disability that necessitates informal infrastructure.

Chavela and Tranquilina thus exemplify a politics grounded in the condition of bodily and environmental vulnerability. They assert value for life that is destitute, deviant, and defenseless, both acknowledging and salving the conditions that perpetuate mass disablement for the racialized urban poor. Invested in the salvaging of life value, Tranquilina's politics of interdependency surfaces most clearly in the novel's violent conclusion. Searching futilely for Ben, Tranquilina and Ana encounter Nacho's lifeless body, recently "wasted" by Turtle: "And then like a déjà vu, Turtle recognized the woman who bent over the boy, removed her cape, a superman's cape, and pillowed it under the boy's mess of black water" (324). Devastated by Nacho's death, Tranquilina soon bears witness to another thoughtless killing. Turtle, mistaken by the Quarantine Authority helicopters as an "undomesticated mammal," is gunned down: "Turtle's chest burned down to her belly. Although she stood in the shower of rain, her face flamed something fierce. She dropped to her knees, quietly, into a puddle of oily water. Someone cradled her, held her as tight and strong as her brother, held all of her together until sleep came to her fully welcomed. We'rrrre not doggggs! Tranquilina roared in the direction of the shooters" (324).

Faced with two lifeless bodies, Tranquilina "[rearranges] the boy in an effort to make him comfortable in his eternal sleep, just as she had done with the other boy lying a few yards away" (325). In this moment she becomes the sum of their fatal entanglements with the cityscape, embodying their injuries in an act of intense empathy: "Absolutely drenched in the black waters of blood and torrents of rain, Tranquilina couldn't delineate herself from the murdered souls because these tears and blood and rain and bullet wounds belonged to her as well" (325).

While scholars like Hsuan Hsu, Sarah Wald, and Alicia Muñoz have interpreted the final scene as a gesture of resistance, prioritizing Tranquilina's "[refusal] to halt" before the Quarantine Authority, I identify it as a reenactment of the famous Pietà, the ultimate gesture of care (325).[50] Instead of adjusting the story to fit a protest narrative I prioritize the apparatus of support that the novel itself highlights. Here Tranquilina transforms into the mourning Mary and gives tribute to bodies considered either invisible or disposable. The representation of violence inflicted upon the racialized urban poor is largely either nonexistent or victim blaming, and those slain at the hands of state-sanctioned violence are rarely paid vigil.[51] This absence of empathy speaks to the systematic devaluation of life that is the work of environmental racism; after all, in the words of Butler, "for [life] to be regarded as valuable, it has to first be regarded as grievable."[52] For Tranquilina the social project of care necessitates abolishing the logic that prioritizes some bodies and some neighborhoods over others, indeed the logic underpinning freeway construction. To move toward care as a social project—a politics of interdependency—we must begin with grief, with the recognition that no subject or landscape is inherently disposable.

While Viramontes's Chicana coming-of-age novel might initially call to mind the ethnic protest narrative or the quintessential narrative of development—the Bildungsroman—it ultimately eschews the agential subject of resistance of Chicana/o cultural nationalism and, relatedly, the subject of self-ownership idealized by ethnic literary studies. It closes with a tableau of grief and interpersonal empathy, an image in accordance with its politics and aesthetics of interdependency: the social project of care and the disabled somatics of place. As such Viramontes's novel solicits alternative paths for ethnic American literary and disability scholarship. It both models and calls for stories that accommodate the debilitating reality of environmental racism and in so doing proffers a transformative disability politics that incorporates considerations of race, neocolonialism, state violence, and urban displacement. Through its critique of state-sponsored infrastructures and its emphasis on informal infrastructures of care, Their

Dogs disarticulates the relation of protest linking ethnic subjectivity and cultural production. Instead it offers an infrastructural imaginary that testifies to the undervalued labor of care and the slow violence of racialized disablement, foregrounding the supporting operations that enable Eastsiders to endure.

NOTES

1. Viramontes, Their Dogs Came with Them, 33, 169. Subsequent references to this novel are cited parenthetically in the text.
2. Narrative prosthesis, according to Mitchell and Snyder, refers to the use of disability as an "opportunistic metaphorical device" in American literature in which the representation of disability operates as a simple narrative shorthand rather than a reflection of disability's lived realities (Narrative Prosthesis, 47).
3. For an extended explanation of the metropolitan growth coalition, see Harvey Molotch's "The City as Growth Machine: Toward a Political Economy of Place," American Journal of Sociology 82, no. 2 (1976): 309–32.
4. Chow, The Protestant Ethic and the Spirit of Capitalism, 40–41.
5. See the chapter "Body as Testimony" in Yaeger's Dirt and Desire. Here Yaeger theorizes a kind of somatic testimony in which bodies operate as living archives.
6. Brady, "Metaphors to Love By," 174.
7. Bullard and Johnson, Just Transportation, 18.
8. See Villa's Barrio-Logos; Rodolfo Acuña's A Community under Siege: A Chronicle of Chicanos East of the Los Angeles River 1945–1975 (Los Angeles: Chicano Studies Research Center, UCLA, 1984); Eric Avila's The Folklore of the Freeway: Race and Revolt in the Modernist City (Minneapolis: University of Minnesota Press, 2014).
9. Goodman, After the Planners, 67; Villa, Barrio-Logos, 71.
10. Meyer, "Sinews of a Super City," 27.
11. Villa, Barrio-Logos, 84.
12. Banham, Los Angeles, 23.
13. Brady, "Metaphors to Love By," 174.
14. Minich, Accessible Citizenships, 35.

15. Saldaña-Portillo, The Revolutionary Imagination in the Age of the Americas and the Age of Development, 9.
16. Yarbro-Bejarano, "Laying It Bare," 277; Minich, Accessible Citizenships, 36.
17. "El Plan Espiritual de Aztlàn." 1.
18. Alaimo, Bodily Natures, 23.
19. Anzaldúa, "El Mundo Zurdo," 218.
20. Ramirez, The Woman in the Zoot Suit, 19.
21. Though Their Dogs portrays Turtle as transmasculine, I use feminine pronouns to remain consistent with the novel.
22. Olivas, "Interview with Helena María Viramontes."
23. Brady, "Metaphors to Love By," 177.
24. Chow, The Protestant Ethnic and the Spirit of Capitalism, 40.
25. In "Fatal Contiguities: Metonymy and Environmental Justice," literary scholar Hsuan Hsu describes the leaky interpenetration of human with environment evident in Viramontes's novel as a type of metonymy, arguing that these "metonymic human-environment relationships" render visible the "human effects of ambient (often imperceptible) environmental harm concentrated in East L.A." (157).
26. Minich, Accessible Citizenships, 34.
27. See Jane Bennett, Vibrant Matter: A Political Ecology of Things (Durham NC: Duke University Press, 2009).
28. Alaimo, Bodily Natures, 2, 16.
29. Garland-Thomson, "Disability and Representation," 524.
30. Bullard, introduction, 10.
31. Bullard, "The Threat of Environmental Racism," 23.
32. Sze, "'Not by Politics Alone,'" 33.
33. Nixon defines slow violence as a "violence of delayed destruction that is dispersed across time and space, an attritional violence that is typically not viewed as violence at all" (Slow Violence and the Environmentalism of the Poor, 2). He particularly focuses on the problem of representation presented by slow violence, as we as a culture seem to respond primarily to instances of spectacular, instantaneous violence. The medium of literature, he argues, is ideal for materializing and narrativizing such slow-acting phenomena and thus inciting us to action.

34. Yaeger, Dirt and Desire, 30–31.
35. Barker and Murray, "Disabling Postcolonialism," 229; Garland-Thomson, Extraordinary Bodies, 26.
36. Erevelles, Disability and Difference in Global Contexts, 27.
37. For the most oft-cited examples of this theory, see Simi Linton, Claiming Disability: Knowledge and Identity (New York: NYU Press, 1998); Tobin Siebers, Disability Theory (Ann Arbor: University of Michigan Press, 2008).
38. Yaeger, Dirt and Desire, 221.
39. Alaimo, Bodily Natures, 2.
40. The official and oft-cited definition of environmental justice, borrowed here from the Environmental Protection Agency, is "the fair treatment and meaningful involvement of all people regardless of race, color, national origin, or income with respect to the development, implementation, and enforcement of environmental laws, regulations, and policies." See Environmental Protection Agency, "Environmental Justice," accessed October 17, 2016, https://www.epa.gov/environmentaljustice.
41. Huehls, "Private Property as Story," 162.
42. Garland-Thomson, "Integrating Disability, Transforming Feminist Theory," 344.
43. Butler and Jackson, "What Makes Performance Possible?"
44. Jackson, Social Works, 36.
45. Brady, "Metaphors to Love By," 181.
46. Brady, "Metaphors to Love By," 178.
47. Dear and Wolch, Landscapes of Despair, 60.
48. Gleeson, Geographies of Disability, 153.
49. See Kittay, Love's Labor.
50. See Hsu's "Fatal Contiguities"; Sarah Wald's "Refusing to Halt: Mobility and the Quest for Spatial Justice in Helena María Viramontes's Their Dogs Came with Them and Karen Tei Yamashita's Tropic of Orange," Western American Literature 48, no. 1 (2013): 70–89; and Alicia Muñoz's "Articulating a Geography of Pain: Metaphor, Memory and Movement in Helena María Viramontes's Their Dogs Came with Them," MELUS: Multi-Ethnic Literature of the U.S. 38, no. 2 (2013): 24–38.

51. The black, brown, and disabled lives lost to state-imposed violence are rarely paid vigil in mainstream media outlets, though social media campaigns like #BlackLivesMatter and #ICan'tBreathe have garnered attention in a number of underground and mainstream spheres and are doing the crucial work of grieving black and brown lives.
52. Butler, "A Carefully Crafted F*ck You."

BIBLIOGRAPHY

Alaimo, Stacy. Bodily Natures: Science, Environment and the Material Self. Bloomington: Indiana University Press, 2010.
Anzaldúa, Gloria. "El Mundo Zurdo: The Vision." In This Bridge Called My Back: Writings by Radical Women of Color, 4th ed., edited by Cherríe L. Moraga and Gloria E. Anzaldúa, 195–96. Albany: State University of New York Press, 2015.
Banham, Reyner. Los Angeles: The Architecture of Four Ecologies. New York: Penguin Books, 1971.
Barker, Claire, and Stuart Murray. "Disabling Postcolonialism: Global Disability Cultures and Democratic Criticism." Journal of Literary and Cultural Disability Studies 4, no. 3 (2010): 219–36.
Brady, Mary Pat. "Metaphors to Love By: Toward a Chicana Aesthetics in Their Dogs Came with Them." In Rebozos de Palabras: An Helena María Viramontes Critical Reader, edited by Gabriella Gutiérrez y Muhs, 167–91. Tucson: University of Arizona Press, 2013.
Bullard, Robert D. Introduction to Confronting Environmental Racism: Voices from the Grassroots, edited by Robert D. Bullard and Benjamin Chavis Jr., 7–15. Cambridge MA: South End Press, 1993.
———. "The Threat of Environmental Racism." Natural Resources and Environment 7, no. 3 (1993): 23–26, 55–56.
Bullard, Robert D., and Glenn S. Johnson, eds. Just Transportation: Dismantling Race and Class Barriers to Mobility. Stony Creek CT: New Society, 1997.
Butler, Judith. "A Carefully Crafted F*ck You: Nathan Schneider Interviews Judith Butler." Guernica: A Magazine of Art and Politics, March 15, 2010. https://www.guernicamag.com/interviews/a_carefully_crafted_fk_you/.

Butler, Judith, and Shannon Jackson. "What Makes Performance Possible?" Lecture, Colorado College, October 2009.

Chow, Rey. The Protestant Ethnic and the Spirit of Capitalism. New York: Columbia University Press, 2002.

Dear, Michael J., and Jennifer R. Wolch. Landscapes of Despair: From Deinstitutionalization to Homelessness. Princeton NJ: Princeton University Press, 1992.

"El Plan Espiritual de Aztlàn." In Aztlàn: Essays on the Chicano Homeland, edited by Rudolfo Anaya and Francisco Lomelí, 1–5. Albuquerque: University of New Mexico Press, 1989.

Erevelles, Nirmala. Disability and Difference in Global Contexts: Enabling a Transformative Body Politic. New York: Palgrave Macmillan, 2011.

Ferguson, Roderick A. Aberrations in Black: Toward a Queer of Color Critique. Minneapolis: University of Minnesota Press, 2004.

Garland-Thomson, Rosemarie. "Disability and Representation." PMLA 120, no. 2 (2005): 522–27.

———. Extraordinary Bodies: Figuring Physical Disability in American Literature and Culture. New York: Columbia University Press, 1996.

———. "Integrating Disability, Transforming Feminist Theory." In The Disability Studies Reader, 4th ed., edited by Lennard J. Davis, 333–53. New York: Routledge, 2013.

Gleeson, Brendan. Geographies of Disability. New York: Routledge, 1998.

Goodman, Robert. After the Planners. New York: Touchstone, 1971.

Hong, Grace Kyungwon. The Ruptures of American Capital: Women of Color Feminism and the Culture of Immigrant Labor. Minneapolis: University of Minnesota Press, 2006.

Hsu, Hsuan. "Fatal Contiguities: Metonymy and Environmental Justice." New Literary History 42, no. 1 (2011): 147–68.

Huehls, Mitchum. "Private Property as Story: Helena Viramontes' Their Dogs Came with Them." Arizona Quarterly: A Journal of American Literature, Culture, and Theory 68, no. 4 (2012): 155–82.

Jackson, Shannon. Social Works: Performing Art, Supporting Publics. New York: Routledge, 2011.

Kittay, Eva Feder. Love's Labor: Essays on Women, Equality, and Dependency. New York: Routledge, 1999.

Meyer, Larry L. "Sinews of a Supercity." Westways 57 (June): 1965, 26–28, 46.

Minich, Julie Avril. Accessible Citizenships: Disability, Nation, and the Cultural Politics of Greater Mexico. Philadelphia: Temple University Press, 2014.

Mitchell, David T., and Sharon L. Snyder. Narrative Prosthesis: Disability and the Dependencies of Discourse. Ann Arbor: University of Michigan Press, 2001.

Nixon, Rob. Slow Violence and the Environmentalism of the Poor. Cambridge MA: Harvard University Press, 2011.

Olivas, Daniel. "Interview with Helena María Viramontes." La Bloga, April 2, 2007. http://labloga.blogspot.com/2007/04/interview-with-helena-mara—viramontes.html.

Ramirez, Catherine S. The Woman in the Zoot Suit: Gender, Nationalism, and the Cultural Politics of Memory. Durham NC: Duke University Press, 2009.

Saldaña-Portillo, María Josefina. The Revolutionary Imagination in the Age of the Americas and the Age of Development. Durham NC: Duke University Press, 2003.

Sze, Julie. "'Not by Politics Alone': Gender and Environmental Justice in Karen Tei Yamashita's Tropic of Orange." Bucknell Review 44, no. 1 (2000): 29–42.

Villa, Raúl Homero. Barrio-Logos: Space and Place in Urban Chicano Literature and Culture. Austin: University of Texas Press, 2000.

Viramontes, Helena María. Their Dogs Came with Them. New York: Atria Press, 2008.

Yaeger, Patricia. Dirt and Desire: Reconstructing Southern Women's Writing, 1930–1990. Chicago: University of Chicago Press, 2000.

Yarbro-Bejarano, Yvonne. "Laying It Bare: The Queer/Colored Body in Photography by Laura Aguilar." In Living Chicana Theory, edited by Carla Trujillo, 277–305. Berkeley CA: Third Woman Press.

19

Neurological Diversity and Environmental (In)Justice

The Ecological Other in Popular and Journalist Representations of Autism

Sarah Gibbons

In "Don't Mourn for Us," a letter to parents of autistic children, self-advocate Jim Sinclair (1993) contests the belief that autism is the barrier behind which lies a "normal" child. Sinclair encourages parents to rethink their belief that autism is an "impenetrable wall" that prevents them from communicating with their normal child. He invites them to stop mourning for a child who is very much alive and to accept that autism is an integral aspect of that child's personality. The disability studies scholar Stuart Murray (2008, 30–31), who also addresses the popular belief that individuals host their autism, considers the detrimental impact of this "autism-inside-the-person" model. The perception that autism involves a parasitic relationship, with the individual acting as a host, has underpinned many theories about autism that position it as a disease as opposed to a set of neurological differences.[1] As Murray (2012, 89–90) suggests, many theories foster the belief that autism must be cured when "all serious research into autism acknowledges that it is a lifelong condition that is built into the fabric of the person who has it," and "as such, it cannot be cured." Many activists and academics, along with the Autistic Self Advocacy Network (ASAN), contest the belief that a cure is desirable (Baggs 2007; Broderick and Ne'eman 2008;

Murray 2012; Sinclair 1993; Yergeau 2010). Yet despite increasing interest in neurodiversity, many believe we are experiencing an autism epidemic.

In this essay I discuss how proponents of the epidemic theory appeal to environmental thinkers by linking rising diagnoses to undesirable changes in our environments. While demonstrating how environmental degradation affects human health and ability is an important aspect of environmental justice, a disconnect exists between the concern that environmentalists express for rising diagnoses of autism and the importance of equal rights that has been the focus of autistic self-advocates and their supporters. To examine the connection between autism discourse and environmentalist discourse I use Sarah Jaquette Ray's (2013) formulation of the "ecological other." Ray explains that mainstream environmentalism has contributed to the exclusion of disabled people in American culture and shows how "the figure of the disabled body is the quintessential symbol of humanity's alienation from nature" as "environmentalism played a significant role in constructing the disabled body, a historical legacy that continues to shape the corporeal bases for its various forms of exclusion" (6). Ray's concept is useful for considering how the language of threat surrounding autism is bolstered by a belief that its development represents the toxic effects of biotechnology companies and consumptive practices.

Guided by Ray's concept of the "ecological other," I examine a selection of North American environmentalist articles and blogs, materials from autism organizations, and two recent documentaries. I examine the language used to articulate connections between autism and our changing environment in these artifacts. I do not engage with the question of whether or to what extent autism has environmental causes. Rather I examine the knowledge translation of research on environmental factors to the general public. Showing how discourse surrounding autism often draws problematic comparisons between the changes represented by ecological devastation and the changing condition of human neurology, I suggest that hypotheses linking environmental toxins and autism tend to be expressed in ways that validate a medical model that frames autism as unnatural. Alicia Broderick and Ari Ne'eman (2008, 468) argue that characterizing autism as a health crisis "draws upon a medicalized disease discourse in which people who have labels of autism are constituted not as neurologically different, nor even as disabled, but rather as diseased, not healthy, or ill." The disease model appears in environmentalist works that position autism as a sign of our worsening ecological condition. I argue that autistic individuals are positioned as ecological others when autism is held up as an example of the toxicity of our contemporary society, and I emphasize the importance of pursuing efforts to link disability rights and environmental justice in a nuanced way.

As I argue that ecological othering presents a significant barrier to acceptance, I build on the work of scholars who have established intersections between disability studies and the environmental humanities. In disability studies, when we differentiate the social model of disability from the medical model, we often use the term environment to refer to built environments. We draw attention to the disabling attributes of buildings and cities, as well as the enabling potential of inclusive design. In our scholarship environment often refers to the social environments that we cultivate with our attitudes toward disability (see Garland-Thomson 1997; Pfeiffer 2002). However, in recent years disability scholars have also examined ecological issues. Some examine the relationship between disability activism and environmental activism (Clare 1999; Taylor 2011). Others examine how exposure to environmental problems in specific localities affects disabled people. Gregor Wolbring and Verlyn Leopatra (2012) have shown that the impact of environmental risks on people with disabilities receives less attention than the impact of risks on other communities. They argue that we need scholarship on the implications of climate change, energy scarcity, and water sanitation for disabled people. As the other scholars in this collection show, we need research that approaches such environmental challenges from the lens of disability studies, as opposed to a medical model that focuses on individual deficits as the site of disability.

Although intersections between disability studies and the environmental humanities have been generative, tensions also exist. As Ray (2013, 37) notes, disability constitutes "the other against which modern environmentalist identity has been formed." In many cultural artifacts disability symbolizes the declining health of an environment. In Disability Rhetoric, Jay Dolmage (2014, 36) explains that one myth surrounding disability is that it is a symptom of the human abuse of nature: "As with the idea that disability is a punishment for an individual or social evil, disability is often used to reflect, even more 'causally,' humankind's degradation and neglect of the natural world and the environment." As a society we project anxieties about humanity's relationship with nature onto bodies we abject. Aligning disability with the declining health of an environment, we stigmatize disabled people.

However, some environmental justice activists might argue that understanding disabilities as symptoms of environmental degradation is imperative. Using disability to measure environmental degradation lends support to the argument that our decisions have material effects. While using disability as an indicator of environmental degradation may appear sound, its eugenic implications are apparent when we consider whether an indicator of environmental health would be the elimination of disability. Although medical technologies have been implemented to reduce the presence of painful disabilities and illnesses in some areas, the often unintended side effects of technological advances can sometimes yield new kinds of painful embodiments; such examples suggest that disability is an ordinary aspect of human life. But as scholars like Rosemarie Garland-Thomson (2005, 1568) argue, even when we know that disability will affect anyone who lives long enough, we are instructed to consider disability as "an exceptional and escapable calamity rather than as what is perhaps the most universal of human experiences." In another context, with the completion of the Human Genome Project, we are taught to read disabilities as errors in the master text of one's genetic code (Wilson 2002). One of the challenges for scholars researching how environmental factors affect human health and ability is retaining a focus on the importance of disability acceptance, an acceptance that involves deconstructing definitions of disability.

Scholars investigating disabilities resulting from exposure to toxins or metal poisoning have created space for a conversation between disability studies and the environmental humanities. The ecocritic Rob Nixon's (2011) work on slow violence speaks to the relationship between environmental toxicity and human health in a political way. Disability acceptance is a central focus for Stacy Alaimo (2010), who examines the narratives of individuals with multiple chemical sensitivity (MCS). Alaimo is careful to avoid reinscribing a medical model of disability that would position MCS as a pathology or deviation. With respect to a model of disability that values deviation, she cautions that many people who are sensitive to chemicals would insist that "not all deviations in this world of toxicants and xenobiotic chemicals should be embraced" (139). Her development of the concept of an openness to deviation involves placing everyone on a continuum of sensitivity to the environment. She advocates "tak[ing] the onto-epistemological condition of chemically reactive people seriously by making the world more accessible for them" (139). She shows how disability studies might consider a more expansive definition of access. While Alaimo's work responds to the struggle for recognition of individuals with MCS, my work pursues a different question of recognition. I engage with the political struggles of autistic adults, whose concerns are often absent from environmentalist writing decrying autism as yet another symptom of environmental degradation.

Bridging disability studies and the environmental humanities reveals too how the medical model shapes environmentalist perspectives on disability and how the discourse of environmentalism is employed to exclude disabled people. Popular environmentalist organizations concerned with the detrimental effects of commercial chemicals and genetically modified foods will cite autism as one of many conditions on the rise because of the practices of unethical companies like Monsanto. Cassady Sharp (2013), writing for Greenpeace, describes a link between glyphosate in Monsanto's Roundup herbicide and rising rates of autism.[2] The March against Monsanto (2013) organization has also drawn attention to autism. Also in 2013 they posted an infographic on social media exhibiting a correlation between the rise in autism diagnoses and the rise in the production of genetically modified foods. The following year March against Monsanto (2014) marked autism awareness month in April on social media by calling for a public outcry over the prevalence of autism, noting that the composition of the national food supply and the Center for Disease Control's vaccine schedule have both changed in the time that rates of autism have increased.[3] People for the Ethical Treatment of Animals (n.d.) similarly used autism to further their cause by using a "Got Autism?" campaign to promote veganism by suggesting a link between autism and cow's milk. Another example of efforts to link autism to poor health and unsustainable practices comes from the celebrity chef Pete Evans, who suggested that the paleo diet could reverse symptoms of autism (Crane 2014). Many experts refuted Evans's claim, but his message was one of many moments in which autism was held up as a sign of our worsening global health. While critiques of Monsanto and other companies are necessary, I am concerned with how popular environmentalism uncritically uses autism to strengthen its arguments.

Many environmental organizations express the same concerns as the charity Autism Speaks. In contrast to ASAN (2014), which understands autism as neurodiversity and suggests that its status as a disability be understood along social lines, Autism Speaks understands autism through a medical lens in which autism represents a series of deficits. By examining how awareness efforts that are invested in curing and preventing autism co-opt the discourse of environmentalism to create a sense of urgency, I suggest that scholars in the environmental humanities and in disability studies can together be critical of these discourses and show how the goal of eradication enacts a eugenic move that positions autistic people as ecological others. Before attempting to save people from autism, concerned environmentalists can first consider whether autistic people are interested in the salvation that research into environmental triggers promises.

Ray (2013) explains that the concept of the ecological other is about cultural disgust; one's physical form becomes evidence of one's allegiance to or disregard for environmental politics. Popular environmentalism presents the body as "the site of negotiation of and resistance to industrial food production" (2). In the fight to combat obesity it is individual bodies, as opposed to systems of production and distribution, that are recognized as targets. While one's weight may be interpreted as evidence of one's commitment to environmentalist values, one's way of interacting with the world has been taken up by an environmentalist lens too. Popular environmentalism may not blame autistic people for disregarding the environment in the same manner in which it blames obese people for unsustainable practices, but I would argue that it exhibits cultural disgust toward autism as a condition through a practice of abstraction. In many popular environmentalist accounts autism is affiliated with the worst offences of biotechnology companies, corporate agriculture, and consumptive practices. For this reason popular environmentalist takes on autism echo the same goals of prevention and cure articulated by charity organizations, which are characteristic of scientific research directions toward autism. The ecological othering of autistic people is made possible by the abstraction that comes with characterizing autism as a disease.

Although the cultural representation of autism is different from the cultural representation of obesity, issues of blame and stigma arise in conversations about autism. While professionals in the mid-twentieth century blamed mothers for autism, suggesting that the parenting styles of "refrigerator mothers" were responsible for their children's behaviors, in the twenty-first century, at least in some circles, blame has shifted to mothers who do not engage in dietary interventions. Jordynn Jack (2014) explains that the memoirs of self-titled autism mothers like that of the American actress Jenny McCarthy suggest that the dedicated parent of an autistic child is one who works hard to eradicate the signs and symptoms of autism through healthy living. In these memoirs, if autistic bodies are the "site of negotiation of and resistance to industrial food production," the mothers are the warriors fighting on the battleground (Ray 2013, 2). The environmentalist rhetoric present in both the accounts of mothers who aim to recover their children from autism and charitable efforts to cure autism positions autism as a disease in need of eradication. Considering the implications of the goal of eradication for autistic people, I chart the absence of the perspectives of autistic people in two documentary works examining environmental triggers for autism.

Sounding the Alarm: Battling the Autism Epidemic (2014) is a documentary exploring the rising rates of autism diagnoses in the United States. It profiles several families, including Bob and Suzanne Wright, who cofounded Autism Speaks for their grandson.[4] As Lei Wiley-Mydske (2014) notes in her review, the film's title uses a familiar and troubling military metaphor to encourage awareness. She also points out that a concern echoed throughout the film is the financial cost of autism. It addresses the issue of inclusion through the story of Kent, who leaves high school and faces the limited prospects available to autistic adults, and John, who opens a car wash to ensure employment for his autistic son and other autistic adults. However, the film's persistent focus on research makes clear that inclusion is a temporary step; the ideal vision of the future promoted by the film is one without autism. Toward the film's close Dr. Christopher McDougle, director of the Lurie Center for Autism, reiterates that discovering the cause of autism is financially imperative. He tells the audience, "If we don't begin to find out how to identify the cause and begin to prevent this disorder, or at least intervene earlier in life so we can alter the lifetime course, it's going to cost society a tremendous more amount of money than it's going to cost by being proactive and addressing it now." The film's lack of acknowledgment of autistic people who strongly object to the normalizing message that autism must be cured undermines the efforts toward inclusion that the film attempts to illustrate. It presents a vision of the eradication of the ecological other, a future that has solved the "problem" of autism.[5] Its message is that greater inclusion is needed until there is a research breakthrough, which is a very different message from that of ASAN and its international partner organizations that present autism acceptance as a goal in its own right. The militaristic logic of Sounding the Alarm is that accepting autism denotes passivity and complacency. The film operates through abstraction; while autistic children and young adults are often present, very few autistic people speak for themselves in this film.[6] Instead fear operates as a rhetorical strategy to encourage attention and raise awareness.

Lori Unumb, the vice president for state government affairs at Autism Speaks, invokes fear as she describes autism to viewers as "an unseen and unprovoked medical disaster" (Sounding the Alarm 2014). She compares autism to a tsunami, warning viewers, "There is a huge autism tsunami that is going to hit the state budgets of all our states." Her characterization of autism as a looming disaster shapes the film's call for research into environmental causation. Wright articulates her belief that while the majority of research on autism points to genetic markers, there must also be an environmental trigger because "there's no such thing as a genetic epidemic and we have an epidemic now." The film visits the offices of autism researchers that describe potential environmental influences. Dr. David Amaral suggests that environmental chemicals such as flame retardants and packing materials like BPA might affect human DNA and increase the risk of autism. Similarly Dr. Irva Hertz-Picciotto emphasizes that research should examine environmental triggers, explaining, "We need to be looking at maternal nutrition. We need to be looking at air pollution, pesticides. We encounter these kinds of exposures in our everyday lives through what we eat, what we breathe, what medications we take." By featuring the voices of scientists alongside militaristic calls to action, the film echoes the rhetorical strategies of environmentalist discourse. The ecocritic Lawrence Buell (2001, 31) defines toxic discourse as "expressed anxiety arising from the perceived threat of environmental hazard due to chemical modification by human agency" and describes how environmentalists like Rachel Carson employ pastoral tropes and cold war rhetoric to convey a sense of threat, framing pesticides as enemies to urge action. While Buell suggests that toxic discourse can bridge environmentalist values and environmental justice, in this case the co-opting of environmentalist discourse to discuss autism results in a call to action against autism itself. The film portrays autism as the enemy that individuals unwillingly host instead of an aspect of their identity.

Many scholars have skillfully critiqued the awareness efforts and research priorities of Autism Speaks (Broderick 2011; Broderick and Ne'eman 2008; Yergeau 2010). My contention is not only that Autism Speaks engages in the practice of ecological othering but that the rhetorical strategies of organizations like Autism Speaks are echoed in environmentalist works that characterize autism as a disease. The Canadian environmentalist David Suzuki's (2011) documentary series The Nature of Things dedicated an episode to exploring potential environmental triggers for autism. "The Autism Enigma" was first aired in 2011, then was re-aired on CBC TV in September 2014. The episode considers rising rates of autism among new Canadians, the impact of dietary interventions, and research into gut bacteria. As it profiles multiple families the documentary presents their situations as tragic not because of a lack of support but, problematically, because they gradually lost their children to autism; throughout the film, interviewees assert that autism takes children away.

Suzuki is a well-respected environmentalist who is known for educating the public in environmental sciences and for criticizing government inaction on climate change, sustainability, and other issues. Since 1979 he has hosted The Nature of Things, a series of documentaries exploring topics in environmental science. He is a reputable international source on environmental issues, whose environmental perspective on autism has the potential to be influential. The question that guides the documentary and that Suzuki (2011) poses, is "Could a change in our microbes affect our bodies and contribute to diseases like autism?" His question, however, assumes that autism is a disease, a perspective that both scientists and activists question. Broderick and Ne'eman (2008) distinguish disability from disease in their characterization of the disease model of autism. Although disability and illness are often related, it is important to recognize that the positioning of autism as an illness has led to misconceptions about the general health of autistic people. The disease model of autism does not take into account how autistic people have identified with the condition, embracing it rather than pushing for its eradication. While many people who develop cancer later in life would not see the eradication of cancer, a life-threatening illness, as a eugenic effort, many autistic people who do not believe their lives are at risk from their diagnosis view the movement to prevent autism as a form of eugenics that suggests their way of being in the world is not valuable.

In "The Autism Enigma" a representative from the Autism Canada Foundation tells viewers, "We have to look at environment now because we know that environment influences our gene expression and we know that if we understand what environmental triggers are influencing autism we can avoid these and maybe consequently reduce the amount of autism that we're seeing" (Suzuki 2011). The organization's vision is "a world in which autism is preventable and treatable" (Autism Canada Foundation 2011). This linguistic construction disguises how reducing the amount of autism means reducing the amount of autistic people, a goal that presupposes autism is undesirable. As Sinclair (1993) argues, "It is not possible to separate autism from the person—

and if it were possible, the person you'd have left would not be the same person you started with." He encourages parents to question whether autism itself is their problem. The Canadian autism researcher Michelle Dawson has similarly objected to the characterization of autism as a problem. In her collaborative work on autism and intelligence, Dawson has shown that researchers have erroneously deemed autistic people unintelligent because they have measured them by neurotypical standards (Dawson et al. 2007; Gernsbacher et al. 2006). Dawson's colleague Laurent Mottron (2011, 35) believes that scholars should move beyond cataloguing autistic deficits; he argues that "by emphasizing the abilities and strengths of people with autism, deciphering how autistics learn and succeed in natural settings, and avoiding language that frames autism as a defect to be corrected, [scientists] can help shape the entire discussion." While Sounding the Alarm and "The Autism Enigma" focus on the loss that autism represents, voices like those of Sinclair, Dawson, and Mottron suggest what would be lost in a future in which autism does not figure.

While the stories of autistic people who require the support of their families and experts to be able to advocate for their needs deserve attention, "The Autism Enigma" excludes the perspective of autistic people and their supporters who would argue that autism is not a medical problem to be solved but a form of neurological diversity that deserves recognition. In their review of Suzuki's (2011) documentary Julia Kitaygorodsky and colleagues (2013) criticize the exclusion of autistic voices. While both documentaries criticize the lack of attention to the environment in autism research, many disability studies scholars criticize instead the lack of attention to quality of life research; as the majority of research is oriented toward producing a world without autism, the everyday challenges of autistic adults are often forgotten. Scott Michael Robertson (2010) argues that research should focus on issues like access to augmentative and alternative communication (AAC), compatible employment opportunities, and social acceptance. Melanie Yergeau (2010) similarly critiques research into causation. She explains that according to the typical autism essay, "the world's population is slowly heading the way of neurological disfigurement—because of vaccines, because of genetics, because of excessive television watching, because of airborne pollutants, because of gluten and casein and artificial sweeteners, because of, quite literally, your mom." Her parodic list derides the sense of fear invoked by contemporary discourse on autism.

As this collection argues, recognizing the detrimental effects of human activity on our environments and their consequences for human health and ability is crucial. However, doing so in a nuanced way is imperative. While many popular environmentalists turn to health to bolster arguments against industrial practices and companies that ecocritics have similarly criticized, positioning the body as a site of environmental injustice can be detrimental when doing so denies the subjectivity of the persons in question. Characterizing autism as unnatural and autistic people as aberrations upholds a problematic idea of natural purity. Many ecocritics gesture toward this issue by referring to how individuals have attempted to justify discrimination and exclusion based on race, gender, and sexuality by insisting that certain social identities are unnatural (Clark 2013).[7]

In closing I would like to turn to Songs of the Gorilla Nation: My Journey through Autism, a memoir by Dawn Prince-Hughes (2004), who suggests that remaining critical of the anthropocentrism that has characterized our disregard for natural environments can translate into greater acceptance toward different kinds of intelligence and ways of being. Songs of the Gorilla Nation weaves together Prince-Hughes's life story with the stories of the gorillas she worked with and studied as an anthropologist. As she explains how gorillas taught her about community, she clarifies that the emergence they facilitated for her was not a recovery from autism, but a way of thinking through it:

> When I speak of emergence from the darkness of autism, I do not mean that I offer a success story neatly wrapped and finished with a "cure." I and the others who are autistic do not want to be cured. What I mean when I say "emergence" is that my soul was lifted from the context of my earlier autism and became autistic in another context, one filled with wonder and discovery and full of the feelings that so poetically inform each human life. When I emerged, I had learned—from the gorillas—far better how I could achieve these things. (3)

Prince-Hughes does not have to overcome her autism to succeed as an anthropologist. As the neurodiversity movement is garnering more support, people are becoming aware of the diverse talents and skills of autistic people. But an interesting aspect of Prince-Hughes's text is her willingness to consider a link between autism and our changing natural environments in a way that avoids abstracting autism into a disease; she is able to consider how environments might influence autistic people while leaving out the assumption that autism is a problem. She explains that she agrees with Elisabeth and Niko Tinbergen, whom she identifies as rarely cited researchers who argue that "modern life, with its unnatural living conditions, chemicals, broken-down social systems, and chronic stress, overstimulates and assaults the human animal, causing some to manifest the biological and psychological matrix we call autism" (Prince-Hughes 2004, 223). Yet in voicing agreement she does not suggest the need for a cure; instead she articulates a hope that autistic people "will be perceived as being as whole as the worlds they sense" (224). I am not suggesting that the theory Prince-Hughes articulates is accurate, but that her work offers insight into how critiquing our persistent use of chemicals and our anthropocentric attitudes can proceed alongside appreciation for the diversity that autism represents; she offers a critique of our approach toward nature while still celebrating the difference that autism signifies.

The neurodiversity movement can offer insight into rethinking an environmentalist perspective on autistic presence. The concept of neurodiversity often appears in media conversations about cognitive difference and the successful employment of many autistic adults in the technology sector. However, the term's connotation of biological diversity is instructive for thinking about autistic presence in relation to environmental issues. Perhaps the value environmentalists place on biological diversity can figure in discussions of neurological diversity too. While characterizing autism as a disease has led to easy correlations between autism and unsustainable environmental practices, perhaps considering neurodiversity from an environmentalist perspective can lead to greater acceptance. While we should recognize the ways environmental health affects human health, we must also attend to the very political definitions of health that adhere around autism and other disabilities. Greater engagement by environmental writers and autistic writers would allow for greater communication of the message that to be both autistic and healthy is not a paradox.

NOTES

I would like to thank Jay Dolmage for his comments on an early draft of this work. I would also like to extend my thanks to the editors of this collection, Sarah Jaquette Ray and Jay Sibara.

1. For example, the belief that autism is a form of mercury poisoning (which still has adherents despite significant research disproving it) is rooted in the idea that autism is hosted.

2. Many articles in the spring of 2013 that discuss the link between autism and Monsanto's herbicide reference Anthony Samsel and Stephanie Seneff's (2013) study, "Glyphosate's Suppression of Cytochrome P450 Enzymes and Amino Acid Biosynthesis by the Gut Microbiome: Pathways to Modern Diseases." This study links the consumption of glyphosate residues to gastrointestinal disorders, obesity, diabetes, heart disease, depression, autism, infertility, cancer, and Alzheimer's disease. Scientists have challenged the study's methodology and argued that the claims are extremely speculative (Goldstein 2014). While some of the critics are Monsanto supporters, environmentalists too have criticized the study (Haspel 2013).

3. Some users strongly objected to the suggested link between vaccines and autism in the comments section by emphasizing that researchers have shown this connection to be false.

4. Bob Wright is a former chairman of NBC Universal, credentials that contribute to the popularity of Autism Speaks. Broderick (2011) describes how the Wrights' charity embraces neoliberal tactics and functions more like a corporation than a disability advocacy organization.

5. One potential technology explored in the film is the use of maternal screening for antibodies that might contribute to the development of autism, with the expressed purpose of making those antibodies nonfunctional. The researchers interviewed do not discuss the ethical implications of this technology, such as whether parents might choose to abort a fetus based on the results of the screening.

6. Many autistic adults argue that Autism Speaks does not represent their interests. The memoirist John Elder Robison (2013) cut ties with the organization following Suzanne Wright's "Call for Action" in November 2013. Wright's comparison of autistic prevalence to a situation in which three million children in the United States went missing or became ill reiterated many of the metaphors to which Robison had objected.

7. Donna Haraway and Anne-Lise François critique the use of terms like natural and pure to oppose advances in biotechnology. François (2003, 50) is critical of GMOs, but she argues that the trend of calling these products "Frankenfoods" betrays "a dangerous fetishization of purity and biological essence fueling the resistance to these newer

technologies." Similarly Haraway "cannot help but hear in the biotechnology debates the unintended tones of fear of the alien and suspicion of the mixed" (qtd. in François 2003, 50).

BIBLIOGRAPHY

Alaimo, Stacy. 2010. Bodily Natures: Science, Environment, and the Material Self. Bloomington: Indiana University Press.

ASAN. 2014. "About." Autistic Self Advocacy Network. http://autistic advocacy.org/about-asan/.

Autism Canada Foundation. 2011. "Mission and Vision." Autism Canada Foundation. http://autismcanada.org/about-us/guiding-principles /mission-and-vision/.

Baggs, Amanda. 2007. "In My Language." YouTube. January 14. https:// www.youtube.com/watch?v=Jnylm1hi2jc.

Baron-Cohen, Simon. 1995. Mindblindness: An Essay on Autism and Theory of Mind. Cambridge MA: MIT Press.

Broderick, Alicia A. 2011. "Autism as Rhetoric: Exploring Watershed Rhetorical Moments in Applied Behavior Analysis Discourse." Disability Studies Quarterly 31, no. 3. http://dsq-sds.org/article/view/1674/1597.

Broderick, Alicia, and Ari Ne'eman. 2008. "Autism as Metaphor: Narrative and Counter-Narrative." International Journal of Inclusive Education 12, nos. 5–6: 459–76.

Buell, Lawrence. 2001. Writing for an Endangered World: Literature, Culture, and Environment in the U.S. and Beyond. Cambridge MA: Belknap Press of Harvard University Press.

Clare, Eli. 1999. Exile and Pride: Disability, Queerness, and Liberation. Cambridge MA: South End Press.

Clark, Timothy. 2013. "Nature, Post Nature." In The Cambridge Companion to Literature and the Environment, edited by Louise Westling, 75–89. Cambridge, UK: Cambridge University Press.

Crane, Emily. 2014. "Celebrity Chef Pete Evans Has Been Slammed for his 2,100 Word Rant on Facebook Claiming the Paleo Diet Can Prevent Autism." Daily Mail, October 1. http://www.dailymail.co.uk/news /article-2775987/Celebrity-chef-Pete-Evans-slammed-2-100-word -rant-Facebook-claiming-Paleo-diet-prevent-autism.html.

Dawson, Michelle, Isabelle Soulières, Morton Ann Gernsbacher, and Laurent Mottron. 2007. "The Level and Nature of Autistic Intelligence." Psychological Science 18, no. 8: 657–62.

Dolmage, Jay. 2014. Disability Rhetoric. Syracuse NY: Syracuse University Press.

François, Anne-Lise. 2003. "'O Happy Living Things': Frankenfoods and the Bounds of Wordsworthian Natural Piety." diacritics 33, no. 2: 42–70.

Garland-Thomson, Rosemarie. 1997. Extraordinary Bodies: Figuring Disability in American Culture and Literature. New York: Columbia University Press.

———. 2005. "Feminist Disability Studies." Signs 30, no. 2: 1557–87.

Gernsbacher, Morton Ann, Michelle Dawson, and Laurent Mottron. 2006. "Autism: Common, Heritable, but Not Harmful." Behavioral and Brain Sciences 29, no. 4: 413–14.

Goldstein, Daniel. 2014. "Tempest in a Tea Pot: How Did the Public Conversation on Genetically Modified Crops Drift So Far from the Facts?" Journal of Medical Toxicology 10, no. 2: 194–201.

Haspel, Tamar. 2013. "Condemning Monsanto with Bad Science Is Dumb." Huffington Post Green, April 26. http://www.huffingtonpost.com/tamar-haspel/condemning-monsanto-with-_b_3162694.html.

Jack, Jordynn. 2014. Autism and Gender: From Refrigerator Mothers to Computer Geeks. Chicago: University of Illinois Press.

Kitaygorodsky, Julia, Maire Percy, Ann Fudge Schormans, and Ivan Brown. 2013. "CBC: The Nature of Things with David Suzuki." Journal on Developmental Disabilities 19, no. 1: 96–102.

March against Monsanto. 2013. "The Rate of Autism Has Increased by 600% in Last 20 Years." Facebook. June 3. https://www.facebook.com/MarchAgainstMonstanto/posts/608525165832674.

———. 2014. "April Is Autism Awareness Month." Facebook. April 1. https://www.facebook.com/MarchAgainstMonstanto/posts/10201714253442926.

Mottron, Laurent. 2011. "The Power of Autism." Nature 479 (November 3): 33–35.

Murray, Stuart. 2008. Representing Autism: Culture, Narrative, Fascination. Liverpool, UK: Liverpool University Press.

———. 2012. Autism. London: Routledge.

Nixon, Rob. 2011. Slow Violence and the Environmentalism of the Poor. Cambridge MA: Harvard University Press.

People for the Ethical Treatment of Animals. N.d. "Got Autism? Learn about the Link between Dairy Products and the Disorder." Accessed November 15, 2014. http://www.peta.org/features/got-autism-learn -link-dairy-products-disease/.

Pfeiffer, David. 2002. "The Philosophical Foundations of Disability Studies." Disability Studies Quarterly 22, no. 2: 3–23. http://dsq-sds.org /article/view/341/429.

Prince-Hughes, Dawn. 2004. Songs of the Gorilla Nation: My Journey through Autism. New York: Harmony Books.

Ray, Sarah Jaquette. 2013. The Ecological Other: Environmental Exclusion in American Culture. Tucson: University of Arizona Press.

Robertson, Scott Michael. 2010. "Neurodiversity, Quality of Life, and Autistic Adults: Shifting Research and Professional Focuses onto Real-Life Challenges." Disability Studies Quarterly 30, no. 1. http://dsq-sds .org/article/view/1069/1234.

Robison, John Elder. 2013. "I Resign My Roles at Autism Speaks." Blogspot, November 13. http://jerobison.blogspot.ca/2013/11/i-resign -my-roles-at-autism-speaks.html.

Samsel, Anthony, and Stephanie Seneff. 2013. "Glyphosate's Suppression of Cytochrome P450 Enzymes and Amino Acid Biosynthesis by the Gut Microbiome: Pathways to Modern Diseases." Entropy 15, no. 4: 1416–63. http://www.mdpi.com/1099-4300/15/4/1416.

Sharp, Cassady. 2013. "6 Reasons to March against Monsanto May 25th." Greenpeace Blogs, May 22. http://www.greenpeace.org/usa/6-reasons -to-march-against-monsanto-may-25th/.

Sinclair, Jim. 1993. "Don't Mourn for Us." Our Voice 1, no. 3. http://www .autreat.com/dont_mourn.html.

Sounding the Alarm: Battling the Autism Epidemic. 2014. Directed by John Block. Blockburger Productions. Electronic Video File.

Suzuki, David. 2011. "The Autism Enigma." The Nature of Things with David Suzuki. Canadian Broadcasting Corporation News Network, December 8. (Video available only in Canada)

Taylor, Sunaura. 2011. "Beasts of Burden: Disability Studies and Animal Rights." Qui Parle 19, no. 2: 191–222.

Wiley-Mydske Lei. 2014. "Film Review of Documentary 'Sounding the Alarm: Battling the Autism Epidemic.'" Autism Women's Network. July 19. http://autismwomensnetwork.org/film-review-of-documentary -sounding-the-alarm-battling-the-autism-epidemic/.

Wilson, James C. 2002. "(Re)Writing the Genetic Body-Text: Disability, Textuality, and the Human Genome Project." Cultural Critique 50 (Winter): 23–39.

Wolbring, Gregor, and Verlyn Leopatra. 2012. "Climate Change, Water Sanitation and Energy Insecurity: Invisibility of People with Disabilities." Canadian Journal of Disability Studies 1, no. 3. http://cjds.uwaterloo .ca/index.php/cjds/article/view/58.

Wright, Suzanne. 2013. "Autism Speaks to Washington: A Call for Action." Autism Speaks. November 11. http://www.autismspeaks .org/news/news-item/autism-speaks-washington-call-action.

Yergeau, Melanie. 2010. "Circle Wars: Reshaping the Typical Autism Essay." Disability Studies Quarterly 30, no. 1. http://dsq-sds.org/article /view/1063/1222.

Section 5　INTERSPECIES AND INTERAGE IDENTIFICATIONS

20

Precarity and Cross-Species Identification

Autism, the Critique of Normative
Cognition, and Nonspeciesism

David T. Mitchell and Sharon L. Snyder

Crip Ecologies and Disability Materialisms

Like many other essays in this collection our work seeks to bring
together scholarship across the fields of ecocriticism, disability,
and queer studies. One of our primary goals is to think through
queer interchanges of environments and bodies in more radical
ways. As work in ecocriticism has so often shown us, we are vulnerable embodied beings who interact with our environments;
thus we experience ourselves and others through a defining
porosity: we are not only affected by the places we inhabit, but
we also leave our imprint on these locations. Marginalized subjects, including disabled people, often experience their lives in
greater proximity to environmental threats such as toxicity, climate change, generational exposures to unsafe living conditions
due to poverty, militarization, body-exhausting labors as in the
case of migrant workers, and more.

Further, we seek to investigate how nonnormative bodies
and minds can reframe what it means to be an environmentalist or "nature lover." Our foray into these arenas of thought
through what we call "crip ecologies" involves an explication of
Mark Haddon's (2003) novel <u>The Curious Incident of the Dog in
the Night-Time</u>. In undertaking this examination we will draw

out an analysis of some of these wanted, unwanted, and even unknowable intimacies with our environments as materials for new transhistorical, cross-cultural, and crip and queer research about human, nonhuman, organic, and inorganic relationships that mark our experiences in the world.

This analysis develops various offshoots of a methodology Tobin Siebers (2013, 291) has theorized as "critical embodiment" and we have termed "non-normative positivisms" (Mitchell and Snyder 2015, 5). We view these two parallel interpretive frameworks as an opportunity to open up approaches to reading disability as an agential, material, and affective embodiment. The argument is that disability studies has forwarded few ways to meaningfully encounter embodiment as part of the productive alternatives that existence in nonnormative bodies offer (Mitchell and Snyder 2015, 2). Since the 1970s disability studies has taken up its analysis of disability as an excluded atypicality from normative modes of social participation. Thus, as Tom Shakespeare (2002, 208) and others have argued, disability can be identified only in relation to disabled people's existence as an oppressed minority but without any alternative value to offer as a product of its social critique.

By intersecting a reading of Haddon's (2003) novel with recent work in the philosophy of new materialisms, we intend to open up investigations into the ways disabled people's alternative interdependent, crip or queer existences provide opportunities to envision an ethics of living that exceeds mere inclusion alongside able-bodied people. In Siebers's (2013, 282) words, the experience of complex embodiment teaches that disability is both affected by environments and changed by the diversity of bodies, resulting in specific knowledge about the ways environment and bodies mutually transform one another.

Within the social model disability has been trapped between two primary lines of argumentation: the first is with regard to oppression and social barriers, wherein disability can be located only as socially excluded (e.g., Oliver and Barnes 2012, 6); the second is with regard to impairment-effects as the necessity of speaking of our bodies as a complicating (even limiting) factor in our lives (Thomas 1999, 34; Wendell 1997, 7, among others particularly in feminist disability studies). Disability studies scholars such as Sarah Jaquette Ray (2013) and Beth Haller (2004) believe Haddon's novel fulfills the criteria of key social model principles. We want to explore the work from a distinctly different point of view, not from the direction of social barriers exposed for autistic people (we don't think this is a primary strength of the novel, as Bartmess [2015] has written) but rather from the point of view of what we can learn about normative cognitive embodiment that the novel critiques. Both of these traditions of thought have proven critical to the innovations of social model thinking; both are necessary to redress social exclusion, marginality, abuse, and neglect (within and apart from the disability rights movement and disability studies proper).

However, the methodological development of "critical embodiment" in Siebers's (2013) terms suggests how ordinary material practices might be critically investigated as a further analytical heuristic for the field. We are caught in our lives and our theories between two zones of negativity without something akin to "complex embodiment." There is no way to identify the creative interdependencies at the foundations of disability alternatives for living in our existing traditions of thought. There is a great need for an ethical methodology from which disabled people can articulate how their lives bring something new into the world that would otherwise go unrecognized. As such, complex embodiment and parallel methodologies such as nonnormative positivism offer pathways to alternative spaces from which to discuss this critical third rail of disability experience.

Flight from Animality

People with disabilities and disability studies have fled from designations of their socially presumed and derided excessive proximity to nonhuman animals (Carlson 2007, 128). Their dubious historical identifications with savage nature—Michael Newton's (2004, 10) "savage girls and wild boys"—and their distancing from Western civilization's most prized capacity of rationality have served as the rhetorical basis of their dehumanization. Darwin's (2011, 32) nineteenth-century paradigm-shifting theory of evolution identified feebleminded and racialized peoples as key evidence of human animal origins. Contemporary bioethicists now identify cognitively disabled infants as "non-paradigm humans" who lack the capacity for the caretaking of others and debate the value of their species status with dogs and other, "less sentient" creatures (Jaworska and Tannenbaum 2014, 243). So it's safe to say that the relationship between disability and animality is a strained one.

This strange-bedfellows relationship has placed disabled persons in one of the most curious situations of scapegoating as their liminal location between human and animal worlds deploy them in contradictory directions: first, in serving as the distinguishing partition between rationality and instinct-driven existence, and second, as sharing a too great proximity to nature. Christopher's cross-species identifications serve as the source of species trouble in Curious Incident in that he is discovered cradling the body of a dead dog in his neighbor's backyard. This act of mourning over the death of a nonhuman individual erroneously identifies him as the killer, suggests a perverse draw of necrophilia for those who exhibit nonnormative behaviors, and bequeaths him an excessive cross-species regard. For Christopher the murder of Wellington is at least tantamount to the killing of a human, but as his Special

Education teacher Siobhan tells him, "Readers [care] more about people than dogs, so if a person was killed in a book, people would want to carry on reading" (Haddon 2003, 5). In other words his story about the death of a dog and his search for the killer will likely cultivate little readerly interest from other humans more invested in animals like themselves. The presumption of normative cognition is that a homology exists within species that does not cross boundaries—like attracts like. Any attraction to unlike suggests something wrong in the individual who would abdicate his desire for humans and more easily locate an affinity with the nonhuman world.

Yet one of the main tasks of the novel is to disprove Siobhan's theory, first by depathologizing Christopher's attachment to animals, and second by creating a successful story about the killing of a dog as its central theme. Consequently the novel is both about Christopher's peculiar affinities as interpretable and also about the process of writing an engaging story. This establishes an equation between the novel's principal themes of nonnormative cognition and creativity.

Christopher begins the story by arguing that dogs have only four moods so they are more reliable signifiers of otherwise inaccessible interior states (i.e., their affective expressiveness matches their exterior presentation more directly than humans'). Dogs, as Christopher points out, are "cleverer and more interesting than some people," and he likes their loyalty and faithfulness to their companions—a quality he longs to experience with the able-bodied world around him (Haddon 2003, 6). In contrast humans talk too much and use subjective and metaphorical expressions such as the mysterious nuances of body language and the varied animacies of facial expressions. Metaphors are, by definition, lies in that they compare two unlike things and require the listener to perform the labor of a difficult crossing of dissociated meaning systems. Consequently Christopher writes a murder mystery rather than a "proper novel" because fiction represents the practice of telling a story about things that did not actually happen (4).

Novels thus represent the publication of formally authorized lies that result in a cascade of untruths. The narrator views this situation as the foundational problem of human interactions: "People are different from animals because they can have pictures on the screens in their heads of things which they are not looking at" (Haddon 2003, 117). In contrast Christopher tries to strictly observe the Latin law of Occam's razor: "No more things should be presumed to exist than are absolutely necessary" (90). Like the prime numbers that organize his chapters, Christopher seeks to arrive at a pure meaning available in the world. This would involve a more direct relationship between signifier and signified in that once a pattern can be discovered you can eliminate the distractions that compete for your attention and threaten to derail meaning with tangential interests. As he explains after hearing he was named after Saint Christopher, "I want my name to mean me" (16). A murder mystery involving the death of a neighborhood dog provides an opportunity to document real-time events and also expose the enigma of a murderer who has killed an individual whose life does not significantly register on humanly determined social scales of value. In other words, the novel sets out to demonstrate that a more direct relationship between actors and actions exists and can be exposed. This tactic places Curious Incident on a par with films such as Errol Morris's The Thin Blue Line in that they explicitly reject the Rashomon-like reality so often revelatory of the floating signifiers that populate postmodern semiotic theory.

Not only does Christopher refuse to observe human hierarchies of value—"People think their brains are special"—but he also finds comfort in the more direct expressive register of simile-based comparisons between himself and machines, particularly computers (Haddon 2003, 118). Throughout the novel he remarks upon the workings of his mind as similar to that of bread-slicing machine (7), a computer that has to be rebooted from time to time (144), a searchable DVD (76), and a film projector (76). The multiplicity of meanings characteristic of data onslaughts in the information age pose significant problems for individuals who are unusually attentive to details, such as those with autism and other cognitive disabilities. The problem in this conundrum would appear at first to be the challenges of an excess complexity of information. The individual with a cognitive disability presumably needs data simplified prior to cognitive processing in order to make more straightforward decisions. However, the problem turns out to be otherwise as the novel unfolds its critique of the limitations of normative cognition.

Resisting the Allure of Speciesism

Near the conclusion of the story Christopher evaluates the murder mystery he has been writing as a failure because "police don't arrest people for little crimes unless you ask them and Mother said that killing a dog was only a little crime" (Haddon 2003, 146). Of course this revelation of normative policing practices resonates with our particular moment of civil unrest in the United States as it introduces questions of species hierarchies in which some lives matter more than others (black disabled lives, for instance) and matter more than those of nonhuman species. As a narrator who might be described as existing on the Autistic Spectrum, Christopher Joseph Boone resists this logic of foundational speciesism taken for granted by the normative human world. In doing so he demonstrates that his attachment to nonhuman lives comes more easily to him and that the human leaves a great deal to be desired as that which is marked as an inherently desirable form of existence. The critique circulates around the ways humans consider rationality (or in contemporary neuroscientific terms, "cognitive processing") a key dividing trait between themselves and those nonhuman bodies over which they believe themselves ordained to exert mastery.

We've already started down the fraught track of what some might call "diagnosing a literary character" by identifying Christopher as one who might be described as existing on the Autistic Spectrum. At a Wang Foundation lecture at George Washington University in 2013 and in his book, The Secret Life of Stories, Michael Bérubé argues against the utility of diagnosing literary characters. As he explains, "we [disability studies scholars] should not diagnose characters" but rather the way narrative elements function in disabled ways (Bérubé 2016, 20). This realignment of disability studies–based analyses in the humanities seeks to reorder analytical priorities and the structural levels of storytelling to which we attend. To do so Bérubé deprivileges the material conditions of impairment—identification of deviant bodies and the pathologizing social interpretations that make them legible—in favor of the analysis of rhetorical and storytelling structures that generatively impair our interpretive approaches for purposeful, normatively sanctioned ends. Since literary characters are fictional creations, diagnosis of their psychological, sensory, and physical traits results in the application of an inappropriate (i.e., medical) register of knowledge about bodies on an invented artistic surface.

Even the novel's author might agree with Bérubé's injunction, for Haddon argues on his website that Christopher is not autistic but rather just a "little odd" (markhaddon.com). We take this line of thinking to exist akin to earlier disability studies arguments that argued the most progressive disability representation would be one in which a character had a disability and yet it meant little to the plot. Characters are characters, and disability should be recognized for what it is: a random occurrence of difference that appears across actively mutating organisms and vulnerable embodiments. However, we're going to risk a plunge into the turbulent sea of diagnosis because we don't believe you can read the novel effectively without undertaking such an effort in a serious manner. More important, we also plan to show that diagnosis is a many-lane highway of critique.

New materialism engages bodies at a more meaningful level than the social model of disability because it refuses to toss the matter of bodily materiality (even experiences of impairment) out of the question of meaning-making itself. Philosophers such as Rosi Braidotti, Elizabeth Grosz, Brian Massumi, Diana Coole, Mel Chen, Samantha Frost, and William Connelly all take up critical materialist approaches to their cultural objects in order to get around the defining impasse of social constructivism that tends to interpret bodies as passively imprinted surfaces entirely scripted by their environments (Massumi 2002, 39). As a contrast new materialists argue for a more agential, lively body that imprints its environment as much as it is imprinted by the forces around it (Coole and Frost 2010, 26; Frost 2012, 162). We're going to argue here that this is fertile ground for future disability studies work.

In addition to beginning with the death of a dog, The Curious Incident also starts with a more traditional lure of making readers think they will be introduced to what it's like to understand the world from an autistic point of view (Mitchell with Snyder 2015, 128). This would be a relatively standard narration of disability if the book kept on this pathway of using internal narrative as a device to raise public consciousness about the difficulties and struggles of people with autism. The novel does do this to a certain extent, and we tend to agree with Bérubé's (2013) critique of Christopher as performing in some kind of ur-autistic role by having every behavioral trait typically associated with autism. At various times in the novel he displays behaviors of qualitative impairment in social interaction, marked impairment in the use of eye contact with others, failure to develop peer relationships, a lack of spontaneous seeking to share enjoyment, marked impairment in the ability to initiate or sustain a conversation with others, lack of varied and spontaneous make-believe play, apparently inflexible adherence to specific and nonfunctional routines or rituals, stereotyped or repetitive motor mannerisms, and persistent preoccupation with parts of objects. Such a catalogue of traits shows up in all standard diagnostic autistic symptom clusters. (Leo Kanner identified all of these "problems" among those with autism in his 1943 essay, "Autistic Disturbances of Affective Contact.") In fact we're somewhat sympathetic to the autistic philosopher Simon Cushing's (2012, 39) argument that autism is a meaningless diagnostic category of loosely connected behavioral traits and should be "junked" in order to start over with an alternative version of neuroatypicality.

Critique of Normative Cognition

However, here we want to argue that we don't believe the novel is significant for its portrayal of autistic behaviors (i.e., the common pursuit of amateur diagnostics so many disability novels fall into as their authoritative value). Instead we want to argue that Christopher's "autism" allows him to invert the unidirectional line of diagnostic interpretation that positions cognitively disabled people as incapable of properly managing their own affairs. The novel systematically diagnoses normative cognition patterns as a primary object of critique through Christopher's assessment of the contemporary overvaluation of rationality (i.e., that which often passes as nonimpaired cognition).

First off, as we suggested earlier, much of Christopher's attachment to nonhuman species undermines the human tendency to adhere to a hierarchical speciesism. The narrator looks to the nonhuman world for evidence of life forms where no life forms are expected to exist (or exist in a meaningful manner). This search involves finding other unexpected contexts where alternative lives thrive. Examples of this artful engagement abound: he believes he would be well suited as an astronaut because he enjoys close confined quarters and isolation from the demands of human sociality (Haddon 2003, 50); he critiques human tendencies to imagine aliens in their own image rather than as ontologically alternative forms of existence, such as beings made entirely of light (69); he watches a Blue Planet video that takes viewers down to the bottom of the Marianas Trench in order discover an entire colony of sulfurous sea creatures where scientists have discounted any possibility of life (80); and he enjoys visiting an open-air zoo for its way of organizing more than two hundred life forms across nonhuman species without ranking of superiority (179).

What all of these alternative investments in nonhuman life forms demonstrate is Christopher's critique of humans who believe God put them on Earth "because they think humans are the best animal" (165). Alternatively Christopher believes in a more agnostic concept of species relations that doesn't privilege humans above other life forms: "Human beings are just an animal and they will evolve into another animal" (165). In fact the most radical reading of the novel might entail an argument that this alternative evolution is already under way, as evidenced by lives such as Christopher's that have grown increasingly reflexive about the nonsuperiority of human actors in relation to nonhuman actors. In her important contribution to postmodernism and primatology, Donna Haraway (1990, 143) argues that humans project their own values onto animal worlds for the ultimate payback of having their own life patterns naturalized and reflected back to themselves as the normative order of things. Such human hubris has resulted in the rampant use of gorillas as justification for heteronormative familial orders and as the experimental military testing grounds for the effects of excessive radiation exposure on ape bodies, to name just two instances (255).

So while Haddon may explain away the significance of his character's differences as mere oddity in the wake of turning down too many requests for charity benefit appearances on behalf of curing autism, the novel helps position autism as an alternative system of devotions to devalued participants (including autism itself). Perhaps even more significant, the novel pursues Christopher's nonspeciesist logic to unravel the ruse of the value of normative cognition. Here is where we see the novel's most significant inroads in the debate about the appropriateness of pursuing diagnostic lines of engagement with literary characters in disability studies. Literary characters are not people, of course, but to ignore the alternative revelations of complex embodiment offered by experiencing the world through more material notions of crip or queer bodies risks losing disability, as the queer studies Foucauldian critic Lynn Huffer (2009, 48) argues, as "a constructive ethical frame that can actually be used as a map for living."

To accomplish this massive undertaking Haddon's novel systematically diagnoses the ways an overvalued normative conception of human rationality (that which makes humans the "best animals") relies on various ruses to construct its seemingly smooth-functioning practice of seamlessly interpreting the world. First, Christopher argues he doesn't like "proper novels" because they are a genre of untruth that imagines things that have not happened but presents them as if they have taken place in the order and the manner in which they are imagined (Haddon 2003, 4). This systematization of thought represented by the novel orchestrates fictional universes in order to reveal principles that nonfictional universes may have difficulty exposing. Second, Christopher hates metaphors because they involve comparing two unlike things and thus are, by definition, lies (15). Third, Christopher interrogates constellations of stars as arbitrary human patterns of meaning-making that persist in time despite the fact that any group of stars could make any random idea or image accessible to the stargazer (125). All of these examples help to solidify that Christopher's mode of cognition refuses to overlook the arbitrary nature of the human imposition of meaning without acknowledging the historical, cultural, and heteronormative relativity of its assignments.

Normative cognition occupies the base of this imposition of order on the universe. To unravel the insufficiencies at the basis of human rationality (or, alternatively, normative cognitive processing) Christopher exposes four falsifying principles: (1) glancing, (2) the human myth of the homunculus, (3) Occam's razor; and (4) Darwinian mutation. Glancing serves as the most basic concept at the heart of his diagnosis of normative cognitive processes. As he explains, humans actively pursue an insufficiency of detail for the sake of coherence: "Most people are lazy. They never look at everything. They do what is called glancing which is the same word for bumping off something and carrying on in almost the same direction, e.g., when a snooker ball glances off another snooker ball. And the information in their head is really simple" (140). For Christopher glancing is a way of seeing without looking at the nuances of an unfolding scene.

As an extension of comparative differences with his own practices of active looking Christopher explains that when a nonautistic person stands in a field he or she may see a field full of grass with some cows standing in it and a sun with a few clouds behind it and a village in the distance. This is the sum total of glancing's superficial engagement with a complex environment over which it positions the viewer as exerting dominion through intentional reductionism. In Christopher's case the process of standing in a field involves an accumulation of nonhierarchized details that flood into his processing center:

> For example, I remember standing in a field on Wednesday, 15 June 1994, because Father and Mother and I were driving to Dover. . . . I went into a field with cows in it and after I'd had a wee I stopped and looked at the field and I noticed these things: 1. There are 19 cows in the field, 15 of which are black and white and 4 of which are brown and white. 2. There is a village in the distance which has 31 visible houses and a church with a square tower and not a spire. 3. There are ridges in the field, which means that in medieval times it was what is called a <u>ridge and furrow</u> field and people who lived in the village would have a ridge each to do farming on. . . . 6. I can see three different types of grass and colors of flowers in the grass. 7. The cows are mostly facing uphill. And there were 31 more things in this list of things I noticed but Siobhan said I didn't need to write them down. And it means that it is very tiring if I am in a new place because I see all these things, and if someone asked me afterward what the cows looked like, I could ask which one. (141–42)

We cite this passage at length because it is the heart of the methodology that Haddon employs in the novel. The argument here is that normative cognition is based on the principle of reductionism in order to keep details at bay and the agential, lively world less dizzying. Alternatively mastery for the sake of exerting dominion is no objective in Christopher's way of cognitively engaging his environment. His cognition process involves opening the floodgates of detail so that scenes can be rendered at highly nuanced levels of particularity. The former results in jettisoning information, while the latter involves an overwhelming level of data gathering.

To further develop this argument Christopher cites the myth of the human homunculus (118), a belief that a small individual exists inside our head and controls our perceptions so experience appears as if we are looking at the world from two windows. As we glance from one scene to another or shift from one idea to another seams appear between the objects or ideas upon which we rest our gaze; the homunculus fills in these seams with random details and associations from prior experience in order to simulate our sensation of a seamless integration of our cognitive fields. These missing details or saccades occur because we "have to keep turning off our brains for fractions of a second while the screen changes" (118). Paradoxically, as Christopher points out, the inability to see this absence results in beliefs in human exceptionalism, for when there is "something they can't see people think it has to be special, because people think there is always something special about what they can't see" (118). Christopher's alternative approach to this "problem" of normative human cognition is to be more aware of cognition's fractional shutdowns. In fact at various points in the novel when he feels threatened or overwhelmed he chooses to shut down his brain as you might reboot a computer. Such shutdowns allow autistic cognition to directly encounter this cognitive absence as an alternative to filling in the seams.

From Christopher's viewpoint these autistic alternatives are not the assertion of his own claims to superiority of cognition but rather a difference that involves an alternative apprehension of the world based upon more material encounters with missing information as one of the bases of the cognitive processing experience. One could argue that the coming evolution of the animal Christopher predicts as slouching toward Bethlehem is on display in scenes such as this, where the challenge is to see if the management of an excess of detail can be accommodated by adaptation of evolving alternative cognition systems, as in the case of autism. In order to keep his brain from jamming like a bread machine processing too many loaves at one time, Christopher fashions himself a version of a cognitive command-and-control center (7). In individuals with autism this cognitive "incapacity" might be characterized as "dysfunctional" (i.e., an ineffective or lower-functioning prefrontal lobe), but the narrator refers to his adapted practice as adhering to the principle of Occam's razor: "No more things should be presumed to exist than are absolutely necessary" (90). The world is already teeming with nuance, and Christopher's alternative approach is to comprehend its defining multiplicity by navigating an excess of stimuli characteristic of the information age rather than adopt the normative practice of reductionism of detail to slow its flow.

Finally these comparisons and contrasts between nonnormative and normative cognitive modes of apprehending the universe follow Darwin's principle of mutation, cited by Christopher as a productive system of miscodings. In order for life to exist things have to make copies of themselves (replication); in doing so they have to make small mistakes (mutation); and these mistakes have to be the same in their copies (heredity; 165). For Christopher the error-driven process that mutation introduces to replication suggests the random nature of species forms: "And these conditions (genetic mutations) are very rare, but they are possible, and they cause life. And it just happens. But it doesn't have to end up with rhinoceroses and human beings and whales. It could end up with anything" (165). In this pure Darwinist scenario of chance the novel places the emphasis on the random nature of human and nonhuman forms that otherwise appear deterministic (i.e., one superior to the other because of the possession of some over-vaunted capacity or another) but in fact prove arbitrary at base. A shifting kaleidoscopic mix of combinations—some of which may be expressed as autism—that disproves our investment in human beings as the best animals of all.

Ultimately Christopher's critique of impossible systematicity exposes the falsity of his own effort at commandeering an orderly world. Rather this goal is one imposed from the outside by the normative experience of reductionist cognition. Ironically he copes with this alternative capacity to exist within a reductionist "scale model world" of his bedroom and his segregated special school by imagining a universe emptied of people (DesJardins 2012, 84). In the film Self Preservation: The Art of Riva Lehrer (2005), the trans, disabled, neuroatypical memoirist Eli Clare explains this impulse thus: "I haven't always felt comfortable around people. For me Nature has been a refuge." Comparably Cal Montgomery (2001, 297), a philosopher of autism (as well as someone diagnosed with the condition), wonders how to develop a disability conversation that includes ways of talking about "people for whom access to human interaction is problematic." Within these autistic and non-normative neurologically related contexts impairment matters as we cannot imagine fashioning more accommodating environments to flourish without them. However, the difference in Curious Incident is Haddon's recognition that diagnosis of cognitive insufficiency has to be inverted toward the presumed desirability of normative rationality in order to allow alternative crip or queer variations to surface with more ethical ways of leading our lives.

Conclusion

Nonnormative positivist analyses of complex embodiment serve as sites for an alternative ethics to be articulated about why disabled lives matter and how we might revise, reinvent, and transform the presumed superiority of normative practices, beliefs, and qualifications of what bodies count. Right now disability studies and disability rights movements find participants caught in the limited horizon of identity by having to argue that disabled people must be allowed to pursue their lives as able-bodied people pursue theirs. This may be so, but in new materialist novels of embodiment such as Curious Incident we want to argue that such a goal is too small and often further solidifies the unchallenged desirability of normate lives.

Crip and queer lives explicated through nonnormative positivisms are those that believe another world is possible. The pursuit of crip ecologies such as this collection offers demonstrate that such worlds will not come into existence unless we vigilantly attend to more visceral engagements with the nuances of disabled lives as viable alternatives—an enrichment of the way alternative cognitions and corporealities allow us to inhabit the world as vulnerable, constrained, yet innovative embodied beings rather than merely as devalued social constructs.

BIBLIOGRAPHY

Bartmess, Elizabeth. 2015. "Review: The Curious Dog in the Night-Time by Mark Haddon." Disability in Kidlit. April 4. http://disabilityinkidlit .com/2015/04/04/.
Bérubé, Michael. 2013. "Narrative and Intellectual Disability." George Washington University Distinguished Lecture in Literary and Cultural Studies. October 29, Washington DC.
———. 2016. The Secret Life of Stories: From Don Quixote to Harry Potter, How Understanding Intellectual Disability Transforms the Way We Read. New York: NYU Press.
Carlson, Licia. 2007. "The Human as Just Another Animal: Madness, Disability, and Foucault's Bestiary." In Phenomenology and the Non-

Human Animal: At the Limits of Experience, edited by C. Painter and C. Lotz, 117–134. Dordrecht, Netherlands: Springer.

Coole, Diana, and Samantha Frost, eds. 2010. New Materialisms: Ontology, Agency, and Politics. Durham NC: Duke University Press,.

Cushing, Simon. 2012. "Autism: The Very Idea." In The Philosophy of Autism, edited by J. L. Anderson and S. Cushing, 17–46. Plymouth, UK: Roman and Littlefield.

Darwin, Charles. 2011. The Descent of Man. New York: CreateSpace Independent Publishing Platform.

DesJardins, Michel. 2012. "The Sexualized Body of the Child: Parents and the Politics of 'Voluntary' Sterilization of People Labeled Intellectually Disabled." In Sex and Disability, edited by R. McRuer and A. Mollow, 69–87. Durham NC: Duke University Press.

Frost, Samantha. 2012. "Fear and the Illusion of Autonomy." In New Materialisms: Ontology, Agency, and Politics, edited by D. Coole and S. Frost, 158–77. Durham NC: Duke University Press.

Haddon, Mark. 2003. The Curious Incident of the Dog in the Night-Time. New York: Vintage Contemporaries.

Haller, Beth. 2004. Representing Disability in an Ableist World: Essays in Mass Media. San Diego: Avocado Press, 2010.

Haraway, Donna. 1990. Primate Visions: Gender, Race, and Nature in the World of Modern Science. New York: Routledge.

Huffer, Lynn. 2009. Mad about Foucault: Rethinking the Foundations of Queer Studies. New York: Columbia University Press.

Jaworska, Agnieszka, and Julie Tannenbaum. 2014. "Person-Rearing Relationships as a Key to Higher Moral Status." Ethics 125: 242–71.

Kanner, Leo. 1943. "Autistic Disturbances of Affective Contact." Nervous Child 2: 217–50.

Massumi, Brian. 2002. Parables of the Virtual: Affect, Sensation. Durham NC: Duke University Press.

Mitchell, David, with Sharon L. Snyder. 2015. The Biopolitics of Disability: Neoliberalism, Ablenationalism, and Peripheral Embodiment. Ann Arbor: University of Michigan Press.

Montgomery, Cal. 2001. "Critic of the Dawn." Ragged Edge 22, no. 3. http://www.ragged-edge-mag.com/0501/0501cov.htm.

Newton, Michael. 2004. <u>Savage Girls and Wild Boys: A History of Feral Children</u>. New York: Picador.

Oliver, Michael, and Colin Barnes. 2012. <u>The New Politics of Disablement</u>. New York: Palgrave Macmillan.

Ray, Sarah Jaquette. 2013. "Normalcy, Knowledge, and Nature in Mark Haddon's <u>The Curious Incident of the Dog in the Night-Time</u>." <u>Disability Studies Quarterly</u> 33, no. 3. http://dsq-sds.org/article/view/3233/3263.

<u>Self Preservation: The Art of Riva Lehrer</u>. 2005. Directed by S. Snyder. DVD. Brace Yourselves Productions.

Shakespeare, Tom. 2002. "The Social Model of Disability: An Outdated Ideology?" <u>Research in Social Science and Disability</u> 2: 9–28.

Siebers, Tobin. 2013. "Disability and the Theory of Complex Embodiment." In <u>Disability Studies Reader</u>, 4th ed., edited by L. Davis, 278–97. New York: Routledge.

Thomas, Carol. 1999. <u>Female Forms: Experiencing and Understanding Disability</u>. London: Open University Press.

Wendell, Susan. 1997. <u>The Rejected Body: Feminist Philosophical Reflections on Disability</u>. New York: Routledge.

21

Autism and Environmental Identity

Environmental Justice and the Chains of Empathy

Robert Melchior Figueroa

This chapter takes an environmental justice approach with an emphasis on recognition justice. The interdependence and co-imbricating nature of recognition justice and distributive justice exist throughout this account; however, emphasizing recognition justice delves far more into the affective, collective, identity, and cultural issues. These issues attract various expressions of robust political inclusion and voice especially when recognition justice receives fuller attention as a form of environmental justice. Specifically regarding autism I explore the meanings of environmental identity, which I have defended is a crucial process for delivering one of the the most effective recognition perspectives in environmental justice studies. The need for recognition emphasis feels like it increases exponentially when I think about the relationship between environmental trauma and environmental identity for autistic advocacy. The entwined relationship between autistic identity and autism advocacy challenges the platitude of empathetic deficiency that is attributed to autism. Alternative meanings of empathy are available from a number of places within the environmental humanities. Drawing from a philosophical understanding of environmental empathy that adjoins critical disability studies, environmental justice emphasizes the voice of political agency, collective experience, and individuated affective impacts. Voices from autistic authors and the autism community, including personal experiences as a parent of an autistic child, provide ways to capture socio-environmental contradictions for autistics and their community. For instance, autistics are medically defined by symptoms of empathetic deficiency and, simultaneously, are noted for having a unique capacity for environmental empathy. Moving testimonies describe astonishing empathetic relations between autistics and nonhumans. We expect these relations to surface in autism literature, and we expect these avenues for empathetic growth to be part of the therapeutic cocktail in the repertoire of autism services. On the other hand, autism is identified by the person's extreme responses to an overstimulating environment. This part of autistic environmental empathy signifies the exhausting challenges produced by an amplified empathy that requires radical retreat and "tuning out." These kinds of contradictions and the socio-environmental problems they create for autistics are represented as chains of empathy. To delink these chains and reconfigure the place of environmental empathy where dimensions of moral agency between autistics (and nonautistics) and the more-than-human-world can transform, I take up Val Plumwood's philosophical conception of the intentional recognition stance. I close with a reflection on the implications for environmental justice studies, in particular how environmental empathy, environmental identity, and environmental justice should be pursued by interweaving environmental humanities with critical disability studies, in this case, critical autism studies.

Recognition and Autism in Environmental Justice

Communities negatively impacted by environmental injustices struggle to reconcile the multiple levels of socio-environmental assault that affects all aspects of life. I refer to this encompassing struggle as "environmental trauma," which contains the central features of trauma respectively found in medical, psychological, and sociological discourses. Thus I include the culmination of external impacts as described in medical trauma discourse, the severely distressing experience to psychological well-being as captured in psychological discourse, and the stigma and marginalization described in sociological discourse.[1] Each of these discourses links to environmental justice, but environmental trauma adds the threats and destruction of nonhumans and relational attachments to place and its inhabitants. Environmental trauma combines these discursive meanings in ethical, political, and ontological contexts to resound the trauma to environmental identity, which I define as the amalgamation of cultural identities, ways of life, and self-perceptions that are connected to a given group's material environment.[2]

Disparities in the distribution and compensation of environmental burdens link directly to the environmental harms and environmental trauma experienced by marginalized communities. Included among those impacted, autistics are commonly considered the embodiment of suspected connections between environmental burdens and disability. Indeed the distributive dimension of justice inundates discussions of autism and environmental justice, ranging from autism clusters to antivaccination advocacy. Addressing health impacts and, by direct causal connections of disparate distribution, ameliorating environmental burdens that disable individuals and communities are rightly premier concerns and purposes of environmental justice. However, the distributive considerations are limited and fail to address oppression surrounding the legacy of the environmental trauma as among the factors to be addressed in understanding the community's environmental heritage—a community-based environmental identity over time.

Autism, as a genetic-environmental condition, ironically what embodiment literally entails, is expressed as an environmental identity, where "identity" is the interfusion with community in the environment. Among a number of experiences from the autistic community (including individuals who have autism and live with autistics in common struggles for the welfare of autistic expression, identity, and inclusion) are that autism resists the normate environmental perception pertaining to appropriate behavior. Our environments are so indelibly socialized as to be socio-environmentally inseparable, involving a whole world of cues, implicit and explicit rules for appropriate behavior. This point is inexhaustibly covered in critical disability studies. Additionally, as new materialist influences indicate, even if we decode "nature's" social construction in its many forms, we still need to overcome the environmental distinction between what are "internal" (reflective, intuitive, affective, cognitive, and bodily experiences) and "external," the normate "outside" (environment, nature, technology, the other, etc.), which presumes a body barrier, a moral barrier, and an identity barrier constructed along oppressive arrangements. Indeed my definition of environmental identity requires emphasis on the point that a fluidity and "porosity of inter-relationality," to use Nancy Tuana's terminology, is entailed when referring to the ethical relationship between the "physical environment" and "identities, ways of life, and perceptions . . . of a community."[3] The use of "community" and "environmental identity" together is intended to heartily contest the concepts that presume innate, atomistic, and nonrelational individual (personal) identities.

In her book The Autism Puzzle, Brita Belli discusses environmental toxins and their relationship (causal as well as community relationships) to autism. The Gallagher family in Brick Township, New Jersey, includes three children, two of whom are autistic. Belli offers this quote from Bobby, the children's mother, reflecting on what she envisions as the outcome of her community's fight to address an autism cluster in connection to a local toxic landfill, a Superfund site:

The only thing I was looking for—and I was hoping the other parents would want [this]—was [for] the children . . . born in Brick Township . . . [to] be able to live in Brick Township for the rest of their lives with their families and have other outlets as they grew older. . . . We should start developing some programs for them so they'll have full lives. I'm not bitter about having children with autism. I'm perfectly fine with raising them until I can no longer walk—but I wanted to have places where I could take them and do things with them and feel like I was in a community of people who were accepting of us.[4]

Recognition justice addresses the ways in which environmental identities are fundamental to understanding and achieving environmental justice through a number of dynamics: the extent to which communities are involved in the discourse of environmental values and practices, the requirement for robust participation and inclusion in environmental decision making, the requirement for epistemic agency and the capacity of communities to "speak for themselves," and respect for lifeways, perceptions, and relations that express the environmental heritage of communities, such as traditional ecological knowledge, local experiences and agency, citizen science, and activism. Thus, as Bobby Gallagher points out, autistic environmental trauma relates to a host of additional environmental justice concerns besides the obviously important and crucial disparate distribution of environmental burdens. What must be included in understanding and resolving environmental trauma for communities is exploration of recognition justice— the site of environmental identity and environmental heritage.

How to transform environmental trauma into an inclusive environmental identity is unanswerable from the distributive environmental justice perspective, and analogous are the failures in the medical model of disabilities in addressing disability identity and recognition justice. Distributive environmental justice would fail to describe the environmental trauma of disability beyond health impacts or access, both absolutely critical and yet unsatisfactory for describing the lived differences, the historical factors, the political voice, and the reconciliation efforts an environmental trauma may require. A purely distributive framework causes the dilemma of autism amelioration, wherein eliminating the environmental cause of the disability should address the environmental trauma of autism by eliminating it and its persons. In an autism cluster "proof" that the water is safe is demonstrated not by data that it meets "healthy levels" of toxins but by showing that autism no longer turns up (or that numbers are reduced to the already alarming national average). Obviously that's a fairly simple way of looking at the genetic-environmental condition of autism, as Bobby Gallagher attests she is not interested in eliminating autism but re-creating environmental opportunities, which I read as transformative opportunities for a positive community environmental identity. The ways she breaks open this oversimplified and reductionist but still puzzling dilemma requires a vision of environmental justice through recognition justice and the social model of critical disability studies.

Autistic Environmental Trauma and the Chains of Empathy

Autistic environmental identity and environmental trauma introduce a relationship wherein sensory perceptions, verbal language acuity, sensory sensitivity, social difficulties, social interactions, emotional and behavioral outbursts, social retreat, differentiated or extraordinarily focused attention span, physical and posture influences, and, yes, differentiated empathetic responses must be recognized and reconciled. While these smack of medical model symptoms that fail to take into account the whole person, they can assist by serving as the channels through which autistic environmental trauma is navigated with amplified environmental identity. Any one of these experiences at any range of magnitudes could describe a single environmental trauma, but for the most part autism includes the entanglement of multiple traumas at multiple magnitudes in many different settings. This entanglement points to the amalgamation of experiences to recognize in autistic environmental identity.

A key component of autistic environmental trauma involves problematizing characterizations of empathetic deficiency embodied by autistics; it literally makes the autistic a problem person in the moral sense. As Patrick McDonagh draws the historical connection, using empathy to distinguish humans and nonhumans (humans from nature) has included definitive views about distinguishing autism by empathetic deficiency on precisely the same grounds as what it means to live a human life. To be human is determined by a normate meaning of empathy that is reductive and innate. McDonagh argues that the meaning of empathetic deficiency is where definitions of nature and definitions of autism overlap.[5] This results in problematizing moral personhood by way of empathetic deficiency and therefore treating autism as the embodiment of one of the most assumed and oppressive threads for human and nonhuman dualism, that between empathy (human) and nature. Simultaneously this problematizes the environment shared by the autistic person who is chained to empathy in a different, far more vulnerable way than normate conceptions of empathy.

In autistic literature we have numerous examples of autism and nonhuman empathy. Titles like The Horse Boy and The Curious Incident of the Dog in the Night-Time and authors like Temple Grandin and Naoki Higashida portray alternative empathetic accounts that reveal the dynamic of assemblages brought on by the environment in which autistics find themselves.[6] These titles and authors call up a backdrop of missing narratives and untold stories about autistics and nonhuman empathy. Like the increasing autistic population and the various autistic industries that follow apace, so the witnessing of environmental empathy between autistics and nonhumans becomes a commonplace on the road to recovery <u>from</u> autism. If you have an autistic child and you are fortunate to find resources by your own limited energy or from any similarly situated parents, you may very likely look for the nearest equestrian center serving disabled children; someone will likely put you on to it. The environmental identity of autistics that includes empathetic advances into nonhuman interaction stirs the recognition of a number of environmental justice perspectives and discloses a vital feature of autistic environmental ethics. The question is the extent to which fascination with autism and nonhuman empathy is dependent upon the fundamental attribution of empathetic deficiency.

The dangerous consistency that requires interrogation is that the common perception of autistic environmental identity as one that involves empathetic exchanges receptive to nonhuman empathy still helps to serve an oppressive deficiency discourse that pertains to both autistics and nonhumans. The appeal of interspecies communication coming from our genetic-environmental notion of autism offers the empathetic engagement desired for reconciling the world's environmental trauma by offering communication through one of our own (human) who is empathetically deficient like you (nonhumans) and can translate our shared plight—like a bridge to resolve the environmental guilt and shame of anthropogenic destruction, or a missing link.

Recognition justice provides us with an opportunity for autistic environmental identities to be an expressed moral agency, but if they are quieted by normate environmental interpretations, then reconciling these environmental traumas cannot proceed very far because they dislodge the environmental identity and reinsert personal identity. Attempting to negotiate these conflicts between environmental identity (wherein autistics are included) and personal identity (wherein autistics are problematized), autistic environmental identity takes on the burden of a slice of the world's environmental trauma, but as a social outsider, an alien, a posthuman of super empathetic responsibility. Consider this in light of the closing question from Naoki Higashida in his book The Reason I Jump:

Q58 What are your thoughts on autism itself?
I think that people with autism are born outside the regime of civilization. Sure, this is just my own made-up theory, but I think that, as a result of all the killings in the world and the selfish planet-wrecking that humanity has committed, a deep sense of crisis exists.

Autism has somehow arisen out of this. Although people with autism look like other people physically, we are in fact very different in many ways. We are more like travelers from the distant, distant past. And if, by our being here, we could help the people of the world remember what truly matters for the Earth, that would give us quiet pleasure.[7]

Stuart Murray's survey of posthuman theses and autism explores several paths of the "the alien thesis" that would read an account like Higashida's "traveler from a distant, distant past" and overlook the greater complexities of embodiment by calling upon unique qualities that autism has for information society. As Murray exemplifies, even when working out the empathy between Temple Grandin and nonhumans, particularly cattle, her description of empathy gets posthuman attention because of the information processing she identifies as her empathetic tool.[8] However, Murray resists the posthuman information-processing account of autistics by asserting that embodiment shifts the post-human fetishizing to a <u>parallel</u> account that retains what Barbara Barnbaum has called "autistic integrity."[9] Autistic integrity defies many psychological assumptions of personal identity–, self–, and other-oriented psychological extension. I explicitly reassert embodiment to this defiance characteristic of autistic integrity and agree with Murray's delinking the posthuman mode of super-empathetic abilities. I invite us to read Higashida's traveler as intended, a simile connecting the empathetic differences that Higashida experiences, posthuman theses notwithstanding. Murray wants to retain respect for current autistic experience and embodiment, which I would describe as an effort to avoid eclipsing the autistic environmental identity into a posthuman information-processing symbol.

Returning to McDonagh's earlier points regarding empathetic deficiency and the oppression of nature, we should consider oppression against collective relations of autism. I'm sure we recall one of the less subtle uses of environmental empathy for autistic oppression and environmental injustice, the "refrigerator mom" characterization. I can only hope this is a passé characterization and we've moved well beyond the very thought of mother-blaming in our many social circles; however, I believe it remains a live reaction both directly and indirectly because of the stigma of failure by those ascribed with a double-edged empathetic authority as it suits us. We gendered empathy along the way. This should be made central in McDonagh's survey of the historical relationship between the empathetic deficiency of autistics and empathetic inabilities, because the gendered manufacturing of empathy reinforces the oppressive human/

nature dualism that ecofeminists like Val Plumwood have thoroughly exposed.[10]

If it is outdated, great; however, it was just over decade ago when my son Soren's autism surfaced enough to exponentially increase the environmental guilt cast against empathetic deficiency. The identification and accountability of his mother, Dawn, as the "first environment" was first directly launched at her by way of the "refrigerator mom" syndrome, linking mother-blaming to the empathetic deficiency by socio-environmental oppressive chains. When "refrigerator mom" becomes passé, "body burden" replaces the crass mother-blaming with another dimension of environmental justice as we rightly turn to endocrine disruptors, implicating mothers environmentally as a biogenetic intermediary, if not the mediating or direct cause, of autism. Thus empathetic deficiency precedes the actual autism experience by identifying the mother as an environmental other able to cause autism by body-mind instantiation as a biosocial transmitter of autism. Combined it suggests a fundamental crisis for environmental empathy. The mother is the legator of the endocrine disruptor inherited by the autistic child, and she is the imprint of empathetic deficiency upon the autistic child. This environmental identity is a moral pronouncement of both mother and child as empathetically deficient around the pivotal environmental heritage of autism. Both mother and child share the relationship of empathy at the depth of inheriting medical or social traits, as it were, but the medical traits are already assumed to be environmental, located in the embodied history of autistic environmental identity. I take Bobby Gallagher's wish to be "accepted by the community" to be disclosing this as just one of the many stigmas that ensue for mothers and autistic children.

Delinking these oppressive chains of empathy requires a reconsideration of autistic environmental identity from an alternative arrangement, a relinking of normate environmental perspectives with autistic environmental empathy. Soon after Soren could walk he took up the hobby of throwing bouncy balls down a wooden stairway and rocks into the stream. Once, when visiting my mother, she set up a small child's pool for Soren, and my relatives quickly observed his rock-to-water throwing interests. With no other children around he was given license to collect and throw as many rocks from my mother's many rock gardens as many times as he pleased. My family's empathetic engagement with Soren's interests were pretty much that of mine and Dawn's: encouragement, he's having fun. It also revealed that one person's hobby may be recognized by another as a symptom of autism: repetitive behavior, uh oh. What is he throwing at? Is he going for splash effect? Is he intrigued by the changes in speed and direction once the rock enters the water? Those questions of purpose, intention, response, and environmental extension to the point of speed and direction of the rocks are eclipsed once the recognition of repetitive behavior takes over. One kind of empathy shifted and transformed another away from the good, the initially appreciated hobby, to problematic behavior and environmental disruption that he may not even care about us or the environment at all. The environmental relation turns from a fun and friendly one to one of observation and surveillance for symptoms related to repetitive behavior, or empathetic disengagement, which pretty much is adjacent to repetitive behavior for autistics, and other symptoms that add up to indicators of environmental trauma. It is easy to see the autistic retreat from human relations; it's an empathetic deficiency that produces the autistic fears of some particular environmental space or individuals within the space. Or perhaps the deficiency is expressed when the autistic refuses to leave the environment, or perhaps when the autistic depends upon the relations within the environment to enjoy the positive engagement of empathy, or perhaps all of these things at the same time with dynamic magnitudes that change as the environment changes and the environmental identity shifts?

All of these questions and observations imply without stating that an environmental empathy exists around our environmental identity, and while empathy narrowed to specific (normate) cognitive capacities of specific individuals according to assumptions about personal identity can shift normate environmental interpretations, recognition of environmental empathy according to environmental identity can also shift normate environmental interpretations. However, the normate preference to define relationships according to personal identity rather than environmental identity is precisely the obstacle to understanding autistic (and nonautistic) environmental identity.

Some months after the visit to my mother's we were in Australia, which allowed Soren (age two) and me to take up a routine of daily beach walks for about six months. Now if you want to talk about license to throw rocks -to water (not into or at but to, as one throws a ball to a companion), we are there. Soren's method was repetition to perfection: stand close to sand and rock shore; scoop wet sand with left hand; taste by licking the sand from hand; and throw sand to the ocean. This could go on, even with interruptions to explore the tidal pools, for a good long time. The reason I bring this up is because the same exact behavior (and licking was always an on-and-off behavior), with an ocean of endless waves, grafts the repetitive behavior onto the repetitive environment. The pattern of Soren's behavior becomes more purposeful from the onlooker's position, as far as fellow beach walkers who spoke to me ever indicated. The grafted repetition extends empathy in the other direction from symptomizing the behavior and downgrading the environmental relationship; instead observations raise questions of how Soren is timing the waves to throw (after licking) the sand. How many waves have to pass between the routine? Does he think he's picking up the same sand every time after a wave? Not just what we think he is projecting but what he _is_ doing in this environmental relationship, his ethical action with the environment. The questions are indicative of the shifting normate environmental perspectives as much as the shifting autistic environmental perspectives, and perhaps here they cross. Or rather these shifts are intersectional with a variety of empathetic conditions. Sure, if I told the beach walkers Soren has autism an "ah ha" would ensue because the normate shifts to deficiency, repetition of an individual who is symptomatic. If the beach walkers did not know what autism is, how could they avoid noting the repetitive behavior? Ironically I didn't tell them because the "official" word was only on the tip of my tongue but wouldn't officially come out for another year. But autism was never mentioned at my mother's either; it was implied by the repetitive behavior observations and implied problem persons, Dawn and Soren. From another point of view maybe beach-walking strangers are less candid about the obvious repetitive behavior, but that's part of the point: that it is behavior fitting normate environmental interpretation, just enough to shift empathetic recognition and leave off speculation of severe abnormality.

This is all very good for the normate environmental interpretation, but is there autistic environmental identity on its own terms? If what is meant by this question is "What is the difference between autistic environmental identity and normate environmental identity?," I would say of both that environmental identity is an aggregate of environmental empathy that defies innatism, genetic determinism, and moral reductionism, _and_ narrows definitions of personal identity. Another way to see this is in light of the human empathetic interactions that Soren enjoys by way of environmental empathy. Part of the reason equestrian therapy for autistics is renowned is that a space is made for the empathetic community by alternative opportunities to express and live in autistic environmental identity without the many normate interruptions. Here the trainers and therapists, horses and children are making possible environmental empathy that is nonverbal, embodied without stigma, and highly relational. As therapeutic, it delivers empathy by every means possible in these environmental relationships, but it also cordons off these opportunities in the therapeutic sector and limits these opportunities in more normate spaces.

The wider opportunities are themselves environmental justice issues, foremost because of privileges to access and explore the alternative opportunities for finding normate shifting and greater environmental empathy. Equestrian therapy played only one part of Soren's exploration. He would spend hours daily catching and releasing crayfish from a park stream; he's always been a companion on hikes; he independently explores the creek, the underside of places for spiders and snakes; he attends wilderness camps; and his exceptional memory makes him an encyclopedic ally of nonhumans. Finding a shrew, he informs the camp counselor that it could win in a battle against a scorpion. Who knew? His vast exploration of nonhumans on the Internet is unsatisfied without their embodiment in a world conducive to his environmental empathy. He would always rather be at Petco talking to another human about the geckos and snakes than do anything with information technology. Having the opportunities and choices, mobility, and resulting independence, he enjoys the privileges that many autistics and their families and advocates cannot afford. But the point is that Soren has been encouraged to seek out and explore his autistic environmental identity, which allowed us to enjoin our own empathy by relocating ourselves in the world of autism, as opposed to being in a world with autism tacked on.

Empathetic Recognition and
Autistic Environmental Justice

The environmental empathy movement in Western environmental philosophy moved from "thinking like a mountain" to the 1990s explorations of ecofeminist philosophers who connected empathetic pathways between environmentally embedded, embodied humans and nonhumans by the common thread that empathy entails ethical action.[11] Plumwood's ecofeminist philosophical work influences a number of the ecofeminist contributions to environmental empathy, but in my reading of this movement her Environmental Culture (2002) absorbs environmental empathy with her account of the intentional recognition stance. It is at this point that she breaks completely with "intentional" meaning as if the nonhuman other has intentional moral agency and embraces an actual intentional capacity that we are able to recognize in nonhuman others and they recognize in us. Plumwood anticipates new materialist appreciations of intentionality by matching cellularity and agency in a manner that conjures autism:

> A simple spectrum or scalar concept like consciousness has the disadvantage, additional to unclarity and obscurity, of having little capacity to recognize incommensurability or difference, and none at all if interpreted in terms of hegemonic otherness. Intentionality can allow us to take better account of incommensurability because there is enough breadth, play and multiplicity to allow us to use diverse, multiple and decentered concepts that need not be ranked relative to each other understanding both humans and non-humans as intentional beings. For example, pheromone-based, sonar-based and pollen-based sensitivities and chemical communication systems such as those used by cells might appear as heterogeneous intentional

capacities that cannot be treated as extensions of the para-digmatic human case, as narrow concepts like consciousness tend to be.[12]

Autistic environmental empathy benefits from Plumwood's assertion because she defies simple spectrum delineations and rankings to intentionality, and for that matter to recognition. To recognize intentionality in the ways Plumwood argues would require being open to multiple expressions of intentionality and accepting that to actually recognize is a moral action. This rein-serts environmental empathy into the context of environmental identity as opposed to standard cognitivist conceptions of per-sonal identity, because Plumwood insists it calls upon a stance in which we are also recognized by nonhuman others. The exchange of empathy is an aggregation of empathy between the inten-tional subjects, achieved not by their individual innate cognitive or affective capacities but from the empathetic recognition made of assemblages between them.

One importance I see in Plumwood's philosophy for critical disability studies is that she provides an entrée to rethinking the normate environmental interpretations to include recognition in ways that undermine the narrow presumptions of personal identity that shrink moral agency. With an alternative intentional agency a reconfiguration of affective and cognitive combinations is expected to widen. Indeed some options of agency may be neither affective nor cognitive combinations. The intentionality is recognized between the moral agents in an environmental relationship. Another Higashida question comes to mind:

Q47 Would you give us an example of something people with autism really enjoy?

We do take pleasure in one thing that you probably won't be able to guess. Namely, making friends with nature. The reason we aren't much good at people skills is that we think too much about what sort of impression we're making on the other person, or how we should be responding to this or that. But nature is always there at hand to wrap us up, gently: glowing, swaying, bubbling, rustling.

Just by looking at nature, I feel as if I'm being swallowed up into it, and in that moment I get the sensation that my body's now a speck, a speck from long before I was born, a speck that is melting into nature itself. This sensation is so amazing that I forget that I'm a human being, and one with special needs to boot.

Nature calms me down when I'm furious, and laughs with me when I'm happy. You might think that it's not possible that nature could be a friend, not really. But human beings are part of the animal kingdom too, and perhaps us people with autism still have some leftover awareness of this, buried somewhere deep down. I'll cherish the part of me that thinks of nature as a friend.[13]

The weaving of Plumwood's insights with critical disability studies promotes an autistic environmental justice approach that works through the assemblages of environmental empathy between a stance of intentional recognition and recognition justice. Returning to the distributive and recognition dimensions of environmental justice, Plumwood already configures the intentional recognition stance adjacent to a primarily human-centered distributive justice without eliminating either dimension of justice or reducing one to the other.[14] The "recognition" in her "intentional recognition stance" is a doubled meaning of recognition as an empathetic recognition and as part of the bivalent (or two-dimensional) environmental justice that entails distribution and recognition in co-original and interpenetrating ways. This feature of Plumwood is often overlooked because Western environmental philosophy, and especially environmental justice, has imposed a wedge between recognition justice existing between humans and recognition justice as the pathway for interspecies environmental justice. Similarly for autistic environmental justice, once the chains of empathy are delinked, more opportunities open for autistics to "speak for themselves." Interspecies environmental justice will require an intentional recognition stance, a reconfiguration of empathy for environmental identity, and co-relational agency.

Recognition environmental justice requires that autistics are more than a subject of study or the bridge between human and nonhuman justice; autistics are self- and community advocates with environmental identities that raise difficult questions for environmental justice. We need to understand the legacy and environmental heritage that is inclusive of and informed by autistics to explore and refine environmental empathy.

NOTES

1. References and examples of environmental trauma in previous writings include Figueroa, "Cultural Losses and Environmental Justice"; Figueroa and Waitt, "Climb."
2. The word material has replaced the word physical as cited in Figueroa, "Evaluating Environmental Justice Claims." The definition is unchanged by this clarification and is the one I prefer.
3. Tuana, "Being Affected by Climate Change, the Anthropocene, and the Body of Ethics."
4. Belli, The Autism Puzzle, 56–57.
5. McDonagh, "Autism in an Age of Empathy."
6. Isaacson, The Horse Boy; Haddon, The Curious Incident of the Dog in the Night-Time; Grandin, Thinking in Pictures and Other Reports from My Life with Autism; Higashida, The Reason I Jump.

7. Higashida, <u>The Reason I Jump</u>, 111.
8. Murray, "Autism and the Posthuman," 64, and Grandin, <u>Thinking in Pictures</u>.
9. Barnbaum, <u>The Ethics of Autism</u>.
10. Plumwood's two major works deserve reference: <u>Feminism and the Mastery of Nature</u> and <u>Environmental Culture</u>.
11. Tracking the threads of the environmental empathy movement is too extensive a project here, but the references are Aldo Leopold, <u>A Sand County Almanac</u>, and the work of Lori Gruen and others mentioned in her "Attending to Nature."
12. Plumwood, <u>Environmental Culture</u>, 179–80.
13. Higashida, <u>The Reason I Jump</u>, 88–89.
14. Plumwood, <u>Environmental Culture</u>.

BIBLIOGRAPHY

Barnbaum, Barbara R. <u>The Ethics of Autism: Among Them, but Not of Them</u>. Bloomington Indiana University Press, 2008.

Belli, Brita. <u>The Autism Puzzle: Connecting the Dots between Environmental Toxins and Rising Autism Rates</u>. New York: Seven Stories Press, 2012.

Figueroa, Robert Melchior. "Cultural Losses and Environmental Justice." In <u>The Oxford Handbook of Climate Change and Society</u>, edited by John S. Dryzek, Richard B. Norgaard, and David Schlosberg, 232–50. Oxford: Oxford University Press, 2011.

———. "Evaluating Environmental Justice Claims." In <u>Forging Environmentalism: Justice, Livelihood, and Contested Environments</u>, edited by Joanne Bauer, 360–76. Armonk NY: M. E. Sharpe, 2006.

Figueroa, Robert Melchior, and Gordon Waitt. "Climb: Restorative Justice, Environmental Heritage, and the Moral Terrains of Uluru-Kata Tjuta National Park." <u>Environmental Philosophy</u> 7, no. 2 (2010): 135–63.

Grandin, Temple. <u>Thinking in Pictures and Other Reports from My Life with Autism</u>. New York: Vintage, 1996.

Gruen, Lori. "Attending to Nature: Empathetic Engagement with the More Than Human World." <u>Ethics & the Environment</u> 14, no. 2 (2009): 23–38.

Hacking, Ian. "Autism Fiction: A Mirror of an Internet Decade." <u>University of Toronto Quarterly</u> 79, no. 2 (2010): 632–55.

Haddon, Mark. <u>The Curious Incident of the Dog in the Night-Time</u>. New York: Vintage, 2004.

Higashida, Noaki. <u>The Reason I Jump: The Inner Voice of a Thirteen-Year Old Boy with Autism</u>. New York: Random House, 2007.

Isaacson, Rupert. <u>The Horse Boy: A Father's Quest to Heal His Son</u>. Boston: Little, Brown, 2009.

McDonagh, Patrick. "Autism in an Age of Empathy: A Cautionary Critique." In <u>Worlds of Autism: Across the Spectrum of Neurological Difference</u>, edited by Joyce Davidson and Michael Orsini, 31–52. Minneapolis: University of Minnesota Press, 2013.

Murray, Stuart. "Autism and the Posthuman." In <u>Worlds of Autism: Across the Spectrum of Neurological Difference</u>, edited by Joyce Davidson and Michael Orsini, 53–72. Minneapolis: University of Minnesota Press, 2013.

Plumwood, Val. <u>Environmental Culture: The Ecological Crisis of Reason</u>. New York: Routledge, 2002.

———. <u>Feminism and the Mastery of Nature</u>. New York: Routledge, 1993.

Ray, Sarah Jaquette. "Normalcy, Knowledge, and Nature in Mark Haddon's <u>Curious Incident of the Dog in the Night-Time</u>." <u>Disability Studies Quarterly</u> 33, no. 3 (2013). Online.

Tuana, Nancy. "Being Affected by Climate Change, the Anthropocene, and the Body of Ethics." In <u>Ethics and the Anthropocene</u>, edited by Kenneth Shockley and Andrew Light. Cambridge MA: MIT Press, forthcoming.

Weil, Kari. "Killing Them Softly: Animal Death, Linguistic Disability, and the Struggle for Ethics." <u>Configurations</u> 14 (2008): 87–96.

22

Moving Together Side by Side
Human-Animal Comparisons in Picture Books

Elizabeth A. Wheeler

Jolena, who has autism, finds she can play at her neighborhood park in the company of her new service dog, Muffet (Szambelan 2009). Involvement with animals is a central way kids with disabilities connect with the world and play an inextricable part in it. This involvement forms the centerpiece in an international canon of picture books. In these books animals form part of what I am calling a "prosthetic community," a cluster of living beings, ideas, resources, and objects that enable disabled children's full inclusion. The human-nonhuman relationships transcend service and companionship, however. These books compare children with disabilities to animals, and different species come to resemble each other. Adults as well as children can use these books as models toward an important goal: recognizing the personhood of animals and children with disabilities and their common membership in the living world. The greater this recognition, the more humans can claim their kinship to nonhuman animals.

One image repeats frequently across this canon of picture books: a child with a disability and an animal moving together side by side. These pictures compare human and nonhuman bodies as they surf, crawl, fly, dance, climb, and play. Their movement represents ingenuity, joy, and, most of all, freedom. At these moments the characters claim their place in the world, expressing their relationship to nature through their bodies. These images usually serve as the climax of the book and the solution to the problem. In this essay I focus on two picture books from this canon: <u>Seal Surfer</u> by Michael Foreman (1997) of Great Britain and <u>Sosu's Call</u> by Meshack Asare (1997) of Ghana.[1]

Moving together side by side, animals and kids with disabilities express a freedom that is not only physical but also political. Human-animal comparisons solve problems. They establish kinship across species. They challenge human domination. They express the interdependence valued in kids' culture, disability culture, and environmentalism. They unsettle social norms. Human-animal comparisons help us rethink our ideas about capability, agency, and belonging (Hediger 2009, 323). As Sunaura Taylor (2011, 201) points out, "The big questions in disability studies seem equally relevant to the animal rights debate: How can we create new meanings for words like 'dependent' and 'independent'? How can those who are seemingly most vulnerable within a society be perceived as also being useful, strong, and necessary?" Human-animal comparisons address another question as well: How can the vulnerability of disabled people be perceived as part of our shared vulnerability on the planet, and the vulnerability of the planet itself, rather than a unique and separate kind of weakness?

Human-animal comparisons also create problems, however. There is the devastating, even genocidal history of comparing people with disabilities to animals. Given this history, kinship across species is often contained as soon as it is expressed. There is also the devastating history of using animals as beasts of burden. Animals often bear the unfair burden of proving the humanity of children with disabilities, just as children themselves bear that unfair burden. In this canon of picture books, including <u>Seal Surfer</u> and <u>Sosu's Call</u>, animals bear the specific burden of proving the masculinity of boys with disabilities. Some of these assertions of masculinity are more traditional; others widen the masculine repertoire to include more vulnerability, flexibility, and cooperation.

In this exploration I have drawn on ideas from animal studies and disability studies since one field affirms the equality of nonhuman animals and the other affirms the equality of people with disabilities. However, I have discovered a problem in bringing these fields together: the ableism, or antidisability bias, in animal studies. The personhood of children with disabilities is still a fragile construct, even among those committed to animal rights.

Ableism in Animal Studies

Disrespect for children with disabilities runs through the philosophical wing of animal studies. This disrespect shows itself in the frequent use of disability as a hypothetical test case for the limits of personhood. The obvious example is Peter Singer, whose Animal Liberation (1975) and Practical Ethics (1979) sparked the field of animal studies. In Practical Ethics his hypothetical examples support the argument for redefining nonhuman animals as persons. Singer pits children with disabilities against animals. Defining personhood as the capacity to make choices and imagine a future, Singer (1993, 118, 171) argues that a chimpanzee qualifies as a person, while some newborn humans do not: "So it seems that killing, say, a chimpanzee is worse than the killing of a human being who, because of a congenital intellectual disability, is not and never can be a person."

Peter Singer is the most notorious example of ableism in animal studies, but he is far from alone. Philosophers often question the limits of the human by invoking hypothetical examples of children, people with disabilities, and children with disabilities. While these philosophers think consciously about race and gender, their comparisons between disability and animality seem unconscious. Although Cary Wolfe (2003, 69, 34, 37) criticizes Singer's ethics as a "utilitarian calculus," he neutrally summarizes Singer's view that "the hydrocephalic child" fails the test of personhood, and uncritically adopts the term "human vegetables" from Luc Ferry. Wolfe compares the struggles for animal, racial, and women's rights but ignores disability justice, even though hypothetical children with disabilities help make his case. Donna Haraway (2003, 3) argues for the importance of human-canine coevolution by making a cognitive impairment joke: "How might stories about dog-human worlds finally convince brain-damaged U.S. Americans, and maybe other less historically challenged people, that history matters in naturecultures?" In The Animal That Therefore I Am, a founding animal studies text, Jacques Derrida (2008, 79) also invokes cognitive disability when he concurs with Descartes that the idea of the animal soul is "the prejudice of children or of 'feeble minds.'"

Over and over rhetorical figures of children and disability appear as animal studies philosophers compare human and nonhuman animals. Why this disparagement in the defense of animal rights? The impulse arises from the relative ranking of human adults, children, people with disabilities, and nonhuman animals. Mel Y. Chen (2012, 89) writes, "In spite of their regular co-occurrence with humans, nonhuman animals are typologically situated elsewhere from humans, as in the linguistic concept of an animacy hierarchy, a scale of relative sentience that places humans at the very top." While they may not be conscious of their preoccupation, animal studies scholars have disability on their minds because animals and people with disabilities are often seen as competing for the bottom rung on the evolutionary ladder.

Children too take part in this fictive competition. The field of child development has its origins in child study, a movement that emerged around 1900 and bore the influence of Darwinism. Children assumed increasing importance for Progressive

Era psychologists like James Sully: "Nearly all the early psychologists articulated the idea that child study mattered because by observing children and 'the lowest races of mankind,' 'we are watching the beginnings of things. . . . Our modern science is before all things historical and genetic, going back to beginnings so as to understand the later and more complex phases of things as the outcomes of these beginnings'" (Blackford 2013, 288). If you add the category disability to the category child, you get an especially fierce contest for the bottom rung of the evolutionary ladder.

I want to contrast this image, the battle royal at the foot of the evolutionary ladder, to the picture book images of children with disabilities and animals moving side by side. These images show that animal rights do not have to come at the expense of disability rights; rather the opposite is true: the greater the social acceptance of disability, the more freedom there can be to claim animal kinship.

The key task is not to establish the correct threshold of personhood. Rather the key tasks are adaptation and cooperation, two organizing principles of disability culture. We work together to make it work. Animals form part of the cluster of support that is a prosthetic community, which epitomizes a disability culture that works well for the people in it.[2] A prosthetic community is a combination of physical objects like wheelchairs and adaptive sports equipment; technologies like text-to-speech synthesizers and news media; service and companion animals; friends, family, and paid caregivers; decent income and health care; disability rights laws; and resources of the creative mind, like brainstorming, fantasy, and activism. These solutions rely on local knowledge in specific ecosystems. The beauty of the prosthetic community is that a disabled person does not have to rely exclusively on one overburdened source of support. The richer the prosthetic community, the more humans with disabilities can compare themselves to animals without risking their status as persons.

The Problem with Human-Animal Comparisons

As things stand, human-animal comparisons create problems. They have justified the subjugation, murder, and incarceration of people with disabilities, ethnic minorities, and colonized populations. This history is so destructive Isabel Brittain (2004) lists "forging links between the character and animals" among "the six pitfalls of disability fiction." Sunaura Taylor (2011, 196) writes, "There is no way to discuss animal metaphors without recognizing the atrocities that they have been used for: the rhetoric of Nazi Germany, of racism, of slavery." Taylor describes the living continuation of this history in her own childhood: "As a child I remember knowing that when my fellow kindergarten classmates told me I walked like a monkey, that they meant it to hurt my feelings, which of course it did. . . . I understood that they were commenting on my inability to stand completely upright when out of my wheelchair—my inability to stand straight like a normal human being" (192). Such animal comparisons are common in the lives of people with disabilities: "When I ask members of the disabled community whether they have ever been compared to animals because of their disabilities, I receive a torrent of replies. I am transported to a veritable bestiary: frog legs, penguin waddles, seal limbs, and monkey arms. It is clear, however, from the wincing and negative interjections that these comparisons are not pleasant to remember" (192).

However, as Taylor (2011, 194–95) argues, being compared to an animal is an insult only in a context where animals endure widespread mistreatment. We can help remove this stigma by advocating for animal and disability rights in tandem. For instance, both factory farm chickens and some disabled children live in cages. Ninety-five percent of laying hens in the United States spend their lives in battery cages, squeezed in too tightly to move. Designed to increase profits, their immobility causes mental and physical disabilities (Friedrich 2014). In Lechaina, Greece, a state-run center for disabled children keeps its residents locked in cages. The cages seemed preferable to strapping the children to their beds, the prior practice, since low staffing levels make it impossible to provide adequate supervision. The center cannot increase staff levels because the European Union and the International Monetary Fund have imposed a hiring moratorium since Greece's economic bailout (Hadjimatheou 2014). The center locks up children not because they are cruel or ableist, but because the prosthetic community lacks resources.

The obvious way to criticize the Greek government is to say that it is wrong to keep children caged like animals, but this criticism misses half the point. It is also wrong to keep chickens caged like animals. Questioning the overall flow of capital—the profit motive in one case and the lack of resources in the other—might increase freedom for both animals and children with disabilities.

Human and nonhuman lives leak into each other if nothing stops them. For Mel Y. Chen (2012, 90) "kinship formations between animals and humans" represent "the unsteadiness of categorical hierarchies and the legitimacy afforded to some of their leakages." Yet "biopolitical governance . . . steps in over and over again to contain these leaky bounds" (129). These picture books reveal both the leakage and the containment, a containment spurred not only by animacy hierarchies but also by the terrible history of comparing people with disabilities to animals. The containing wall comes down harder for some children than others, depending on the degree of stigma and the age of the child. Small children are free and encouraged to imitate various animals. However, while an older child may swim like a seal or fly like a bird, she cannot eat like a pig or crawl like a dog without courting insult.

I found no picture books that compared a child with a cognitive disability to an animal; the deep stigma attached to cognitive disability prohibits that human-animal comparison. However, I did find many picture books comparing children with physical disabilities to animals, including the two I feature here. Michael Foreman and Meshack Asare are distinguished and prolific writer-illustrators. The human-animal leakages in Seal Surfer and Sosu's Call happen in literal cascades of water. Both books take place in Atlantic fishing villages, one in Cornwall in western Britain, one in Ghana in western Africa.

The SuperCrip and the Beast of Burden

Taylor (2011, 201) is right about the key question "How can those who are seemingly most vulnerable within a society be perceived as also being useful, strong, and necessary?" The next question, however, is "Useful to whom?" Animals and kids with disabilities become heroes by proving their usefulness to human society, and thus their right to exist. The burden of proving one's own personhood gives rise to two mythological figures: the SuperCrip and the Beast of Burden. In disability studies the SuperCrip signifies a hero with a disability who performs astonishing and admirable feats. The SuperCrip never acts for himself alone; he exists to inspire or admonish others. Usually the story contains elements of magic realism, falling silent on the adaptations required to achieve seemingly miraculous feats. The SuperCrip is a close cousin to the idea of passing, which in the case of disability refers to doing more than you really can in an effort to meet social expectations.

I am using the term Beast of Burden to signify a nonhuman animal who bears the burden of triangulating relationships between humans (Chen 2012, 129). Families often triangulate their relationships through animals, "deflecting to pets or routing through pets emotion and communication intended for other family members" (Melson 2003, 37). Animals also perform this type of emotional labor in public, and the triangulation can work to the advantage of kids with disabilities. For instance, a pet or service dog can deflect attention away from the disability and give the child a different story to tell. In My Buddy, a picture book about a service dog for a boy with muscular dystrophy, the narrator testifies, "Before Buddy, I didn't like to go places. People stared at me. Now people look at us—and ask about my dog" (Osofsky 1992, n.p.). These picture books frequently transfer the focal point from the disability to the nonhuman animal. In other senses too kids with disabilities use animals to leverage greater status for themselves.

This canon of picture books showcases a particular variety of triangulation: animals establish the masculinity of boys with disabilities. They enable traditionally masculine actions like physical courage and outdoor adventures. In Sosu's Call and Seal Surfer the protagonists are the sons and grandsons of fishermen who establish their belonging in the male line of the family through their sojourns outdoors. Of the twelve picture books I found featuring animals and kids with disabilities that had the same protagonist for the entire story, all the main characters were boys.

Human-animal partnerships allow boys with disabilities to become like the independent, adventurous heroes of so many classic picture books, from Harold and the Purple Crayon to Where the Wild Things Are (Spitz 1999, 189). Apparently animal help does not foreclose independence in the same way human help does. The narrator of My Buddy says, "Before Buddy, Mom and Dad helped me. Mike and other friends helped, too. But friends sometimes get tired of helping. And I wanted to do things on my own" (Osofsky 1992, n.p.). A dog's help doesn't count as a form of dependence. Doing things with Buddy equals doing things "on my own."

Seal Surfer: The Prosthetic Community

Foreman's (1997) Seal Surfer concerns Ben, his grandfather, and their shared love of the ocean. The book takes place among the surfers and fishermen of St. Ives, Cornwall. One of Britain's most distinguished and prolific writer-illustrators, Foreman grew up in the fishing village of Pakefield, Suffolk, and now divides his time between London and St. Ives (Carey 2011; "Michael Foreman" 2014). Seal Surfer glows with intimate knowledge of the British coastline, its steep cliffs, waves, and seasons. Ben's rich prosthetic community includes a wheelchair, crutches, and an adaptive surfboard. While Ben's surfing prowess represents to some degree a SuperCrip need to impress the viewer, the story leaves plenty of room for physical vulnerability and interdependence.

Leigha McReynolds (2013, 118) writes that the introduction of an animal body in a prosthetic relationship allows disabled human characters "to thrive in an embodiment that exists beyond the ableist myth of an impermeable, bounded self." Permeability and boundlessness characterize Seal Surfer, from the leakage between animal and human identities to the immersive water-colors. The interdependence of the prosthetic community extends to a larger sense of interdependence with the natural world. The ocean seems boundless, and so does the boy's ability to connect with nature. The watercolor illustrations render a translucent sea, the human and seal characters visible within it and sharing its colors. In traditional portrayals men's bodies are impermeable and women's bodies leak. Seal Surfer's paintings of the sea permeating Ben's body may indicate a new masculinity in the making.

Ben's disability is only one small part of this big picture. Foreman expresses this relative importance literally in the book's first two pages, set in the spring. While the text describes the grand-son and grandfather collecting mussels and spotting a seal who seems to be injured, the opening picture focuses on something else: the larger natural world all three mammals share. The big picture is a spectacular landscape in bright, layered watercolors reminiscent of Monet. The massive rocks are not gray, but built out of purple, turquoise, ochre, and chartreuse, resolving into a deeply observed re-creation of Britain's west coast.

The two human figures and the seal are tiny in this landscape, which might seem to diminish them. Instead, however, these proportions establish their belonging and naturalize the boy's disability. We see the three figures from far above; as the picture book scholar Perry Nodelman (1988, 150) observes, "Figures seen from above become part of an environment, either secure in it or constrained by it." Seal Surfer emphasizes the security rather than the constraint. Ben's comfort outdoors and his ability to collect mussels with his grandfather show his belonging in this family of fishermen. Indeed the book never shows physical constraint. For instance, "Ben and his grandfather carefully climbed down to a rocky beach" (Foreman 1997, n.p.). The picture, however, doesn't show that careful climb. The boy is already lying down on a tall rock near the shoreline, his crutches lying next to him. At the very top right of the picture, on the tall, jagged cliffs, sits a wheelchair.

How did the boy get from his wheelchair down rocky cliffs on his crutches? The picture refuses to answer that question. Instead it takes the boy's presence in nature for granted. Ben wears shades of blue and green, like the sea and the grass. The light from the sea turns the wheelchair shades of purple, blue, and pink, like the rocks next to it. The text never refers to the mobility equipment shown in the pictures. In another form of naturalization, the colors of the wheelchair and crutches always match the landscape: gray like the sea wall of the harbor in the evening, pink like the sunset, transparent blue like the spring ocean. The adaptive equipment is so tiny in the vast landscape it might seem inconsequential, but young children love to scan pictures for the tiny details irrelevant to adults.

These opening pages suggest the kinship between humans and seals through physical likeness and a transfer of focal point. The second two-page spread moves down to a closer view of the seaside rocks, where Ben looks at the seal again and sees "a flash of white. A newly born seal pup nuzzled her mother" (Foreman 1997, n.p.). He lies propped up on his elbows on one flat rock, just as the baby seal lies propped on her flippers on the next. From the left corner of the picture Ben and his grandfather stare in awe at the newborn seal. Ben's body juts out diagonally, his feet facing the viewer. Nodelman (1988, 136) explains, "A character on the lower left with his back turned to us will receive the most sympathy, for his position is most like our own in relation to the picture." The glance curve moves up Ben's body to his intent, smiling face, then across his sight line to the seals in the right-hand picture. The viewer identifies first with the boy, then with the seals.

Ben's connections run many ways, from his grandfather, the seals, his human friends, and his multiple assistive devices to his love for the ocean. His prosthetic community includes his peers. The second beach summer starts with Ben on a typical Saturday at Surf School. As usual the book emphasizes Ben's abilities rather than his disability: "He was a strong swimmer, and after much practice he and the other new surfers were ready to catch some waves" (Foreman 1997, n.p.). Ben walks across the sand to the water in a line of four students. The author draws Ben's crutches in subtle, thin lines. The boy next to Ben is chatting to him while carrying Ben's board along with his own. Because the boys are talking and because there are four kids and four boards in a row, Ben's disability is inconspicuous. The other boy's help seems completely casual and natural. This casual familiarity also appears in a picture of the third spring. The grandfather is dead and gone, but a group of three friends cluster around Ben's wheelchair, looking at the sea from the high cliffs. Ben moves comfortably from the companionship of family to friendships with peers.

The prosthetic community also includes a variety of adaptive equipment available to a First World child, especially one covered by Britain's National Health Service before the recent austerity cutbacks. It is helpful that Seal Surfer shows a child with a physical disability moving among different types of equipment, since such ambidexterity confuses many people. It can even lead to accusations of fraud. The book makes it clear that different technologies work for different uses and seasons. Even the other kids' nonadaptive surfboards could be seen as prosthetics, since humans cannot surf without them. Tim Jordan (2011) has argued that the surfboard could also be seen as a companion species. He concedes that the surfboard does not have changes of expression or body language, "yet a board does react back and can be part of joy" (272).

Ben and the young seal share a physical likeness and the same sport. The book reaches its climax as the boy and the seal pup, now grown, surf a huge wave together. The wave absorbs nearly the whole picture from top to bottom, the crest curling along the top edge. Foreman captures the moment just before the wave breaks and the white water falls on the two surfers. From the steep angle it looks as if the water is going to break hard, on them and on the viewer. The boy and the seal share kinship as amphibious mammals. Both of them move adequately on land but more elegantly in the sea. Both of them fish. Their bodies and wakes are parallel as they surf down the same wave. On his board

Ben is horizontal and tripedal, like the seal. His webbed gloves are like flippers. The angle of the surfboard echoes the shape of the seal's snout, and the boy's blue and gray wetsuit echoes the seal's colors. This animal comparison does not disparage the boy, neither does his resemblance to a female animal. On the contrary the comparison establishes his fluency in the ocean environment. He belongs in the natural world.

Their shared vulnerability before the power of the ocean also creates parallels between the seal and the boy. So does their elders' assumption that they can be independent despite danger. Like the young seal who braves his first winter storms, Ben hits a big wave that pushes him into a rock. The wave smacks him off his surfboard. Just as Ben was concerned for the seal's safety, the seal is concerned for his. Ben is sinking into the depths when the young seal rescues him. "Sunlight shone through the water onto Ben's face as the seal pushed his body up. With a final heave she flipped Ben onto his board. He held on, and the next wave carried him to shore. His friends crowded around to make sure he was all right" (Foreman 1997, n.p.).

In the rescue the seal becomes a kind of feral service animal, but not an overburdened one. This pairing of traits shifts the meaning of feral, which loses its connotation of savagery, and service, which loses its connotation of obedience. In the picture the seal hoists Ben onto his board while his three human friends paddle close to the pair, concern evident on their faces. This prosthetic community means that the seal does not have to act alone to make the boy independent or valuable to his peers. Nor does the animal have to integrate the boy into human society. That integration has already happened. The seal is just doing a favor for another surfer. It is a friendship of equals.

Ben's surfing and other ocean adventures reinforce his masculinity. In seal surfing, fishing, and hunting mussels, Ben's proficiency with marine animals brings him closer to a respected elder, his grandfather. We also see him move into his grandfather's role. At the end of the book Ben assumes his late grandfather's old fishing spot below the sea wall in the harbor. More elders, the fishermen of his village, look on as Ben greets the young seal, now mature. She doesn't look like Ben anymore; now she looks like his grandfather. "Ben cheered as he saw the once young seal—now as whiskery as Granddad—with her young pup" (Foreman 1997, n.p.). On the last page of the book Ben imagines himself as a male elder: "And maybe one day he would lie on the cliff tops with his own grandchildren and together they would watch the seals." Ben's three grandkids lie on a rock like seal pups, propped up on their elbows. Ben sits next to them, his crutches leaning behind him. He will continue the male line of the family, and subsequent generations will continue their relationships with the seals. Ben's prosthetic community allows a connection to nature sustainable over the seasons and years. In a translucent Atlantic he thrives and takes risks.

Sosu's Call: Social Change and the Prosthetic Community

Sosu's Call depicts a new prosthetic community in the making, symbolizing the social changes in Ghana over the past twenty years. The picture book reflects how children with disabilities have moved out of the margins and into public life worldwide. Sosu's Call is a SuperCrip story wherein a mobility-impaired boy's relationship to an animal helps him move into a wider world. With the encouragement of his dog, Fusa, the protagonist Sosu performs a heroic rescue, gains status in his coastal village, and leaves his previous isolation behind. Asare is one of Africa's best-known children's authors and the book has won many awards, including the 1999 UNESCO first prize for Children's Literature in the Service of Tolerance. In 2002 a jury from thirteen African countries chose Sosu's Call as one of the twelve best African books of the twentieth century (Gray 2002, 10). These prizes acknowledge not only Asare's talent but also the increasing prominence of disability rights in Africa.

The Ghanaian disability activism of the 1990s forms the context for Sosu's Call. Asare's picture book appeared in 1997, in the midst of a twelve-year struggle culminating in the passage of the 2006 Ghana Persons with Disability Act (Quayson 2007, 205; Anthony 2011, 1073). The Act has enabled access to quality education, health care, employment skills, small business capital, barrier-free buildings, social life, voting, and public office.[3] In this political context Sosu's bravery consists not only in his physical feats but also in his request for inclusion. Like the real-life Ghanaian disability activists of his day, Sosu makes the news. When the TV and radio journalists come to his house and ask him what he would like most, he says he wants to go to school.

At the end of the story Sosu heads to the local school in his new wheelchair, an emblem of the changes at work in Ghana. "Prior to the 1990s, very few students with disabilities in Ghana were included in regular education classrooms"; Ghana's Education for All policy has now opened the school doors (Alhassan 2009, 116). According to Christie Yaghr, a Ghanaian Deaf and disability community leader, "The new educational measures in Ghana have indeed improved the lives of children with disabilities. This is because these measures have opened the chance for children with disabilities to go to school. It is unlike the past where nobody paid attention or gave recognition to the importance of their education."[4]

Unlike Ben in Seal Surfer, however, Sosu's education and equipment cannot be taken for granted. It is still unusual for children with physical disabilities in rural Ghana to attend their local schools. In a postcolonial nation like Ghana, rural schools lack accessible buildings and special education teachers. The cost of wheelchairs is prohibitively high. According to Yaghr, parents "cannot purchase wheel-chairs for them to commute to and from school," and "government funding for wheel-chairs for persons with disabilities is either not enough, absent, or [for] a selected few who are rather well to do." The happy ending of <u>Sosu's Call</u> represents a best-case scenario rare in the real world.

The desire to be useful motivates Sosu's heroism. This goal respects Ghanaian tradition and overturns Ghanaian prejudices. <u>Sosu's Call</u> refutes two of the attitudes that frustrated and delayed passage of Ghana's Persons with Disability Act. The Ghanaian disability studies scholar Ato Quayson (2007) details these ableist attitudes. The first is the idea that people with disabilities have received a divine curse and can alter others' luck. The second is the idea that people with disabilities have no useful labor to offer and can survive only as disparaged beggars. On the streets of Accra live people with motor impairments much like Sosu's: "The vast bulk of beggars on intersections and street corners are persons with various kinds of disability, thus making the link between the two almost natural in the minds of the nondisabled. Indeed, a local Akan saying, 'e ti se bafa ne fom' (it is like the cripple and the ground), which is used to convey the inseparability between the two entities, derives from the observation that persons with severe motor impairments are often seen dragging themselves on the ground, begging for alms at street corners and elsewhere" (206). <u>Sosu's Call</u> evokes these stereotypes in the process of overturning them. Although Sosu's family supports him, several illustrations show him sitting like a beggar, alone and idle on the ground outside the family house (Asare 1997, 6, 10, 16). Sitting in his yard, Sosu asks himself, "What good is a boy without a pair of good, strong legs?" (7). The repetition of this image conveys the dullness of his existence. Sosu appears in the left-hand observer position with which the viewer identifies, wearing a bright orange shirt that makes him stand out as the protagonist. Thus the viewer identifies with Sosu's idleness and exclusion and sees them as problems rather than the inevitable results of his disability.

By contrast a flashback shows Sosu in an active and capable role with his father in their fishing canoe. Father and son stroke their oars in parallel lines, embodying the smooth passing of the fishing livelihood from father to son. They are out in the peaceful lagoon, the space of men's work and the "kind mother" to the village that supplies many delicacies (Asare 1997, 3). However, two older men in another canoe pull up beside the father and son, saying, "We don't think it is wise to bring that boy of yours out here. It is unlucky enough to have the likes of him in the village. We doubt if the Lagoon Spirit is pleased to have him sitting here as well! We think you must keep him in your compound" (9). Thus the reader learns that Sosu wasn't always idle and excluded. One stigma has led to another in a vicious circle. A disabled person is excluded from useful labor because he is considered bad luck. Then he is stigmatized because he is idle.

Usefulness is a central virtue for Ghanaian children. "No child is useless" is a slogan of Education for All (EDIN and the National Bureau for Students with Disabilities, 2009) An eldest son, Sosu would normally take a central role in caring for his family as he grows into manhood. As a Ghanaian special educator explains, it is a huge loss if a child cannot grow up to take care of his parents: "I think the role of the child right from the beginning is to grow up and to look after the adult. . . . We have a saying in Ashanti, literally it means 'I have cared for you for all your teeth to grow so now you care for me for all my teeth to drop out.' . . . So if you have a child who is not going to be successful or they are not going to be able to do that then that is a really big loss, that is a massive loss" (Anthony 2011, 1078). Sosu finds a way to fulfill his social role, taking care of the old and the very young and thus proving his usefulness.

Like the other books in this canon, Sosu's Call depicts an animal and a child with a disability whose bodily movements resemble each other. Side by side they solve a problem, and that solution leads to a new vision of inclusive community. However, the containment of the human-animal comparison is stronger here than in Seal Surfer. The stronger containment is necessary because of the greater stigma attached to resembling a dog rather than a seal, but also because of the different social context. In a poor nation where wheelchairs are rare and most people with physical disabilities beg and drag themselves across the ground, dignity is more fragile. Therefore it is more important to contain the animal resemblance. The postcolonial racist legacy of comparing Africans to animals also casts its shadow on the comparison of a Ghanaian boy to his dog. For example, Vivian Yenika-Agbaw (2008, 114–16) criticizes the charity Heifer International for trumpeting in its publicity, "A goat saved an African child," and describes the outrage across Africa when an African village was exhibited at a German zoo in 2005.

Nonetheless Sosu's Call depicts an African boy who saves his village and establishes his human worth by moving like a dog and following a dog's lead. Breaking the barriers between human and nonhuman animals also breaks down barriers for human beings with disabilities. Initially, however, movement is a ground for difference between Sosu and the dog Fusa: the dog is allowed to leave the family home, but Sosu is not. Like many Africans, Sosu's family lives in a house surrounded by a wall, and the yard within the wall hosts domestic activities. On the third double-page spread of the book, Sosu sits on the ground right outside his house. He is looking up at the narrow patch of world he can see above the wall when Fusa comes bounding into the yard. Fusa has accompanied Sosu's brother and sister to school: "The dog was always back puffing and its eyes shining with the satisfaction of having been outside! It was this more than anything else, that made him envious" (Asare 1997, 7). The dog has the free range of the village denied to Sosu.

On the day "all of that changed," however, Sosu's body language starts to resemble the dog's, and this resemblance continues throughout their rescue of the villagers. Their shared movements indicate when they become a team. Sosu has nearly always appeared in the lower left corner, where viewers identify with him. Now Fusa joins him, and viewers can identify with the pair. Both dog and boy stretch their neck up and out, looking at the coconut palms "as their tops bent and swayed desperately in the wind" of a sudden, violent storm (Asare 1997, 17). In the next double-page spread both dog and boy pull back in alarm as "the old wooden gate shot across the yard like a massive kite!" (19).

Sosu and Fusa figure out together how to respond to the storm. Fusa's help is not physical; rather theirs is a thinking partnership. The book next shows the two figures against a plain white background, emphasizing the internal nature of their brainstorming. "Something had to be done. And fast. But what could he do? The only other people in the village at this time were those who were too old and frail to do anything. There were many like that in the village. Often, they were left with very young children. They could all be trapped and drowned if the sea continued to rise" (Asare 1997, 21). Fusa's listening seems to pull a good idea out of Sosu's mind, as often happens in creative partnerships. While Fusa looks at him with "a knowing and reassuring look in its eyes," Sosu hits on the idea of crawling to the drum shed and drumming. His drumming will notify the working adults to return to the village and rescue those trapped by rising floodwaters (21).

Fusa becomes a human's working partner like dogs throughout the centuries, including service dogs. Stephen Kuusisto (1998, 177). says of his guide dog, Corky, "although we move as one, we are more than that. Guide dogs and their human partners must each trust the other's bravery and judgment." Fusa supports and shares Sosu's bravery and judgment: "The look in Fusa's eyes did not only say that it knew where to find the drums. It also said, 'Don't be afraid! We will be all right!'" (Asare 1997, 22).

Sosu becomes a hero by moving on all fours like a dog. In the book's climactic picture he and Fusa head for the drum shed on all fours, "leaning into the howling wind and sloshing through churning water" (Asare 1997, 23). The boy and the dog resemble each other in their poses and earthy colors. The viewer too is down at ground level. Sosu lifts one hand in the air while Fusa raises the corresponding paw. The dog looks back at the boy reassuringly and wags his tail, their communication in synch despite the stress of the storm and the need for swift action.

Sosu acquires the dog's freedom to roam, and his entrance into wild nature signals his new freedom in human society as well. When he crawls out of the family compound to the drum shed, he infiltrates the forbidden world of work. Alerting the adults about the flood, Sosu saves the lives of the village's children and grandparents. By rescuing those "too old and frail to do anything" he demonstrates that he himself is neither frail nor incapable.

In this village joining the human community means joining the outdoor world. To be fishing in the sea or lagoon is to be a man. When the men in the canoe say that Sosu displeases the Lagoon Spirit and must stay at home, they exclude him from the nature at the center of their working world and spiritual worldview. However, when the churning tide of water spills into his yard, the sea comes to him. Crawling through that tide Sosu joins the useful world of men in water. However, he doesn't do the same job as the men who come running home to carry the grandparents and babies out of the flood. In the crisis he invents a new job that a young man with a disability can do, and thus widens the definition of useful labor.

Floods often enter this village on its narrow strip of land between the sea and the lagoon. The villagers accept the inevitability of flooding in their ecosystem. Their vulnerability is part of the social contract. Sosu comes into this shared vulnerability instead of being seen as helpless in a way separate and different from the rest of his society. His rescue forms part of the natural cycle of humans responding to their wetland home. He embodies nature in his drumming. At first he is uncertain because he has never played a drum before. Then he becomes the voice of nature, bringing the villagers running to him because he enacts the story of the storm with his hands:

> But suddenly, the storm, the pounding waves of water, the young children, the sick, the old, the animals, the crashing fences and snapping trees, all came rushing to him like moving pictures!
> So he struck the drum harder and faster until he heard it above the shrieks and howls of the wind:
> Belem-belen-belem! Bembem-bembem-bembem! (Asare 1997, 27)

At his moment of human acceptance, Sosu's body language stops resembling the dog's and he comes up off the ground. Through his partnership with Fusa other humans learn that Sosu is capable in the same way his dog already knows he is. The men realize that Sosu has drummed the call that brought them home in time to save the village. "He was soon riding on strong shoulders, with Fusa leaping into the air to reach him!" (33). In the last two spreads Sosu talks to the press and receives his wheelchair while his family and neighbors cluster behind him. He is seated up high with the dog on his lap or next to his chair. Fusa seems to have become his pet rather than his partner. Thus the animal-human comparison is paradoxical in Sosu's Call. Moving like an animal has enabled Sosu to become a useful and respected member of his village, yet the resemblance must be left behind for other humans to accord him full dignity. The book has to break the association between him and the ground in order to cut the ties between disability, begging, and uselessness.

Sosu's Call is not just a SuperCrip story about individual accomplishment. It also tells the story of a village that can change its mind. The book refutes the stereotype of African villages as immune to change. Yenika-Agbaw (2008, 34) writes, "The representations of West Africa in children's books seem to make Africans' efforts to modernize invisible to all who are not there." She asks, "Should African children accept every single tradition that has been handed down to them by their elders?" (50) Sosu's village is not the stereotypical one where children follow every tradition, even the most destructive ones. Instead tradition and modernity come together, represented by the village chief, who presents the gleaming new wheelchair. The last pages of Sosu's Call shows the chief in his traditional robe, bracelets, and headwear, shaking Sosu's hand as the boy sits in his new chair. The chief joins Sosu on the left page, where he has so often been alone, and a half-circle of villagers stand behind him.

A collective exclusion becomes a collective inclusion. Celebrating their survival at a village festival, everyone finally wears the same bright colors as Sosu, and the same bright umbrellas cover them all. Sosu has joined the human community—or rather they have joined him. It is fitting that the chief presents the wheelchair, since chiefs had been "unwitting guardians of prejudice toward disabled persons" (Quayson 2007, 207). The last page shows elements of Sosu's new prosthetic community: his family, neighbors, and leaders; his wheelchair; and his dog. Infrastructure changes have also taken place. The text tells us that a smooth new wheelchair-accessible path now leads from Sosu's house to the school. We might also consider the journalists' microphone and camera as part of Sosu's prosthetic community, since the news coverage has enabled all the other changes.[5] In Sosu's struggle, as in others, media coverage contributes to human rights.

Through his bodily movements Sosu forms a creative partnership with an animal, embodies the power of nature, and infiltrates the human community—even though his bodily movements were the original basis of his exclusion. The animal and human worlds resemble each other. Nonetheless the story must disavow this resemblance for Sosu to take his place in the human community. The disability-positive message at the happy ending of Sosu's Call contains the leakage. Yet the animal-human comparison floods into the middle of the text and creates the fertile ground for that happy ending.

Freedom of Movement

Sosu and Ben find their freedom with nonhuman animals in wild nature. It's just too bad they have to work so hard for it, and that the animals do too. Their adventures demonstrate their skill and bravery. The problem is the need to prove their worth, to readers and other characters. Sosu and Ben, the dog Fusa and the young seal, have to perform SuperCrip athletic feats and heroic rescues to demonstrate their personhood. Appreciation for animals, both wild and domestic, often comes in stories of gratitude for their service to humans. It isn't enough for animals to exist for themselves. Similarly kids with disabilities face the task of meeting the benchmarks adult humans set. In Ben's village in Britain the benchmark is self-fulfillment; in Sosu's village in Africa the benchmark is service to the community.

As boys with disabilities, Sosu and Ben also bear the burden of demonstrating their masculinity. Both boys come from fishing villages where physical courage and outdoor adventures are prerequisites for joining in male elders' pursuits. However, the animals enable two different kinds of masculinity, one quite old and the other quite new. In the older kind, traditional masculinity steps in to erase and replace disability as the standard of personhood. If you can prove you are traditionally masculine, your disability no longer threatens your status as a person. The newer kind of masculinity, however, is a masculinity-with-disability that widens the gender roles to make more room for vulnerability, partnership, and adaptability at work and play.

In their moments of freedom, however, child and animal have nothing to prove to each other. They have learned to trust each other's judgments through partnerships in play and problem solving. That trust is more important than the world's judgments. Children with disabilities and animals belong together in the natural world. Surfing and responding to floods, both boys dive deeply into their watery ecosystem. The vulnerability of disability is no different from our shared vulnerability before the power of water. Animals and humans work together to save lives, and this cooperation could extend to saving the ocean itself.

For Ben and Sosu getting out into nature requires a robust human world. Wheelchairs, individual feats, and service animals can't do the trick on their own. It takes a prosthetic village to raise a child with a disability. Seal Surfer sports a prosthetic community so rich it can afford to take nature access for granted. <u>Sosu's Call</u> displays the kind of social change necessary for kids with disabilities to come outside into the world. In a diverse prosthetic community people with disabilities don't have to lean so hard on service animals that they become beasts of burden.

The greater the climate of social acceptance, the more children with disabilities can claim their resemblances to animals. In <u>Sosu's Call</u> and <u>Seal Surfer</u> bodily movement forms the basis of the human-animal comparison. The dog and seal have tremendous freedom of movement, and this range of motion transfers metaphorically to the boys. Their resemblance to animals does not signify lower status but the freedom to roam. Many animals and children with disabilities lack this freedom. If we opened the cages, we would see the capabilities for joy, problem solving, partnership, and adventure we find in these picture books.

NOTES

1. A complete list of these picture books appears after the bibliography.
2. For the concept of the prosthetic community I draw from Leigha McReynolds (2013), who expands the definition of a prosthetic beyond an inanimate object to a network of relationships between beings. McReynolds defines a "prosthetic relationship" as "the joining of two living bodies in order for one or both of the bodies to perform a specific task, where both bodies share agency in the performance" (116).
3. Christie Yaghr, email, November 30, 2014.
4. Christie Yaghr, email, November 30, 2014.
5. I owe this insight to my colleague Mary Elene Wood.

BIBLIOGRAPHY

Alhassan, Awal Mohammed. 2009. "Teachers' Implementation of Inclusive Education in Ghanaian Primary Schools: An Insight into Government Policy and Practices." <u>Advances in Social Science Research Journal</u> 1, no. 2: 115–29.

Anthony, Jane. 2011. "Conceptualising Disability in Ghana: Implications for EFA and Inclusive Education." International Journal of Inclusive Education 15, no. 10: 1073–86.

Asare, Meshack. 1997. Sosu's Call. Accra: Sub-Saharan Publishers.

Blackford, Holly. 2013. "Raw Shok and Modern Method: Child Consciousness in Flowers for Algernon and The Curious Incident of the Dog in the Night-Time." Children's Literature Association Quarterly 38, no. 3: 284–303.

Brittain, Isabel. 2004. "An Examination into the Portrayal of Deaf Characters and Deaf Issues in Picture Books for Children." Disability Studies Quarterly 24, no. 1. http://dsq-sds.org/article/view/841/1016.

Carey, Joanna. 2011. "Michael Foreman: Life through a Line." Guardian, March 4.

Chen, Mel Y. 2012. Animacies: Biopolitics, Racial Mattering, and Queer Affect. Durham NC: Duke University Press.

Derrida, Jacques. 2008. The Animal That Therefore I Am. Edited by Marie-Louise Mallet. Translated by David Wills. New York: Fordham University Press.

EDIN and the National Bureau for Students with Disabilities. 2009. In Their Own Words: The Real Story of Disability in Ghana. VSO Media.

Foreman, Michael. 1997. Seal Surfer. San Diego: Harcourt Brace.

Friedrich, Bruce. 2014. "The Cruelest of All Factory Farm Products: Eggs from Caged Hens." Huffingtonpost.com, March 16.

Gray, Eve. 2002. "An African Century." Bookseller, August 23. http://www.thebookseller.com/feature/african-century.

Hadjimatheou, Chloë. 2014. "The Disabled Children Locked Up in Cages." BBC News Magazine, November 13. http://www.bbc.com/news/magazine-30038753.

Haraway, Donna. 2003. The Companion Species Manifesto: Dogs, People, and Significant Otherness. Chicago: Prickly Paradigm Press.

Hediger, Ryan. 2009. "Crossing Over: (Dis)ability, Contingent Agency, and Death in the Marginal Genre Work of Temple Grandin and Jim Harrison." In Animals and Agency: An Interdisciplinary Exploration, edited by Sarah E. McFarland and Ryan Hediger, 321–39. Leiden: Brill.

Jordan, Tim. 2011. "Troubling Companions: Companion Species and the Politics of Inter-relations." NORA: Nordic Journal of Feminist and Gender Research 19, no. 4: 264–79.

Kuusisto, Stephen. 1998. Planet of the Blind. New York: Delta.

McReynolds, Leigha. 2013. "Animal and Alien Bodies as Prostheses: Reframing Disability in Avatar and How to Train Your Dragon." In Disability in Science Fiction: Representations of Technology as Cure, edited by Kathryn Allan, 115–27. New York: Palgrave Macmillan.

Melson, Gail F. 2003. "Child Development and the Human-Companion Animal Bond." American Behavioral Scientist 47: 31–39.

"Michael Foreman." 2014. Walker: Picture Book Party. http://www.walker.co.uk/contributors/Michael-Foreman-2741.aspx.

Nodelman, Perry. 1988. Words about Pictures: The Narrative Art of Children's Picture Books. Athens: University of Georgia Press.

Osofsky, Audrey. 1992. My Buddy. Illustrated by Ted Rand. New York: Square Fish, Henry Holt.

Quayson, Ato. 2007. Aesthetic Nervousness: Disability and the Crisis of Representation. New York: Columbia University Press.

Singer, Peter. 1993. Practical Ethics. 2d ed. Cambridge, UK: Cambridge University Press.

Spitz, Ellen Handler. 1999. Inside Picture Books. New Haven CT: Yale University Press.

Szambelan, J. P. 2009. "Dear Dad: A Story about a Girl with Autism and Her Dog." YouTube, April 26. https://www.youtube.com/watch?v=s5XvxOOsUZE.

Taylor, Sunaura. 2011. "Beasts of Burden: Disability Studies and Animal Rights." Qui Parle: Critical Humanities and Social Sciences 19, no. 2: 191–222. http://www.jstor.org/stable/10.5250/quiparle.19.2.0191?seq=1#page_scan_tab_contents.

Wolfe, Cary. 2003. Animal Rites: American Culture, the Discourse of Species, and Posthumanist Theory. Chicago: University of Chicago Press.

Yenika-Agbaw, Vivian. 2008. Representing Africa in Children's Literature: Old and New Ways of Seeing. London: Routledge.

PICTURE BOOKS

Asare, Meshack. 1997. Sosu's Call. Accra: Sub-Saharan Publishers.

Davis, Patricia A. 2000. Brian's Bird. Illustrated by Layne Johnson. Morton Grove IL: Albert Whitman.

Foreman, Michael. 1997. Seal Surfer. San Diego: Harcourt Brace.

Harter, Debbie, illustrator. 2000. The Animal Boogie. Vocals on accompanying CD by Fred Penner. Oxford: Barefoot Books.

Kluth, Paula, and Patrick Schwarz. 2010. Pedro's Whale. Illustrated by Justin Canha. Baltimore: Paul H. Brookes.

Herrera, Juan Felipe. 2004. Featherless/Desplumado. Illustrated by Ernesto Cuevas Jr. San Francisco: Children's Book Press, Editorial Libros para Niños.

Hudson, Charlotte. 2006. Dan and Diesel. London: Red Fox.

Lears, Laurie. 1999. Waiting for Mr. Goose. Illustrated by Karen Ritz. Morton Grove IL: Albert Whitman.

Martin, Bill, Jr., and John Archambault. 1987. Knots on a Counting Rope. Illustrated by Ted Rand. New York: Henry Holt.

Osofsky, Audrey. 1992. My Buddy. Illustrated by Ted Rand. New York: Square Fish, Henry Holt.

Senisi, Ellen B. 2002. All Kinds of Friends, Even Green! Bethesda MD: Woodbine House.

Stockham, Jess. 2008. Having Fun! Just Like Us! Swindon, UK: Child's Play.

Stryer, Andrea Stenn. 2007. Kami and the Yaks. Illustrated by Bert Dodson. Palo Alto CA: Bay Otter Press.

Source Acknowledgments

"Risking Bodies in the Wild: The 'Corporeal Unconscious' of American Adventure Culture," by Sarah Jaquette Ray, originally appeared in Journal of Sport and Social Issues 33, no. 3 (2009): 257–84.

"Bringing Together Feminist Disability Studies and Environmental Justice," by Valerie Ann Johnson, in Barbara Faye Waxman Fiduccia Papers on Women and Girls with Disabilities, Center for Women Policy Studies, 2011. http://www.ungift.org/doc/knowledgehub /resource-centre/BFWFP_Bringing_Together_Feminist_Disability _Studies_and_Environmental_Justice_Valerie_Ann_Johnson.pdf.

"Lead's Racial Matters," by Mel Y. Chen, originally appeared in Animacies: Biopolitics, Racial Mattering, and Queer Affect (Durham NC: Duke University Press, 2012) and is reprinted by permission of the copyright holder, Duke University Press. All rights reserved.

"Defining Eco-Ability: Social Justice and the Intersectionality of Disability, Nonhuman Animals, and Ecology," by Anthony J. Nocella II, originally appeared in Earth, Animal, and Disability Liberation: The Rise of the Eco-Ability Movement, edited by Anthony J. Nocella II, Judy K. C. Bentley, and Janet M. Duncan (New York: Peter Lang, 2012).

"The Ecosomatic Paradigm in Literature: Merging Disability Studies and Ecocriticism," by Matthew J. C. Cella, originally appeared as "Editor's Choice: The Ecosomatic Paradigm in Literature: Merging Disability Studies and Ecocriticism" in ISLE 20, no. 3 (2013): 574–96.

"Bodies of Nature: The Environmental Politics of Disability," by Alison Kafer, originally appeared in Feminist, Queer, Crip (Bloomington: Indiana University Press, 2013) and is reprinted with permission of Indiana University Press.

"Meditations on Natural Worlds, Disabled Bodies, and a Politics of Cure," by Eli Clare, originally appeared in Material Ecocriticism, edited by Serenella Iovino and Serpil Oppermann (Bloomington: Indiana University Press, 2014) and is reprinted with permission of Indiana University Press.

Contributors

Stacy Alaimo is a professor of English and Distinguished Teaching Professor at the University of Texas at Arlington. Her essays appear in Queer Ecologies, Prismatic Ecologies, Material Ecocriticism, Thinking with Water, and the PMLA. Her books include Undomesticated Ground: Recasting Nature as Feminist Space (Cornell University Press, 2000), Bodily Natures: Science, Environment, and the Material Self (Indiana University Press, 2010), and Exposed: Environmental Politics and Pleasures in Posthuman Times (University of Minnesota Press, 2016). She coedited Material Feminisms (Indiana University Press, 2008) and edited Matter, a volume for the Gender series of Macmillan Interdisciplinary Handbooks (2016). She is currently completing the book Composing Blue Ecologies: Science, Aesthetics, and the Creatures of the Abyss.

Matthew J. C. Cella is an associate professor of English at Shippensburg University of Pennsylvania, where he also teaches courses in the Disability Studies Program. He is the author of Bad Land Pastoralism in Great Plains Fiction (University of Iowa Press, 2010) and the editor of Disability and the Environment in American Literature: Toward an Ecosomatic Paradigm (Lexington, 2016). His research has been published in a range of journals, including ISLE, Journal of Rural Studies, Great Plains Quarterly, and Western American Literature.

Mel Y. Chen is an associate professor of gender and women's studies and the director of the Center for the Study of Sexual Culture at UC Berkeley. Animacies: Biopolitics, Racial Mattering, and Queer Affect (Duke University Press, 2012), which won the Alan Bray Memorial Award, explores questions of racialization, sexuality, disability, and affective economies in animate and inanimate life. Other writings appear in Women's Studies Quarterly, Discourse, Amerasia, Medical Humanities, GLQ, and Journal of Literary and Cultural Disability Studies. Chen coedited the special issue of GLQ titled "Queer Inhumanisms" (with Dana Luciano) and currently coedits a Duke University Press book series entitled Anima (with Jasbir K. Puar).

White, disabled, and genderqueer, **Eli Clare** happily lives in the Green Mountains of Vermont, where he writes and proudly claims a penchant for rabble-rousing. He has written two books of essays, Brilliant Imperfection: Grappling with Cure (Duke University Press, 2017), from which in an earlier version "Notes on Natural Worlds, Disabled Bodies, and a Politics of Cure" is drawn, and Exile and Pride: Disability, Queerness, and Liberation (South End Press, 1999), and a collection of poetry, The Marrow's Telling: Words in Motion (Homofactus Press, 2007), and has been published in many periodicals and anthologies. He speaks, teaches, and facilitates all over the United States and Canada at conferences, community events, and colleges about disability, queer and trans identities, and social justice. Among other pursuits he has walked across the United States for peace, coordinated a rape prevention program, and helped organize the first Queerness and Disability Conference.

Robert Melchior Figueroa is an associate professor of philosophy at Oregon State University. He pursues a philosophy of environmental justice that extends across numerous domains: Latinx issues, climate refugees, indigenous environmental heritage, critical tourism studies, resettlement communities, environmental colonialism, environmental discrimination, and discriminatory environmentalism across a multitude of cases around the world. Since 2003 Rob has been thinking through critical autism studies and environmental justice as he works with his autistic son, Soren. Despite many efforts and advocacy work, it was Rob's two-year-old daughter, Nyomi, who taught him to rethink his efforts to be in the autistic world. His chapter debuts writing from this world. He coedited Science and Other Cultures: Issues in the Philosophies of Science and Technology (with Sandra Harding; Routledge, 2003). He is currently completing two books on the philosophy of environmental justice.

Kelly Fritsch is a disabled feminist and a Banting Postdoctoral Fellow in Women and Gender Studies at the University of Toronto. Her postdoctoral research develops crip and feminist technoscience by tracing the political and affective economies of war, imperialism, and disability to examine body enhancement and capacitation technologies such as prosthetics and personal assistive and adaptive devices. Fritsch holds a doctorate in social and political thought from York University and is a coeditor of Keywords for Radicals: The Contested Vocabulary of Late Capitalist Struggle (AK Press, 2016).

Sarah Gibbons is a PhD candidate in the Department of English at the University of Waterloo. Her research at the intersection of disability studies and the environmental humanities considers how the knowledge translation of scientific research in a variety of media genres impacts public understandings of autism. She is an assistant editor and social media coordinator for the Canadian Journal of Disability Studies.

Kim Q. Hall is a professor of philosophy and the director of gender, women's, and sexuality studies at Appalachian State University. She is the guest editor of "New Conversations in Feminist Disability Studies," a special issue of Hypatia: Journal of Feminist Philosophy, and the editor of Feminist Disability Studies (Indiana University Press, 2011). Published articles include "Toward a Queer Crip Feminist Politics of Food" in philoSOPHIA: A Journal of Continental Feminism and "No Failure: Climate Change, Radical Hope, and Queer Crip Feminist Eco Futures" in Radical Philosophy Review.

Valerie Ann Johnson is the Mott Distinguished Professor of Women's Studies and director of Africana Women's Studies at Bennett College. Her research, conducted in Costa Rica, Zimbabwe, Tanzania, the Seychelles Islands, and the United States, centers on gender, bioethics, disability, the health of women and girls, and environmental justice. In North Carolina she researches African American foodways. At present she is working with Karima Jeffrey (Hampton University) on an edited volume of science and speculative fiction by and about black women and girls. Johnson chairs the North Carolina African American Heritage Commission, serves on the state's Historical Commission and the Ms. Committee of Scholars, and is on the board for Scarritt Bennett Center in Nashville, Tennessee—a nonprofit education, conference and retreat center. Activist work includes serving on the Board for the North Carolina League of Conservation Voters and membership in the North Carolina Environmental Justice Network. Johnson also serves on the Steering Committee for the Anna Julia Cooper Center at Wake Forest University.

Alison Kafer is a professor of feminist studies at Southwestern University, where she also teaches in the race and ethnicity studies and environmental studies programs. She is the author of Feminist Queer Crip (Indiana University Press, 2013).

Jina B. Kim is a Consortium for Faculty Diversity postdoctoral fellow in the Program in Critical Social Thought at Mount Holyoke College. She received her PhD in the departments of English and women's studies at the University of Michigan, Ann Arbor. Her research interests are in the areas of contemporary multiethnic U.S. literatures, feminist disability theory, women-of-color feminisms, and urban environmental justice. In 2012 she received the Irving K. Zola Award for Emerging Scholars in Disability Studies.

Anita Mannur is an associate professor of English at Miami University. She is the author of Culinary Fictions: Food in South Asian Diasporic Culture (Temple University Press, 2009) and has published widely on food and culture. She is starting a new project on toxic narratives in the Global South.

Mary E. Mendoza is an assistant professor of history in the Department of History and the Program in Critical Race and Ethnic Studies at the University of Vermont. An environmental and borderlands historian, she is currently working on her first book, which explores the intersections between the natural and the built environments along the U.S.-Mexico border from a transnational perspective. She also thinks and writes more broadly about race, justice, and intersectionality in the field of environmental history.

David T. Mitchell and **Sharon L. Snyder** are the authors of Narrative Prosthesis: Disability and the Dependencies of Discourse (University of Michigan Press, 2000) and Cultural Locations of Disability (University of Chicago Press, 2006). They are also the creators of four award-winning films about disability arts, history, and culture: Vital Signs: Crip Culture Talks Back (1995), A World without

Bodies (2002), Self Preservation: The Art of Riva Lehrer (2005), and Disability Takes on the Arts (2006). Together they coedit the Corporealities book series for the University of Michigan Press, founded the Committee on Disability Issues in the Profession at the Modern Languages Association, and curated "The Chicago Disability History Exhibit" for the 2006 Bodies of Work: Disability Arts and Culture Festival. Their newest book, The Biopolitics of Disability: Neoliberalism, Ablenationalism, and Peripheral Embodiment (University of Michigan Press, 2015), is a meditation on alternative ethical maps for living evolved within crip and queer experiences. They have a new short film on disability memorialization of the victims of the T4 program in Germany, Disabled People and the Holocaust (2015). They both teach at George Washington University.

Anthony J. Nocella II is a community organizer and assistant professor of sociology and criminology, peace and conflict studies, women and gender studies, and environmental studies at Fort Lewis College. He is the executive director of the Institute for Critical Animal Studies, the national co-coordinator of Save the Kids, and a cofounder and editor of the Peace Studies Journal. Nocella has published over twenty-six books and fifty book chapters and essays and is the editor of the Radical Animal Studies and Total Liberation book series with Peter Lang Publishing.

Sarah Jaquette Ray is an associate professor of environmental studies at Humboldt State University, where she also leads the Environmental Studies Program. She is author of The Ecological Other: Environmental Exclusion in American Culture (University of Arizona Press, 2013) and coeditor of Critical Norths: Space, Nature, Theory (University of Alaska Press, 2017). She is working on a book project, "Climate Justice Pedagogies: Affect, Action, and the Anthropocene," and a coedited project, "Latinx Environmentalisms: Cultural Histories and Literary Traditions."

Julie Sadler is a white disabled editor and writer living in Toronto. Born with a cardiac birth anomaly, she writes from her experience with the medical system. She is an independent scholar researching issues of trauma, disablement, and structural violence.

Cathy J. Schlund-Vials is an associate professor of English and Asian/Asian American studies at the University of Connecticut, where she is the director of the Asian and Asian American Studies Institute. She is the author of Modeling Citizenship: Jewish and Asian American Writing (Temple University Press, 2011) and War, Genocide, and Justice: Cambodian American Memory Work (University of Minnesota Press, 2012). Her work has appeared in a number of collections and journals, including Modern Language Studies, Amerasia, Life Writing, American Literary History, and positions. She has coedited a number of collections, including Disability, Human Rights, and the Limits of Humanitarianism (Ashgate, 2014), Keywords for Asian American Studies (2015), "Recollecting the Vietnam War" (special issue of Asian American Literary Review, 2015), "Interrogating the Perpetrator" (special issue of the Journal of International Human Rights, 2015), and Asian America: A Primary Source Reader (Yale University Press, 2017). She is president of the Association for Asian American Studies.

Siobhan Senier is an associate professor of English and the James H. and Claire Short Hayes Chair in the Humanities at the University of New Hampshire, where she teaches courses in Native American literature, women's studies, and sustainability studies. She is the editor of Dawnland Voices: An Anthology of Writing from

Indigenous New England (University of Nebraska Press, 2014) and dawnlandvoices.org. Her other publications include Voices of American Indian Assimilation and Resistance (University of Oklahoma Press, 2001) and essays in American Literature, American Indian Quarterly, Studies in American Indian Literatures, MELUS, Disability Studies Quarterly, and Resilience: A Journal of the Environmental Humanities.

Jay Sibara is an assistant professor of English at Colby College. He is currently revising a book manuscript, "Imperial Injuries: Race, Disability, and Environment in Narratives of Resistance to U.S. Empire." His work has appeared in MELUS (2014). Before joining the faculty at Colby, Sibara worked at Harvard Law School's Center for Health Law and Policy Innovation on projects to improve access to care for low-income people living with HIV/AIDS. He received his doctorate in English with a certificate in gender studies from the University of Southern California. A member of the Access Initiative of the Association for the Study of Literature and Environment, Sibara collaborated on the development of the organization's disability access and accommodations policy.

Natasha L. Simpson is a graduate student in the Community Development Graduate Group at the University of California, Davis. Simpson's most recent position was as the Disability and Food Justice Fellow at Phat Beets Produce in Oakland California, where she created a political education curriculum at these intersections for the community as well as for members of the organization; Simpson is additionally a member of a Sins Invalid's leadership development program for queer, gender-nonconforming, and/or people of color with disabilities. She received her BA in Women and Gender Studies at San Francisco State University.

Víctor M. Torres-Vélez is a visiting assistant professor of anthropology at Western Oregon University. He is a critical medical anthropologist by training, specializing in the intersections between environmental justice movements, disease, and biomedicine. His interdisciplinary theoretical expertise and interests include political ecology, development theories, theories of social change, transnationalism, science and technology studies, and contemporary and classical theory. His regional focus is Latin America and the Caribbean. He has published essays in Souls: A Critical Journal of Black Politics, Culture, and Society and Centro Journal and is currently working on a book entitled "Tainting the Land, Wounding the Body: Health, Environment and Antimilitarism in Vieques, Puerto Rico."

Traci Brynne Voyles is an assistant professor of women's studies at Loyola Marymount University. She is the author of Wastelanding: Legacies of Uranium Mining in Navajo Country (University of Minnesota Press, 2015), which was selected by the Border Regional Libraries Association for the Southwest Book Award. Her research interests revolve around environmental justice, environmental history, feminist theory and gender studies, ecofeminism, and comparative ethnic studies. Her current book project explores the environmental and cultural history of southern California's Salton Sea.

Elizabeth A. Wheeler is an associate professor of English and environmental studies and the lead developer of the Disability Studies Minor at the University of Oregon. Her book, HandiLand: The Crippest Place on Earth, will be published in the Corporealities: Discourses of Disability series at the University of Michigan Press. Handiland looks at contemporary young adult and children's literature to trace the emergence of young people with disabilities into nature, school, work, and other public spaces. Her scholarship has appeared in ISLE: Interdisciplinary Studies in Literature and the Environment, Children's Literature Quarterly, and the anthology Afrofuturism in Time and Space. Her depression, migraine, and chronic pain also appear with some frequency.

Index

Underlined page numbers indicate illustrations.

death world, 351
"defects," 244
de Haro, Mercedes García, 488–89
de Haro Camacho, Jesús, 488–89
Deleuze, Gilles, 59
delusion, 153–54
Department of Agriculture, U.S. See USDA (U.S. Department of Agriculture)
Department of Defense Appropriation Act, U.S., 306
Department of Labor, U.S., 475, 478, 483, 489
Department of Natural Resources, U.S., 242
Derrida, Jacques, 597
Desai, Jigna, 395
Desert Solitaire (Abbey), 50–51, 205–6, 210, 211–12, 235n10
deviance, xiii, 67n16, 144, 149–50, 155, 535
diabetes, 250, 272, 286n22, 547n2
diagnosis, xiv–xv; of autism, xi, 532, 536, 539, 562; of literary characters, 560–61, 564
Díaz, Bernabé Alvarez, 491
Dickens, Charles, 125, 135–36n57
diet, 414
dietary deficiencies of migrant laborers, 486–87
Dietrich, Kim, 123–24
differences, 143–45
disability: activism, 86, 87, 141, 160–61, 174, 249, 609; animal rights and, x, 238–39n45,

597, 598, 599–600; brilliant imperfection of, 250, 264n1; Brundtland Commission on, 422–23; as a burden, 333, 334n2; construction of, 48, 55–56, 67n16, 67n19, 149–50, 190; contexts of, 1, 56, 173, 174, 179, 185–86; deconstruction of, 158–64; definitions of, 47–48, 78, 90n6, 158, 160–64, 333; depoliticization of, 407–8, 412–13, 415; empowering ability of, 314, 315, 325, 327, 328–32; eradication of, 150, 258–59, 538–40; medicalization of, 173–74, 348, 415, 419n7; medical model of, 222, 464, 533–34, 535, 577–78; social model and, 9, 169, 173–79, 197n3, 464, 554–55, 561; in Their Dogs Came with Them, 513–16, 519
"Disability, Connectivity, and Transgressing the Autonomous Body" (Gibson), 59–60
Disability, Queerness, and Liberation (Clare), 233
Disability and the Global South (Erevelles and Livingston), 272
disability counternarrative, 190
Disability Employment Opportunities Job Fair, 88–89
disability justice, 404; environmental justice and, 80; food justice and, 403, 405, 408, 412–13, 415, 416–17; sustainability and, 423
Disability Rhetoric (Dolmage), 534

disability rights movement, 160–61, 174, 238–39n45, 570

disability studies, ix–x, 1; definition of, 79; difference and, 143–44; ecocriticism and, 169, 173–74, 175, 182; environmental studies and, ix–xv, 2–3, 61–63, 201–2, 533–36; risk culture and, 33, 54–55, 59–60, 61–62, 63–64n4; social model and, 554–55, 556; as a special education field, 163. See also feminist disability studies and environmental justice

disability theory, x

disabled somatics of place, 511–12, 514, 515, 516, 524

disablist presence, 40, 49, 53, 54, 66n12

disaster relief, 84–85

Discovery Channel, 67n18, 156–57

discrimination, 74–75, 87–88, 149

disease, definition of, 161–62

displacement, 31, 172, 343, 515–16, 519–20, 524

dissent, 144, 155

distanced warfare, 292, 294, 305, 306

diversity: biological, xi, 16, 196n1, 258–59, 546; cultural and ecological, 282, 283; neuro-, xi, 16, 537, 545, 546

DNA, 540

Dolmage, Jay, 534

dolphins in captivity, 146–47

domesticity, 108, 129, 396

domination, 43, 148, 163, 263

"Don't Mourn for Us" (Sinclair), 531

Dorn, Michael, 61

double bind of disability, 36–37, 39

double consciousness, 81–82

double negative. See litotes

Douglas, Mary, 64n7

Dow Chemicals, 384

Duffin, Lorna, 458

"dumb," 158–59

Dumit, Joseph, xiv, 372

Earth, Animal, and Disability Liberation (Nocella et al), 141

Earth Charter, 74–75

East Los Angeles, 16, 502, 504, 505. See also Their Dogs Came with Them (Viramontes)

eco-ability, x, 8, 141, 143–44, 150–51

ecocentrism, 169–70, 172

ecocriticism, 3, 9, 169, 170, 195, 206–7, 212, 544

ecofeminism, 67n17, 74, 196n1, 210–13, 588

"Ecofeminism and the Politics of Reality" (Vance), 210–13

The Ecological Other (Ray), 16

ecological others, 16, 273, 435, 532–33, 534, 537–38, 541

ecology, x, 30, 45, 141, 143, 294; literary, 170, 182, 185, 186, 188, 195; queer, 223

economization of life, 368–69, 370–71, 376

ecopsychology, 52–53

ecosomatic paradigm, 9; background and overview of,

Human Genome Project, 535
human-nonhuman nature interactions, 225–29, 232–33
"human vegetables," 597
Hurricane Katrina, 84–85
Hussein, Saddam, 345
hydroelectric development, 191–
92, 194, 197–98n6

identity: adventure culture and,
31, 32, 36–37; Chicana/o, 509,
515–16; environmental, 574,
575–79, 580–84, 585, 586–87,
589, 591, 591n2; exceptionalism and, 82; personal, 581,
582, 585, 588–89; risk culture
and, 41–42, 44, 46, 47
"Identity in Mashpee" (Clifford),
286n19
immigration: disease and, 454,
476; restriction of, 42, 44, 142
Immigration Act of 1924, 44
Imperial Irrigation District (IID),
461–62
imperialism, 12–13, 14; Iraq
and, 338–39, 341, 343, 345,
346–48, 351; lead toxicity and,
104, 108, 132n19, 134n41;
risk culture roots in, 43, 45, 47;
UXOs and, 296
Imperial Valley, 459–64; drainage infrastructure of, 448–
49, 461–63, 466; farming in,
460–63, 464; and "perpetual
bondage" of water, 459, 466
imprisonment of disabled people, 157–58
Imrie, Rob, 196n1, 213–14

inclusion for autistic persons,
539–40
indigenous liberation movements, 283
indigenous people. See Native
Americans
indigenous studies, xi; disability
and, 276, 282; sustainability
and, 282–84
Indio, 456, 458
individualism, 1–2, 39–40, 43,
57, 62, 82, 143–44
individualization, 370–71, 375–
76
industrialization: of food production, 439, 442, 537, 538;
invalidism and, 456, 463; risk
culture and, 46–47, 50–51, 88;
sustainability and, 427; toxicity
and, 101–2, 113
industrial tourism, 50–51, 205–6
informal support systems, 517–
25
infrastructure, public, 513, 516–
18, 520–21, 524–25
In My Language (Baggs), 227–28
institutional failure, 314, 320,
321
institutionalization of disabled
people, 142–43, 144, 455
Instituto Nacional de Migración,
488
insurgents, 350, 355n32
integrity, x, 427–28, 431, 438,
507; autistic, 582
intelligence quotient (IQ), 121,
135n48, 143, 364, 366–67
intentionality, 588–89

Wargo, John, 315–16
warnings, product, 95
Warrior Marks (Walker and Parmar), 79
wastewater, 460–63, 466
Wayne, Leslie, 112
Waziyatawin, 283
weapons testing in Vieques, 315–16
weight discrimination, 86–87
Weihenmayer, Erik, 39, 221–22
welfare erosion, 521
Wendell, Susan, 55–56, 414
the West, health seekers and, 451–52, 453–58
Western framework and natural world, 259–61
Westways, 506
wheelchairs: becoming and, 60; compared to cars, 58, 205; in Ghana, 609–10; motorized, 205–6, 207–8; nature access for, 66n11, 201, 212, 214–16, 218, 220, 237n27; in Seal Surfer and Sosu's Call, 604–5, 606, 609, 616–17
Wheeler, Elizabeth A., x, xii, 12, 18–19, 20
White, Evelyn, 202
white domesticity, 108
White House Task Force on Childhood Obesity, 87
white phosphorous, 350, 355n32
Whole Access, 216–17, 222, 238n30
"Why Is China Poisoning Our Babies?" (Harris), 111, 133n27
Wildavsky, Aaron, 64n7

wilderness: the body and, 34–37, 40, 46, 54–59, 61, 62, 66n11, 67n16; construction of, 3, 20–21, 48, 61; environmentalism and, 29–32, 64nn5–6; ideal plot, 31, 34, 62, 66n13; inaccessibility of, 57–58; movement, 30–32, 33–34, 41–48; myth, 33, 40, 54, 56, 58, 66n11, 225, 394; preservation, 42, 43, 62, 63nn1–2. See also nature
"Wild Men from Borneo," 261
Wiley-Mydske, Lei, 539
Williams, Lynice, 76
Wisconsin, 243
Wolbring, Gregor, 534
Wolch, Jennifer, 521
Wolfe, Cary, 596–97
Wolfe, Patrick, 271
women: cooking and, 432–33; environmental devastation and, 323; invalidism and, 456–58, 469n33; wilderness and, 63n2. See also feminism; feminist disability studies and environmental justice; feminization; women's politicization in Vieques
women's politicization in Vieques, 313–33; background of military activities and, 315–17; hegemony, reification, and subjection and, 317–21; issue confrontation and, 321–25; legitimation crises and, 325–28; overview of, 313–15, 332–33

Woodlot Revolt, 279
World Bank, 113
world order, 351
World Trade Organization, 102
Wright, Bob and Suzanne, 539–40, 547n4, 547n6

xenophobia, 45

Yaghr, Christie, 609, 610

Yellow Peril, 107
Yenika-Agbaw, Vivian, 612, 616
Yergeau, Melanie, 544
Young Citizens for Community Action (fictional entity), 509

Zafar (character), 391, 397
Zepeda, Marcelo, 481–82
zones of dependence, 521
Zumaya (character), 514

www.ingramcontent.com/pod-product-compliance
Lightning Source LLC
Chambersburg PA
CBHW022344280326
41935CB00007B/64